*T*he Supervisory Process in Speech-Language Pathology and Audiology

*T*he Supervisory Process
in
Speech-Language Pathology
and Audiology

Jean L. Anderson, Ed.D.

Department of Speech and Hearing Sciences
Indiana University
Bloomington, Indiana

A College-Hill Publication
Little, Brown and Company
Boston   Toronto   San Diego

College-Hill Press
A Division of
Little, Brown and Company (Inc.)
34 Beacon Street
Boston, Massachusetts 02108

Library of Congress Cataloging-in-Publication Data

Anderson, Jean L., 1920–
    The supervisory process in speech-language pathology and audiology.

"A College-Hill publication."
Includes bibliographies and index.
1. Speech therapy—Study and teaching—Supervision.
2. Audiology—Study and teaching—Supervision.
I. Title. [DNLM: 1. Audiology.   2. Organization and Administration.
3. Speech Pathology.   WM 475 A547s]
RC428.A53   1987   616.85′5′007   87-26174

ISBN 0–316–03959–4

Printed in the United States of America

To the many supervisors who have contributed so much to the profession of speech-language pathology and audiology

C • O • N • T • E • N • T • S

Appendices 325

Subject Index 397

Author Index 405

P · R · E · F · A · C · E

Although supervision has long been a component of the profession of speech-language pathology and audiology, the study of the supervisory process has been largely ignored until recently. In the past few years, however, there has been a surge of interest which has resulted in published articles, convention presentations, continuing education offerings, books, and activities of the American Speech-Language-Hearing Association (ASHA). This book will make a statement about where the profession stands in its implementation of the supervisory process as a major influence in the preparation of future speech-language pathologists and audiologists and the delivery of service to clients. It will propose a continuum of supervision, offered as a framework upon which supervisors and their supervisees may place themselves as they work together, and through which they can examine, "dissect," and discuss the process. It is hoped that the presentation of this continuum and the accompanying material will encourage members of the profession to view the supervisory process as an important and appropriate area for self-study. Additionally, it is hoped it will help make clearer the many questions that exist about the effectiveness of supervisory methodologies and will stimulate active research to seek answers to those questions.

This book has been written mainly for the many people in speech-language pathology and audiology who have been or may be plunged into the role of supervisor without opportunity to think about it or study it. Speech-language pathologists and audiologists often become what I call "overnight supervisors"—one day a clinician, the next a supervisor. Many are thrust into the role without preparation, sometimes without much choice, and nearly always without much role definition from the organization for which they work or within themselves. Often they have little opportunity to talk with anyone about supervision and are forced to draw upon their own past experiences as supervisees, positive or negative, as a source for the development of their own techniques and methodologies. I hope that this book will help them and all other supervisors to make supervision manageable. I hope that it will encourage them to think about the process and to increase their knowledge of themselves and their supervisory procedures. I hope supervisors will perceive supervision as a process that can and must be studied, just as we expect our clinicians to study the clinical process. I hope, too, that student supervisees in educational programs will study the book and that it will serve two purposes for them—to help them understand their role as supervisees, and to prepare them for the time in the not-too-distant future when they will probably be supervisors themselves.

This book has been "happening" to me since long before I began seriously to put the words on paper. A series of events led to my interest in the supervisory process, but a few of them stand out as probably the most significant. The first was my own introduction into supervision, when I, too, became an overnight supervisor of a student in a school practicum assignment which was not defined and for which there were no guidelines.

The second experience, and possibly the most significant, was the opportunity to serve as a state supervisor of speech-hearing-language programs in a department of education. In this position I was able to spend several days a week for several years observing and talking with speech-language pathologists in the schools, program supervisors, and administrators as well as university personnel. Often I talked with clinicians who were serving as supervisors of "student teachers" with little or no guidance from universities about their responsibilities, and I learned about their questions. My experiences in this position led me first to a concern about the number of "leaderless" programs, that is, those in which there was no leadership from a person within our discipline. My attention first focused on this administrative aspect—what the ASHA Committee on Supervision was later to call *program management*. However, that attention soon turned to the *process*, later termed *clinical teaching* by the ASHA Committee. My interest in the process came as a result of the dawning realization that, when visiting and observing first- or second-year, or even more experienced clinicians I could often guess correctly where they had done their "student teaching," as the school practicum experience was then called, because of the obvious modeling that took place. Through this realization, I became aware of the impact that the teaching aspect of supervision has on the development of professionals and the significance of that impact on their future clients. In other words, I began to ask myself these questions: If each generation of clinicians does exactly what its supervisors do, where are we going in terms of the kind of service we will deliver to our clients in the future? Is there something in this teaching aspect of supervision that makes the difference between clinicians who become clones of their supervisors and clinicians who are able to go beyond their supervisors and become the independent, autonomous clinicians that we profess to produce in our educational programs? Is there something in the supervisory experience that makes the difference and, if so, what is it?

The third important influence on my developing concern about how we, as a profession, were dealing with the supervisory process came when I had the privilege of becoming the chair of the first ASHA Committee on Supervision of Speech Pathology and Audiology. It was through the data-gathering done by the Committee that I fully realized the magnitude of the profession's lack of recognition of the importance of this process which affects all of us at some time. Further, the enormity of our neglect of the dedicated and frustrated members of the profession who were serving in the important role of supervisor became clear and was well documented by the first position statement of the Committee (ASHA, 1978a).

The fourth event was the opportunity to develop a doctoral-level program at Indiana University in which students could study the supervisory process, learn to prepare other supervisors, and conduct research on supervision. The interaction with the students in that program and the research we completed have been an important dimension of my own development.

Thus, a long journey that began with the sudden assignment of a student in the school practicum those many years ago has culminated in the struggle to produce this book. In the words of Alice in Wonderland, I have become "curiouser and curiouser" about the dynamics of the process, and about what I call the professional/political issues that have prevented, or at least not encouraged, the study of this important facet of our profession.

I make no claim for having found the answers to all the questions. Certainly I do not wish to proclaim that this book provides the answers for everyone. I only hope that it provides some encouragement for others to ask more questions about supervision—individually as supervisors or collectively as a profession. The book has become a statement of what I believe to be important in the supervisory process. Some of it is supportable by data, some by consensus, some by common sense. Not everyone will agree with what I say. None of it should go unchallenged, for we have only begun to scratch at the complexities of the process.

It was my somewhat nebulous objective at one time to produce a book that would bring together a spectacular review of what has been written in all the helping professions about supervision. This effort would have resulted in a lengthy tome that would not necessarily have been definitive for, alas, I have learned that many of those disciplines to which I had thought to turn—assuming that they had discovered the answer to the mystery of supervision—are not much better off than we are. Therefore, I have included only that material from other professions which is pertinent to specific points. I have drawn particularly, as will be seen, on the work in education by Blumberg, Cogan, and Goldhammer. But . . . a funny thing has happened on the way to getting this book on paper! We have begun to develop a body of literature of our own over the past few years. It is literature that ranges over a broad continuum of importance and quality, but nevertheless it is ours, and it is developing rapidly to answer our own questions.

A few clarifications are necessary for the reader. One is related to the title, which includes "audiology." Why, you may ask, is a speech-language pathologist writing about supervision in audiology? The answer is that I believe the supervisory *process* is the same for the two areas of practice within the discipline. Differences, if they exist, will be more related to the position of supervisor and supervisee on the continuum, or to such factors as the differences between the needs of supervisees in the diagnostic process and in the therapeutic process. Not all audiologists will agree with me, but nevertheless I hope there will be much in this book that they will find useful.

Another clarification is necessary in relation to some of the examples provided in the book. My own professional background is in the schools, the school practicum, and the university program, so many of the examples come from those settings. I wish to emphasize here, however, as I do throughout the book, my unwavering belief that the *process* of supervision has more commonalities than differences across sites and situations. Therefore, readers are invited to apply the examples to their own experience.

The reader who is looking for statistical validation for the effects of any method of supervision will be disappointed with this book. So will the reader who is looking for unequivocal support for "*the* way to supervise." Neither will be found here, nor in any other source. Despite my confidence in the value of the approach to the supervisory process presented in this book, I am the first to acknowledge that it has not been validated. It is an approach which makes sense to me and which is actually used by many supervisors now, whether or not they conceptualize it in the same way I do. The methodology proposed herein should be "weighed and measured" carefully, however, to determine its validity.

We are, I think, in a wonderful period of evolution in the study of the supervisory process. It is my wish that this book will contribute to that evolution.

A▪C▪K▪N▪O▪W▪L▪E▪D▪G▪M▪E▪N▪T▪S

How can I acknowledge the influence of the many people who have shaped my thinking, offered encouragement, challenged my statements, and contributed ideas over a professional lifetime? It is a pleasant but difficult endeavor, which surely cannot include all the people who have been important to me and whose influence can be found in this book.

I must mention first those indomitable women whom I met when I became a state supervisor of speech and hearing programs: Elizabeth MacLearie, Martha Black, Geraldine Garrison, and Gretchen Phair—fighters in those early days for better services in the schools, for better preparation of students, and for better supervision of the school practicum, which they believed would result in better services to school children. The work of Ruth Becky Irwin of Ohio State University, a pioneer in the study of supervision long before many people thought it important, helped me realize that it was a process that could and should be studied. The late Betty Ann Wilson of Purdue University and I held many discussions about supervision, and I learned much from her. Adah Miner shared her time and her expertise with me during a memorable visit to Seattle in 1973. Bill Diedrich's scholarly approach to the clinical and supervisory processes stimulated my thinking. There are many others whose ideas melded into mine in those years, for I found, as I began to talk and write and hold conferences about supervision, that there were many others who were interested but who had not found a forum or a sounding board for their concerns and interests. All of these people contributed to my knowledge of the issues and increased my understanding of the needs.

I cannot even begin to document the impact of the interest, cooperation, and support of all of my colleagues in the Department of Speech and Hearing Sciences at Indiana University—administrators, academic faculty, and especially the supervisors. Without them I could never have had the freedom or the opportunity to study and experiment and teach in an area which was not taken very seriously by many others at the time I began. Only because of them has this book been possible.

And now my students. It is something of a cliché for authors to thank their students for what they have learned from them. In my case, it is more than a cliché. When we began to develop the training program in the supervisory process at Indiana University, there was no text, no background of research upon which to build, no course content except what could be drawn from other disciplines. What we did have was a group of wonderful, thoughtful, inquisitive, questioning doctoral students who were willing to experiment along with me, who could tolerate the uncertainty and recognize the need that I saw, and who could successfully incorporate the study of the supervisory process into the regular doctoral program of the department. I have continued to have that very special kind of student to this day. I have never before been able to thank them collectively for what they have done for me and for the developing study of supervision. I take that opportunity now.

Christine Strike and Ronald Gillam, two doctoral students who became interested in applying their knowledge about single-subject and ethnographic research methodologies to the study of the supervisory process, have added a dimension that would not have been possible without them. I thank them for a contribution that should encourage the research we need so much.

Other people require special thanks. Chapters were read and valuable suggestions made by Judith Brasseur, Susann Dowling, Mary Dragoo, Elizabeth McCrea, Kathryn Smith, and again, Christine Strike. Their feedback and their support have been unbelievably helpful. Sandra Ulrich of the University of Connecticut had a major impact on the book through her meticulous reading and thoughtful suggestions. I appreciate her support and her friendship. I am also grateful to Marie Linvill and Susan Altman of College-Hill Press for their encouragement and patience.

Several people have typed various portions of this book—Glenda Washburn and Sherleen Goodlette at the early stages, and Peg Miller, who carefully brought the whole project to completion.

Finally, thanks go to my sister, Arda Landergren, for her special support and assistance during the long period in which I have been writing this book. We are both happy that it is completed!

*I*ntroduction

Speech-language pathologists and audiologists have been involved in supervision since the beginning of the profession. Indeed, supervision seems to have been the one component that has affected everyone in the profession at some time.

ASHA Committee on Supervision in
Speech-Language Pathology and Audiology, 1978a

Carl Rogers (1957), over 25 years ago, could have been talking about supervision when he maintained that the training of future counselors and therapists was characterized by a rarity of research and a plentitude of platitudes. Sixteen years later, Cogan (1973), talking about supervision of teachers, stated that supervisors need to be prepared to live with partial knowledge, and in 1980 Froehle and Kurpius discussed an assumption about supervision which they called "a humbling one indeed. . . it derives from continual discovery that someone has been there before; that there are no new breakthroughs in the supervision domain" (p. 51). Boyd (1978) said that the time is right for development and refinement of supervision of counselors and called for greater clarification of what is involved in supervision.

Speech-language pathology is in a position similar to the other helping professions. The ASHA Committee on Supervision has stated, "We have no data to indicate that supervision makes a difference in the effectiveness of clinicians at any level of training or in the employment setting. We also have no knowledge of critical factors in supervision methodology" (ASHA, 1978a, p. 480). Realistically, this is the state of the art today as well. This fact should not, however, keep supervisors from questioning, experimenting, analyzing, and when they realize they have only raised more questions, trying again. Luft (1969) suggested that there has always been unevenness in theory and application. "Man could sail long before he understood the aerodynamics of hull and wing. . . . If our current knowledge is limited, spotty, contradictory and foolish, that at least tells us where we are, and everyone is invited to improve on it" (p. 33). This may be the underlying theme of this book if there can be one. The combined efforts of a great many people are needed to clarify and validate this process in which so many are involved—and *everyone is invited*!

DESCRIBING SUPERVISION AND SUPERVISORS

Before proceeding to a study of supervision, it is necessary to differentiate between the *clinical* process and the *supervisory* process. The clinical process, as defined in the report of the Committee on Supervision of the American Speech and Hearing Association (ASHA, 1978a), is "that interaction that takes place between the clinician and the client" (p. 479). The supervisory process is defined as "the interaction that takes place between the supervisor and the clinician and may be related to the behavior of the clinician or the client or to the program in which the supervisor and clinician are employed" (ASHA, 1978a, p. 479). This interaction between clinician and supervisor is superimposed upon the clinical process. At some point in the total process the clinician changes roles and becomes a supervisee, a process that requires different objectives, insights, and behaviors. The clinician then must play two roles interchangeably—clinician to the client, supervisee to the supervisor. Figure 1–1 represents the levels of the clinical and the supervisory processes and illustrates the transitional area where the clinician interchanges roles.

Tasks of Supervisors

The ASHA Committee Report (ASHA, 1978a) divides the tasks of supervisors into two categories, *clinical teaching* and *program management*. The report defines each category as separate aspects of the role while stating that each supervisor's job description may include behaviors from each category.

> Clinical teaching is defined as the interaction between supervisor/supervisee in any setting which furthers the development of clinical skills of students or practicing clinicians as related to changes in client behavior. Traditionally this interaction has consisted of observation and conferences.

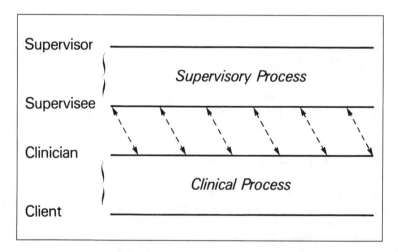

FIGURE 1-1. *LEVELS OF THE CLINICAL AND SUPERVISORY PROCESSES*

The conferences may include such components as objective setting, positive or negative feedback, information giving, questioning, joint problem solving, and planning for clinician and client change. Program management is defined as those activities that relate to the administration or coordination of programs, for example, scheduling, budgeting, program planning, employing, or dismissing personnel. (p. 479)

Emphasis on Clinical Teaching

The discussion in this book will center mainly on clinical teaching, although many of the principles to be presented are applicable to program management. Clinical teaching, as defined previously, should be the core of the supervisory process in any setting. It may receive a greater emphasis in the educational program, but it is also the procedure through which continuing growth and development of clinicians is implemented after they enter the work force. Clinical teaching is certainly an essential and crucial component of any program, even though program management may become the predominant responsibility of the supervisor of a service delivery program. A minimal amount of space will be spent here on details of administration or program management. The basics of organization and administration will be learned more effectively from the extensive literature, coursework, and pre- or in-service offerings developed by professionals for whom the study of management is a speciality. Volumes of literature are available, some of which are cited in the references in this book. Coursework, in-service workshops, and conferences are readily available to most persons who wish to prepare themselves for administrative roles or who find themselves in such positions without appropriate preparation.

A further reason for concentrating on clinical teaching is the current interest in this category of supervision and the fact that it has not been dealt with extensively in the past by the profession. This is true despite the fact that clinical teaching appears to be the major responsibility of a large percentage of the professionals who are supervisors in speech-language pathology and audiology—those who supervise in educational programs, or in off-campus practicum or Clinical Fellowship Year (CFY) situations. Additionally, it appears that the clinical teaching component may be neglected in the service delivery setting in favor of program management tasks because of the pressures of time, or because of a lack of information and preparation for clinical teaching which may make it more threatening than the more structured administrative activities (Anderson, 1974). For these reasons, this book will be devoted to the goals, objectives, and methodologies inherent in the clinical teaching process.

Titles of Supervisors

The Committee on Supervision also clarified terminology about the persons who supervise. The Committee's report states that, although the individual who carries out the tasks of supervision "may be called supervisor, coordinator, consultant, chairperson, head clinician or clinical teacher, among other titles," the term *supervisor* was used in their report as a generic label for individuals who may operate under any of those titles in any of the places where speech-language pathology and audiology takes place (ASHA, 1978a, p. 479). The title of supervisor has been used in that manner in most of the literature up to this point, and will be used in the same way here. It is assumed that this person will have an educational background in speech-language pathology or audiology prior to becoming a supervisor. The topic of supervision by persons with other professional backgrounds will be discussed in a later chapter.

SETTINGS FOR SUPERVISION

A brief description of the framework in which speech-language pathologists and audiologists and their supervisors function will set the stage for further consideration of the supervisory process. Settings in which they may work are described and duties will be discussed briefly.

The primary mission of speech-language pathologists and audiologists is the provision of clinical services to individuals who have communication disorders. These professionals are prepared for colleges and universities where their experiences include clinical work with communicatively handicapped individuals. This clinical phase of their preparation is supervised by certified personnel in programs operated on-campus by the college or university or in off-campus settings. The professionals prepared in this way ultimately provide services to the communicatively handicapped in a variety of settings—schools, clinics, rehabilitation centers, hospitals, nursing homes, private practice, and other agencies and institutions.

At any point in their professional careers these speech-language pathologists and audiologists may also become supervisors. They may be employed in educational programs or in service delivery settings.[1]

Educational Programs

In college and university programs, supervisors facilitate students' application of academic learning to the clinical setting and monitor their clinical work in the interest of optimal service to current and future clients. Most of this applied teaching takes place in campus clinical programs operated by colleges or universities in conjunction with their academic programs. Supervisors in such programs operate within a number of different frameworks, depending upon the particular organization or program in which they are employed. Some are full-time supervisors employed for that purpose alone, whereas for others, supervision is only a part of their responsibilities, which may include clinical work, teaching, administration, or research.

---

[1]It is recognized that many service delivery programs are located within university programs, but for purposes of this book the terms *educational program* and *service delivery program* are used to differentiate function of the programs—preparation of students or service to clients.

Off-Campus Practicum

The off-campus practicum, where students are assigned to service delivery settings to obtain clinical experience, is part of the total educational program. Some colleges and universities use off-campus sites more extensively than others, but to meet ASHA requirements, all students must have at least one assignment to a site other than the campus program. Two types of supervisors are involved in this off-campus experience. One is the on-site supervisor, whose primary responsibility is the provision of clinical services to the clientele of his or her employing agency. This person assumes the additional role of supervisor for a particular student(s) from the college or university for an allotted time. The other type of supervisor involved in the off-campus practicum is employed by the college or university to serve as a liaison between the campus program and off-campus personnel. The university supervisor performs a variety of tasks, ranging from site selection and assignment of students to on-site observation, and has different degrees of responsibility for the supervision and evaluation of the student, depending upon the structure of the total educational program and the nature or proximity of the off-campus site.

Service Delivery Settings

In settings where the main objective of the organization is the delivery of services to clients, supervision is the process through which these services are planned, monitored, evaluated, and improved. The functions of supervisors in these settings vary greatly and may include, among other duties, maintaining quality of services to clients through program organization and management, monitoring and evaluating services, and being responsible for the on-going professional development of the speech-language pathologists and audiologists employed in the agency. Such supervisors may also be directly or indirectly involved with students who are assigned to their programs by the college or university for off-campus practicum experience, with persons completing the Clinical Fellowship Year, or with paraprofessionals.

The Clinical Fellowship Year

Many speech-language pathologists and audiologists supervise their colleagues during the Clinical Fellowship Year (CFY). The CFY is a year of employment, usually the first year, in which a speech-language pathologist or audiologist is supervised by an individual who holds the Certificate of Clinical Competence (CCC) from ASHA. The CFY experience is assumed to be a supervised internship and is one of the requirements for the granting of the CCC from ASHA. Program supervisors or other speech-language pathologists who hold the CCC may be asked to supervise persons who are completing a CFY in their own or in another program. In these cases, contact between supervisor and supervisee is usually more intermittent than in the other situations.

ASHA's Membership and Certification Handbook contains the requirements for the CFY and lists the responsibilities of supervisors (ASHA, 1985c).

Other Types of Supervisory Settings

Some supervisors function at the state or regional level, mainly in education or health departments. Their roles may be administrative, regulatory, or consultative, and may affect the individual speech-language pathologist and audiologist indirectly more often than directly, although this varies.

Another supervisory setting exists where supportive personnel (paraprofessionals or aides) are employed to work with speech-language pathologists and audiologists in delivery of services. When assigned a paraprofessional, a speech-language pathologist or audiologist automatically assumes the role of supervisor in relation to the work done by the aide with clients. ASHA has provided guidelines for supervisors in these situations (ASHA, 1981).

Some speech-language pathologists and audiologists may find themselves in a supervisory position with professionals from other disciplines. For example, speech-language pathologists or audiologists may become supervisors in rehabilitation centers where they are responsible for physical and occupational therapists and their work, or they may find themselves in interdisciplinary settings where their function is to work with supervisors from other disciplines to meet organizational objectives.

COMPLEXITIES OF THE SUPERVISORY PROCESS

Clearly, everyone in speech-language pathology and audiology participates in the supervisory process at some time, either as supervisor or supervisee. It is obvious that the "web of supervision" is a complex one, wherein professionals may be involved in many different types of supervisory interactions throughout their careers or at any one time. The nature of the interactions varies greatly across situations and time.

For example, in educational programs supervisors may supervise students whose clinical experience ranges from none to several semesters, be university supervisors for off-campus sites, and perhaps supervise CFY speech-language pathologists or audiologists in their own or another setting.

Student clinicians may be engaged in the supervisory process at any one time with several different supervisors in their educational program. The supervision may be done on a one-to-one basis or in a group. At the same time, they may be assigned to an off-campus site, adding the site supervisor and the university coordinator of the practicum to the list of individuals with whom they interact. Or the off-campus site may be the single assignment for a particular period of time, often becoming the most intensive supervisory experience of the student's entire program.

In the service delivery setting a variety of supervisory relationships are possible. In some programs a speech-language pathologist or audiologist may be appointed supervisor of the other professionals on the staff. Such supervisors may work with beginners or with professionals who have had many years of experience, with practicum students, CFY candidates, professionals in other disciplines, or paraprofessionals. In all settings, however, there is a high probability that speech-language pathologists and audiologists will work in places where their immediate supervisor or administrator is from another profession. In a hospital or clinical setting, the speech-language pathology and audiology program may be directed by a doctor, a physical or occupational therapist, a nurse, or a business manager. In a school setting, the supervisor may be a director of special education, a principal, or another administrator. The range of possible interactions in such settings is broad. For example, a speech-language pathologist or audiologist working in a school program may interact with one or more of the following: a program supervisor, a CFY supervisor, a state/regional supervisor, several principals, and a director of special education. Realistically, it must also be stated that speech-language pathologists and audiologists often work in places where little or no supervision is provided, thereby creating another set of issues.

In summary, before becoming certified professionals (that is, holding the CCC), speech-language pathologists or audiologists may have been supervised by many different supervisors within the clinical program on campus, by one or more off-campus practicum supervisors, and by a program supervisor or colleague during the CFY. After obtaining the CCC, they may interact with a program supervisor, a state or regional supervisor, a person whose training is in another discipline, or in some form of peer supervision. They may in turn supervise individuals in the CFY, students in an off-campus practicum, or supportive personnel, and may at some point become a supervisor in an educational program, a service delivery setting, a state or regional agency, or in an interdisciplinary situation.

An additional complexity is that nearly every person who is a supervisor is also a supervisee to someone, thus necessitating a change of role similar to that shown in Figure 1-1 for the clinician/supervisee.

CHARACTERISTICS OF SUPERVISORS—DEMOGRAPHIC DATA

It has always been difficult to obtain demographic data about supervisors in speech-language pathology and audiology. Although ASHA annually asks members to indicate their primary and secondary activity on their membership application, the total number of professionals who are participating in some form of supervision has never been clearly documented. ASHA figures gathered in September 1986 indicate a total membership of 49,878. Of these members, 39,769 responded to a survey which identified their primary and secondary activity. Data indicate that 3.1 percent of the respondents listed supervision as their primary activity. A secondary activity was reported by 17,761 of the respondents; 19.5 percent of those individuals indicated that the secondary activity was supervision (Shewan, personal communication, 1987). Fein (1984), reporting on a similar survey, stated that 3.7 percent of respondents listed supervision as a primary activity while 30 percent spent at least one hour per week in supervisory activities. Pickering (1985) extrapolated from figures distributed by the Council of Graduate Programs in Communication Sciences and Disorders and estimated that over 5,000 individuals were "engaged in some clinical supervision within or external to the 300 educational programs" (p. 15). This does not begin to identify the total number of those who are engaged in part-time supervision, that is, those professionals involved in supervising students in off-campus practicum, CFY candidates, or supportive personnel.

Despite the problems in identifying supervisors, several surveys have provided some descriptive data from certain settings which will be reported here. Black and her colleagues (1961), in an early survey of 40 state and 101 county- or city-level supervisors of school programs, found an almost equal distribution of men and women in supervisory positions. As for educational level, the majority (80 percent of state and 73 percent of local school supervisors) held master's degrees plus additional graduate work; 14 percent of local and 8 percent of state supervisors held the doctorate degree. Others held only the master's degree without additional work. These figures included about 39 percent whose area of specialization was not speech-language pathology or audiology, that is, they were general school administrators or special education directors.

Anderson (1972), in a later survey of 211 (93 full-time, 118 part-time) supervisors of school programs, all with educational backgrounds in speech-language pathology or audiology, found that 36 percent were male and 64 percent were female. Most frequently indicated title for full-time personnel in the study was supervisor; for part-time it was coordinator. Of full-time supervisors, 90 percent had master's degrees, 6 percent had bachelor's degrees, and 2 percent had doctorate degrees. Of the part-time personnel, 13 percent had bachelor's degrees, 83 percent had master's degrees, and 2 percent had doctorate degrees.

University and college supervisors employed as coordinators or liaison with the off-campus supervisors of school practicum were the subject of another survey by Anderson (1973a). Of the 144 programs responding to the survey, 131 (91 percent) employed university supervisors who were speech-language pathologists or audiologogists to supervise the school practicum and 9 percent reported a supervisor from education. Of 131 supervisors who were speech-language pathologists, 61 percent had master's degrees, and 28 percent had doctorate degrees. Seventy-one percent held the CCC from ASHA in speech pathology, 1 percent in audiology and 15 percent in both. Rank was reported as follows: instructor, 29 percent; assistant professor, 46 percent; associate professor, 13 percent; professor, 8 percent. Seventy-two percent of these practicum supervisors also supervised in the clinic operated by the educational program. Sixty percent taught courses in organization and administration of public school programs, and 76 percent taught other classes. Fifty percent had other academic responsibilities and 36 percent reported some administrative duties.

Although Anderson's study was not designed to obtain information about the school clinicians who serve as on-site supervisors in the school practicum, some descriptive data about them resulted from the survey. On-site supervisors were reported to be selected by the student teaching department in education and/or the speech pathology department on the basis of subjective judgment by the university supervisor(s) on such factors as personality, willingness to work with students, competency as a clinician, intellectual curiosity, availability and location, type or quality of program, compatibility, temperament, and stability. Fifty-one percent of the programs required school clinicians who supervised the practicum to have ASHA certification, 16 percent required recent training, 59 percent required experience as clinicians, and 41 percent required a master's degree.

The data on educational levels or requirements are mainly of historical interest because current ASHA standards recognize supervision only when done by certified professionals, that is, those holding master's degrees. Thus, the number of programs requiring a master's degree and ASHA certification would presumably be higher now because of the upgrading of ASHA certification requirements for speech-language pathologists and audiologists, as well as for program accreditation for universities.

A survey by Schubert and Aitchison (1975) of clinical supervisors in 204 colleges and universities revealed a profile of the supervisor in these settings as between the ages of 26 and 39 (60 percent), female (63 percent), employed less than six years in their present position (70 percent), employed full-time (86 percent), and holding a master's degree (60 percent). Approximately 73 percent of the supervisors in this study had less than five years of paid professional experience as a clinician and approximately 94 percent had less than five years paid experience as an instructor in speech-language pathology and audiology before becoming a supervisor. Sixty-six percent of the respondents did not have tenure in their positions and 35 percent indicated that it was not possible for them to receive tenure. Eighty percent were voting members of their faculty.

Schubert and Aitchison also identified some interesting gender comparisons. More of the female respondents were between the ages of 26 and 32 (48.42 percent of females, 20.54 percent of males) whereas 28.65 percent of males and 13.29 percent of females were over 45 years of age. Men had been employed longer in their present positions than women, but spent less time in supervision and more time in academic teaching and administration than the women respondents. There were major differences in salary, with women being paid less than men. Also, 71.35 percent of the males and 16.77 percent of the females held doctoral degrees. More males than females held tenure and voting privileges in their departments. More females (47.78 percent) than males (23.78 percent) considered supervision to be a profession in itself. From these results two types of supervisors can be visualized—the older male faculty member holding a doctoral degree, tenure, and voting privileges who supervises as part of his total responsibilities and the female who is younger, has less security in the job, holds a master's degree, and has less involvement in the academic program (for example, voting, teaching, and administration). Ten years later, Kennedy (1985) identified similar patterns.

Supervisors of the CFY were described by Schubert and Lyngby (1977). They reported that the CFY supervisor is likely to be employed in the setting where the CFY takes place, but may travel up to 30 miles to observe or consult. The supervisor is likely to have had three or more years of professional employment and an equal number of years of supervisory experience, some of the prior experience being only that of supervising Clinical Fellows.

These studies are far from complete in describing all the persons who serve as supervisors. It is not clear in these surveys if the respondents include audiology supervisors or are limited to speech-language pathology. No demographic data have been published about off-campus supervisors in places other than the schools or about supervisors in hospitals, private clinics, or other places where speech-language pathology and audiology services are provided. Neither are there data on people involved in the supervision of paraprofessionals.

PURPOSES OF SUPERVISION

Of course, supervision is not a process that is unique to speech-language pathology and audiology. Supervision exists wherever individuals work together in any type of hierarchical structure where one person has authority, influence, or power over another to accomplish the objectives of the system in which they are operating or to ensure adequate service to clients. Professionals in the helping professions—psychologists, counselors, medical educators, and social workers, among others, also utilize supervision in their training programs, as they endeavor to pass on information from teacher to student. Because of the lack of attention to supervision in the speech-language pathology and audiology literature, those who are interested in supervision have often turned to other areas for guidance.

A perusal of the literature from education, business management, counseling, social work, and other disciplines where supervision is utilized reveals various perceptions of its purpose. Blumberg (1980) identified the goals of supervision in education as the improvement of instruction and the enhancement of the personal and professional growth of teachers and stated that these two goals are interdependent. Mosher and Purpel (1972), also writing about supervision in education, said that the goal is a very simple one which is common to all professions and occupations—to make sure that other persons do a good job.

Statements of the purpose of supervision are often embedded in discussion of roles, tasks, or components. Van Dersal (1974) believed that the goal of a supervisor is to work "with a group of people over whom authority is exercised in such a way as to achieve their greatest combined effectiveness in getting work done" (p. 10). Tannenbaum (1966) stated that the components of supervision in business organizations are (1) planning, (2) organizing, (3) controlling, (4) communicating, (5) delegating, and (6) accepting responsibility.

These statements refer mainly to the organizational-based supervisor in the work setting. Others have looked at the purposes of supervisors in preparing people to work in their profession. Mosher and Purpel (1972) called it "teaching teachers to teach" (p. 3). In discussing what they call applied training in such fields as education, counseling, social work, and psychiatry, Kurpius, Baker, and Thomas (1977) proposed that the supervisor conceptualizes, implements, controls, and manages this application of information. Brammer and Wassmer (1977) said that supervisors assist students in applying counseling theories, principles, and methods to their own clients. For Dussault (1970), the purpose is both teaching and evaluation, which are formally different though they may be performed by the same person.

Vargus (1977), in reviewing many years of literature on supervision in social work, said that nearly all writers describe the roles of the supervisor as administrator and teacher and generally mention one of the following goals of supervision: (1) to assure that agencies provide adequate service, (2) to help workers function to fullest capacity, and (3) to help workers achieve greater professional independence and autonomy.

Purposes in Speech-Language Pathology and Audiology

References to the purposes of supervision in speech-language pathology and audiology are found also in statements of role and task. Villareal (1964), in reporting on a conference called by the American Speech and Hearing Association to discuss guidelines for supervision of the clinical practicum, cited the report of one sub-committee at the conference when he wrote, "The role of an effective supervisor should transcend the mere monitoring of the student's clinical activities. It should include the informal teaching of clinical content, the demonstration of clinical techniques, and the mature counseling of the student in relation to his clinical training" (p. 14). Van Riper (1965) said that students are turned into clinicians through supervision. A group of supervisors of school programs (Anderson, 1970) stated, "The major roles of the supervisor are to manage, evaluate and innovate programs for the communicatively handicapped children and youth within the community. At all times the welfare of children with speech, hearing, or language disorders is the reason for the supervisor's activities" (p. 152). Turton (1973) said, "Supervision can be viewed as a process wherein one person is responsible for changing the knowledge and skill level of another" (p. 94).

Supervision is the act of overseeing the application of particular procedures for given tasks, according to Halfond (1964). 'More specifically, supervision is a process in which the direct application of information about communication disorders is reviewed by the supervisor and student clinician. Supervision also implies the giving of direction and maintenance of controls" (p. 442).

Ward and Webster (1965b), in discussing the training of clinicians, said that "Clinical supervision is conceived as an interactive process between student and supervisor in which both are working together to find the most productive ways of effecting the diagnostic or therapeutic relationship" (p. 104).

Writing about supervision in audiology, Rassi (1978) defined clinical supervision as clinical teaching and said, "Its aim is to teach a student in a one-to-one situation how to apply his academic knowledge in a practical clinical setting as he functions in that setting. The ultimate goal is to transform the student into an independent clinician" (p. 9).

Personal definitions often reveal the boundaries of individual thought about the purpose of supervision. The author has obtained interesting insights about the personal parameters of supervision for many individuals by asking participants at the beginning of workshops and conferences to write their definitions of supervision. The range is as wide as might be expected. Examples of these definitions are as follows:

"Help the clinician improve his/her clinical skills."

"All things to all people."

"Supervisors would evaluate clinicians to see what is needed to improve their therapy."

"He should know the clinician and the work they do so that he can give suggestions as to improvement of weaknesses and encouragement of strengths."

"She is responsible for stimulating, encouraging, and guiding each of those supervised to become more current professional individuals."

"Would compliment each worker but would suggest improvements in techniques, philosophy, interactions, or wherever needed."

A DEFINITION FOR SPEECH-LANGUAGE PATHOLOGY OR AUDIOLOGY

It is clear that there are a variety of personal concepts built in to all of the statements about the purposes of supervision and the role of the supervisor, with some common threads running throughout. To add to this array, the following definition/description of the supervisory process is offered as the basis for the remainder of this book.

> Supervision is a process that consists of a variety of patterns of behavior, the appropriateness of which depends upon the needs, competencies, expectations, and philosophies of the supervisor and the supervisee and the specifics of the situation (task, client, setting, and other variables). The goals of the supervisory process are the professional growth and development of the supervisee and the supervisor, which it is assumed will result ultimately in optimal service to clients.

SUMMARY

Supervision in speech-language pathology and audiology is a pervading and complex entity of the profession. Although it is accepted that a great number of individuals are involved in supervision, demographic data are limited. The stated purposes of supervision vary with individuals; however, this book is based on the premise that the objective of supervision is to develop independent professionals who can provide optimal services to individuals who have communication disorders.

Historical Background

It takes a great deal of history to produce a little literature.

Henry James
Life of Nathaniel Hawthorne (1879)

History is perhaps of most interest to those who have lived through it. Many speech-language pathologists and audiologists today seem to be relatively unaware of what happened in the profession prior to their entrance into it—and for a vast majority of them that entrance was not too many years ago. This writer is a strong advocate of the trite, but surely true, concept that if we don't know where we've been we won't know where we want to go. It is tempting to indulge in reminiscences about the days when the climate was not so encouraging for those who were interested in the supervisory process, who wished to see the profession recognize the importance of the process, who believed that the skills of supervisors were vital in the development of clinicians, and who were willing to "make waves" in calling these concerns to the attention of the rest of the profession.

Pages could be written, and have been, about the lack of attention to supervision, about the low status of supervisors in many programs, about policies of the Publications Board of ASHA which for some time prevented the publication of research on the supervisory process in the journals of the association, about the lack of preparation and accountability, about the lack of strong research on the clinical and supervisory processes, and about many other issues. The writer, in an earlier statement, called supervision the "neglected component of the profession" (Anderson, 1973b, p. 4); and, indeed, it was for many years. These and many other issues have been documented by the ASHA Committee on Supervision in a *Special Report: Current Status of Supervision of Speech-Language Pathology and Audiology* (ASHA, 1978a), and by Culatta and Helmick, 1980, 1981; Oratio, 1977; Rassi, 1978; and Schubert, 1978. Readers are urged especially to make themselves familiar with the report of the Committee on Supervision for a comprehensive understanding of the issues that had existed up to that time.

Rather than dwelling on the deficiencies already documented elsewhere, this chapter will turn to the actions that have taken place over the past years as the profession has gradually changed attitudes toward the study of the supervisory process. The writer would not wish to be accused of being overly optimistic about the professional "climate" as it relates to supervisors and the process in which they are engaged, because there is still much to be done. Much has happened in a relatively short time, however, and it seems important as a background for future chapters to document the evolution of the profession's attention to the issues of supervision, at least as reflected in the literature.

EARLY ATTENTION TO THE CLINICAL PRACTICUM

Even the earliest literature documented an awareness of the need for clinical practicum. Paden (1970) reported that the charter membership of the organization that was to eventually become ASHA included individuals interested in teaching, research, and clinical practice in speech correction. Thus, even in those early, faltering efforts to develop the profession there was a recognition of the need for applied teaching. The first volume of the *Journal of Speech Disorders*, the publication of the newly formed American Speech Correction Association, listed six areas of graduate study required for certification, including clinical practice, and indicated that the course of study usually covered one year (two terms) and sometimes two years (Blanton, 1936). In 1938 the organization, in formulating changes in membership requirements, decreed again that members must hold the B.A. degree in "speech correction" and that the educational programs must include clinical practice. (Paden, 1970)

DEVELOPMENT OF SUPERVISION

Treatment of the clinical practicum was rather casual in those early days. Although the requirements obviously implied indirectly the need for supervision of the practicum, guidelines for the practicum or for supervision as it is now perceived seemed to be nonexistent. This contrasts sharply with current requirements for supervised practicum and the concentration of time spent in supervision that characterizes educational programs today.

When clinical practicum and supervision were mentioned in the earliest journals of the profession, it was usually in connection with membership requirements in ASHA, not in terms of content or process. Occasionally, an author or a member was identified as a supervisor in a school or clinic program or a state department of education. In fact, in the early days when only one person was employed in a school system to develop a program for communicatively handicapped children, he or she was often given the title of supervisor or director, even when probably providing direct services, sometimes the only direct service being offered.

As far as has been determined, the first use of the word *supervisor* in the early speech pathology literature was in a discussion of a bill introduced into the Senate that would authorize the U.S. Commissioner of Education to allot money to states for the education of physically handicapped children (as the speech and hearing handicapped were classified at that time). It was also designed to empower the Commissioner to formulate qualifications of "teachers, supervisors, and directors" and to suspend payments to states that did not comply, "thus assuring adequately trained teachers for physically handicapped children, rather than political appointees" (Robbins, 1937, p. 32). Federal programs did not begin with Public Law 94-142! A later volume indicated that the bill did not pass, thereby, it is assumed, relieving the Commissioner of an awesome responsibility (Robbins, 1939). Milisen (1939), one of the early advocates of the provision of clinical services, suggested a plan for school programs whereby a classroom teacher within a building would be responsible, after minimal in-service education, for speech improvement and speech correction. He called the person responsible for training of and monitoring the work of that appointed teacher a "speech correction supervisor." In 1939, ASHA membership requirements included "active present participation in actual clinical work in speech correction or in administrative duties immediately concerned with the supervision and direction of such work" (Robbins, 1939, p. 78). Most university and service programs at that time were small, often consisting of one person. One can only speculate about the nature of the supervisory or administrative duties, but can be certain that these duties were much less complex than they are today.

As the profession and its organization began to grow, the concept of two levels of membership or certification developed. In 1942 the qualifications for Associate Membership included a requirement for clinical clock hours—at least 200 clock hours under supervision. This clinical work, according to an amendment to the By-Laws, was to consist of observation and actual experience with clinical cases, the operation of laboratory and clinical equipment, the planning of case programs, objective reporting of case records, the operation of a speech clinic, and proper professional relationships with members of other professions. Competencies, approached from a somewhat negative perspective, were covered in one sentence—"The clock hours of experience should cover a variety of cases, so that the Associate will have had sufficient professional background to know his shortcomings, and to know when to seek expert guidance from Professional Members and Fellows" (ASHA, 1942). Was this the beginning of the belief that the purpose of supervision is to point out weaknesses, not strengths? Or that somewhere there is a supervisor who has all the answers?

Qualifications for Professional Members, therefore supervisors, were as follows: "A Professional Member should be a person prepared to give counsel, to head speech clinics, do diagnosis of speech defects, be expert in speech therapy and able to instruct others in this art and science. He should have initiative and resourcefulness, should understand and be able to apply objective approaches to problems in this field" (ASHA, 1942). Although the competencies were not specific and measurable, they were official and they led the way to stronger requirements that have changed as the profession has grown.

The following years found the young association changing its membership qualifications frequently, always accommodating levels of membership which implied, sometimes directly, sometimes not, the need for supervision. In 1946, for example, associate members were described in the By-Laws as persons "qualified on an ethical basis who have not, however, completed a professional education in the field of speech correction and are, therefore, not recommended as qualified by the Association to do speech corrective work beyond the apprentice level" (ASHA, 1946, p. 54). Were these the first paraprofessionals? The use of the word *apprentice* is interesting in relation to subsequent discussion of styles of supervision in this book. *Clinical* members were qualified to act as clinical technicians *under the guidance* of more completely trained individuals. *Professional* members were considered "qualified to supervise others in the correction of defects" (ASHA, 1946, p. 55). No specific qualifications were given for this ability to supervise others, so one must assume that level of training and amount of experience were the prime criteria for the Professional Member/Supervisor—not too different from later years, as will be seen.

During the 1940s and 1950s, the profession was building its scientific base, and accumulating a body of knowledge in normal development and disorders of communication. At the same time, it was developing standards for educational programs and certification in the American Speech and Hearing Association. As Butler (1980) points out, "The supervisory practices of thirty years ago may not have been as formalized or as data-based as today's practices, but there was supervision, indeed. Many of us who received our initial training in those years were fortunate to receive both clinical and academic instruction from the same individual, translating from class to clinic, principles and methods of delivering services to speech, language and hearing disordered adults" (p. 8).

The literature for those years reveals the struggle of the young profession to come to grips with the best way to prepare future clinicians. "Long before the general 'competency' movement of other professions in the 1960's, ASHA and its membership supported the concept of establishing training goals and in recognizing levels of expertise through the CCC. The foresight thus demonstrated by the Association's leaders significantly shaped our profession. It has not only permitted, but required, that those who serve the public in any one of a number of work settings. . .do so with a common core of knowledge and a recognized level of competency" (Butler, 1980, p. 8).

Impact of Needs in School Programs

The interest in more meaningful clinical practicum, and consequently, its adequate supervision, seems to have developed in great part as a result of the rapidly growing number of school programs where the bulk of the services to the communicatively handicapped was provided at that time. Throughout the late 1940s and into the 1950s, there were "stirrings" in the literature about the need for more "coursework" in clinical practicum and "practice teaching" in preparing people to work in the schools (Carrell, 1946). Also of concern was the need for establishing programs in schools to provide services to communicatively handicapped children and in universities to prepare professionals to deliver those services (Chapman, 1942; Hawk, 1936; Miller,

1948). Others at that time were writing about the components of programs for preparing "speech correctionists" for the schools and a struggle was occurring to establish requirements for school certification that would satisfy both departments of education and departments of speech pathology (Brown, 1952; Irwin, 1948, 1949, 1953; Mandell, 1952).

Backus (1953), in discussing preparation of clinicians for working with children, made the first reference to the quality of the supervision being provided, when she asserted:

> For too long professionals' training consisted largely of courses dealing with etiology of speech and hearing disorders. Courses called 'methods of therapy' provided few laboratory experiences for students. What laboratory experiences there were consisted mostly of therapy with adult clients; when clinical practice with children was available, it was largely unsupervised. When the word 'supervision' was used it represented too often only a paper requirement. Where provisions have been made for staff to supervise clinical practice, far less attention has been paid to qualifications of persons performing that function than to qualifications of persons doing diagnostic and research work. (pp. 195–196)

Not until 1957 did ASHA change its requirements so that the required 200 clock hours of clinical practice could be divided between the clinical setting and the public schools. Even before this, some states had established certification requirements for speech pathologists who planned to work in the schools. These requirements were closely patterned after those for classroom teachers and, therefore, included "student teaching," now more commonly labeled "school practicum" (Shefte, 1959). MacLearie (1947) reported the results of a survey on student teaching and suggested recommendations for such experiences—the first attempt at concrete guidelines to be found in the literature.

Although this discussion of school programs may appear to be irrelevant here, it seems clear in reading the early literature that feedback to universities about the needs in school programs, where most of the services were then being delivered, had an impact on the clinical practicum, and therefore, indirectly on supervisory needs.

SUPERVISION ON THE MOVE

This early slow start in recognizing the importance of the supervisory process is probably understandable. Speech pathology and audiology were in their early youth as a profession. The view of supervision glimpsed in the early membership requirements reflected the superior-subordinate perception of the supervisory process which predominated at that time in other areas where supervision existed. The building of a new profession required attention to basic foundations as well as to multitudinous professional issues. Perhaps a certain amount of time and a certain stage of maturity were necessary before the complexities of the supervisory process could be addressed.

Whatever one perceives as the reasons, it is obvious that there has been a very slow evolution of knowledge, interest, and activities related to the supervisory process. A review of relevant events reveals that each decade brought contributions that led to the current status.

A brief overview of these events—the developing literature, ASHA activities, organizations—will be given here in the interest of a perspective on the historical background. Details of the literature will be given later in appropriate sections.

For those who have been involved in these efforts, it should be rewarding to realize how much has been accomplished; for those who have not been involved, it may help them to understand the present.

The Decade of the 1950s

Although the profession appeared to be occupied with other issues during the 1950s, some important groundwork was laid. The word *supervisor* began to be more common in the literature.

The Literature

In what appears to be the first dissertation to investigate any aspect of the supervisory process in speech-language pathology and audiology, Shefte (1959) reported on the rapidly developing interest in communicatively handicapped children in the schools in the 1950s. The need for services accompanying this development placed responsibility on the colleges and universities where professionals were being prepared to work in the schools. Shefte describes clearly the parallel emergence of standards set by state departments of education and the American Speech and Hearing Association which college and university programs then made efforts to meet. She traces the development and expansion of educational programs for therapists (current terminology at that time), particularly in terms of the experiences that were provided for those who were to work in the schools. She points out the concerns about the nature of clinical practice and student teaching, and the attempts being made to define its parameters more specifically. The dissertation documented the degree of importance of certain aspects of the student teaching program as viewed by supervisors and therapists. The author provided guidelines which were urgently needed at the time in the development of this aspect of college and university programs. Many supervisory issues emerged out of these concerns.

At about this same time, Elizabeth MacLearie, supervisor in the Ohio Department of Education and a pioneer in promoting better services in the schools, published an appraisal form for speech and hearing personnel to be used by supervisors or administrators. MacLearie (1958) pointed out the fact that improvements in speech and hearing programs must come primarily through improvement of the therapist. "Supervision is of no value unless it brings about learning situations. Assessment made as objectively as possible is the first step toward improvement. The appraisal should be equally acceptable to the supervisor and to the speech therapist" (p. 613).

Organizations of Supervisors

A significant activity during the 1950s was the organization of two supervisor groups—the Council of Speech and Hearing Consultants in State Departments of Education and the Council of Coordinators and Administrators of Language, Speech and Hearing Services in the Schools. These groups meet at the time of the annual convention of ASHA but have remained independent organizations. Both groups have been called upon for assistance in implementing ASHA-directed activities toward strengthening programs in the schools. Furthermore, the early members of these organizations sowed the seeds of interest in the supervisory process.

The Decade of the 1960s

The 1960s saw a growing concern about the direction of the profession, including continuously increasing requirements for education and certification. Discussion of issues surrounding the clinical practicum became more specific. Many of the stated concerns were clearly supervision issues, although not always verbalized as such. The involvement of the federal government in funding the preparation of personnel to work with handicapped children brought further attention to the quality of college and university programs.

The Literature

The literature of this period began with a report of a nationwide study of speech and hearing services in the schools, which was supported by the U.S. Office of Education and conducted by the Research Committee of ASHA. Published as *Monograph Supplement #8 of the American Speech and Hearing Association*, it was a landmark document (ASHA, 1961). Not only did the survey divulge the first comprehensive data about school programs; once again, concern about this segment of the profession focused on the content and supervision of the clinical practicum in the university and its implication for the quality of services provided later in the schools. It also provided data about the supervision of school programs at the time, descriptive information about local and state supervisors, a listing of their activities, and their professional responsibilities and relationships (Black, Miller, Anderson, & Coates, 1961). Additionally, the survey revealed insufficiency of staff for supervision of practicum in college and university programs as a major problem. A substantial number of practicing clinicians reported deficiencies in their clinical practicum. And, once again, the student teaching (school practicum) experience received attention when state supervisors expressed a need for more frequent and more comprehensive supervision of this experience (Irwin, Van Riper, Breakey, & Fitzsimmons, 1961).

Regarding supervision in school programs, Darley and Hanley (1961) stated, "The facts concerning present operating procedures suggest significant lack of uniformity in the carrying out of supervisory responsibilities. Practices with regard to direct observation and guidance of clinicians vary widely, some relatively inexperienced clinicians reporting that they receive only token supervision.

There are indications that some supervisors do not receive information of sufficient scope and detail to permit effective program evaluation and enlightened program planning" (p. 126).

Soon after this, specific comments about supervision began to appear in the literature. In a discussion of the status of the profession, Perkins (1962) identified several concerns related to supervision and made the strongest statement up to that time about its inadequacies. Perkins believed the profession suffered in comparison to other clinical professions because the sponsored experience required for certification at that point "is far from being the same as closely supervised clinical work" (p. 340). He further stated that the quality of supervision of clinical practicum was questionable and, for the first time, pinpointed the problem of status of supervisors. "An appointment to supervise trainees in our profession is not yet a coveted mark of distinction" (p. 340). And later, "Agreed, funds are not available in most institutions for thorough supervision of all student clinicians by highly qualified professionals. But if we have specialized skills that are essential to success in our profession, how else can they be imparted except through careful guidance?" (p. 344).

More evidence of interest in the practicum came in the 1960's, when a seminar was conducted by ASHA on *Guidelines for Supervision of Clinical Practicum in Programs of Training for Speech Pathology and Audiology* (Villareal, 1964). Sponsored by the Vocational Rehabilitation Administration, the proceedings of the seminar were reported in an ASHA publication which revealed that the participants concerned themselves with "clinical practicum, that part of professional training in which the information gleaned from courses on speech and hearing disorders and methodology for assessment and therapy is translated into the skills and competencies of the speech and hearing clinician" (p. 9). Issues discussed by the participants were the nature and distribution of clinical practicum, the nature of supervision of clinical practicum, characteristics and qualifications of the clinical supervisor, and the nature of students' educational needs. The report is interesting reading in light of today's concerns since many of the issues discussed in 1964 are the same as those discussed today.

In the same year, Kleffner (1964) reported on another conference on *Guidelines for the Internship Year.* Held prior to the date when standards for the new Certificate of Clinical Competence were to go into effect, this seminar addressed the issue of specific criteria for supervision of the first year of professional experience, an experience that developed into the Clinical Fellowship Year (CFY). Topics of discussion were the intern (even though this terminology was rejected early in the report), the supervisor, the supervision, the environment, and the components of the experience. The report clearly identified many issues which are current, particularly in the CFY. In the conclusion of the report, Kleffner makes a very cogent statement about supervision, carrying the concern into the employment setting:

> Thus far in the report, supervision has been viewed only in relation to
> the internship year. In the broader professional perspective, this view of
> supervision is unnecessarily narrow. If we provide supervision only for

the purpose of guiding and monitoring the work of inexperienced clinical personnel, we have failed to capitalize on a most important source of strength and growth in the profession. It is clinical foolhardiness, at the very least, even to imply that supervision should cease as soon as nine months of supervised experience is completed. The place of supervision in a clinical program is *changed* rather than *diminished* as those being supervised gain in experience. As the experience of the staff increases, so does the opportunity for creative contribution by the supervisor to the program and to the client. None of us is so adept, so experienced, and so insightful in our clinical endeavors that we cannot stand to gain from the insights into clinical tasks which the overview of a supervisor—clinical consultant—makes possible. Clinical supervision is a necessary and desirable component in any truly comprehensive clinical service program. (p. 20)

In the first major article devoted solely to issues of supervision of the practicum, the status of supervision was addressed by Halfond (1964), who proposed that the supervisory process is one of the more crucial aspects of professional education in speech-language pathology and audiology but that "supervision, which serves in the transition from academic proficiency to professional application, is either downgraded or neglected. There is evidence that supervision is a stepchild in the educative process" (p. 441). The author continues with a thorough treatment of supervisory principles and methodologies from his point of view and finishes with a plea for the profession to attend to the supervisory portion of the training process and its value in the provision of better clinical services.

The role of the clinical supervisor was described by Van Riper (1965) as one of the most important of all functions in the educational program. "It is in our personal interaction with the students we supervise," he said, "that we are able to have our most important impact" (p. 75). Later, Erickson and Van Riper (1967) preface a detailed account of a plan for student observation of demonstration therapy with the following statement:

We must remember that in training clinicians we not only teach; we also nurture. The teaching and nurturing of clinical understanding and skills pose perhaps a greater challenge than do any other of the tasks which face us as we prepare students for careers in speech pathology and audiology. Some of our students have taught us only too well that mere academic knowledge of normal and disordered communication, although prerequisite to competent clinical work, by no means ensures competency. (p. 33)

In addition to these occasional statements about supervision, the 1960s produced reports of conferences on supervision in the schools (Anderson & Kirtley, 1966) and of the school practicum (Kirtley, 1967). The members of the Research Committee of the California Speech and Hearing Association undertook an extensive study of the supervised school experience in their own state and made recommendations based on the data collected from college supervisors, master clinicians (on-site school clinicians who supervised the school practicum), and former students (Flower, 1969; Rees & Smith, 1967, 1968).

At about this time, Miner (1967) coordinated a seminar at an ASHA convention in which a detailed discussion of the elements of supervision was presented. Miner listed the following items which she called eight elements of "quality supervision" of clinical practicum:

1. Understanding and utilizing the dynamics of human relationships which promote the growth of the student clinician.

2. Establishing realistic goals with the student clinician which are clearly understood by both student and supervisor.

3. Observing and analyzing the teaching-learning act involved in the therapy procedures.

4. Providing the student with the necessary "feedback" which will enable him to become increasingly self-analytical.

5. Knowing and using a variety of materials, methods, and techniques which are based on sound theory, successful practice, or documented research.

6. Recognizing and setting aside the supervisor's personal prejudices and biases which influence perception and develop rigidity in order that the subjective task of evaluation may become as objective as possible.

7. Challenging and motivating the student clinician to strengthen his clinical competency without the supervisor's assistance.

8. Appreciating the individual differences among student clinicians to such an extent that supervisory programs and practices may be radically altered to suit his needs. (pp. 471–472)

Hatten (1966) was the first to actually investigate the components of the supervisory conference in a dissertation study which will be reported later. This pioneer dissertation was never published but identified some important variables in the supervisory process. Additional publications in the 1960s regarding supervision were that of Brooks and Hannah (1966) and O'Neil and Peterson (1964), who discussed specific supervisory techniques. Stace and Drexler (1969) reported on a survey of supervisors of student interns, "young professionals" as they labeled them, in private speech and hearing centers.

The Decade of the 1970s

The 1970s brought an unprecedented surge of activity in the literature, in ASHA activities related to supervision, and in the general interest shown by the profession.

The Literature

Compared with previous periods, the 1970s were extremely productive in terms of the literature on supervision. Conference proceedings and reports (Anderson, 1970; Conture, 1973; Turton, 1973) were printed and circulated.

Several dissertations were completed during this time (Caracciolo, 1977; Dowling, 1977; Engnoth, 1974; Goodwin, 1977; Hall, 1971; Ingrisano, 1979; Pickering, 1979; Smith, 1978; Underwood, 1973). Articles directed toward the supervisory process, some based on the previously listed dissertations, were published in *Asha* (Anderson, 1973a, 1974; Caracciolo, Rigrodsky, & Morrison, 1978a, 1978b; Culatta, Colucci, & Wiggins, 1975; Culatta & Seltzer, 1976, 1977; Dowling, 1979a; Gerstman, 1977; Oratio, 1978, 1979a; Pickering, 1977; Schubert, 1974; Schubert & Aitchison, 1975). The *Journal of Language, Speech and Hearing Services in the Schools* published papers about supervision in the schools (Anderson, 1972; ASHA, 1972) and on the school practicum (Baldes, Goings, Herbold, Jeffrey, Wheeler, & Freilinger, 1977; Monnin & Peters, 1977; O'Toole, 1973). A few articles on supervision in speech-language pathology and audiology were published in other journals (Dowling, 1979b; Irwin, 1975, 1976; Irwin & Hall, 1973; Irwin & Nickles, 1970; Oratio, 1976; Schubert & Laird, 1975; Till, 1976). During this time there were also several presentations at ASHA conventions, most of which have remained unpublished. Three books on supervision were published in this decade—two on supervision of speech-language pathology (Oratio, 1977; Schubert, 1978), and one on audiology supervision (Rassi, 1978).

Organizations

The two organizations of state supervisors and school program supervisors continued to function, meeting at the time of ASHA conventions. Main activities of this period were joint problem-solving about situations unique to each group and a great amount of input to ASHA and the U.S. Office of Education, which would come to fruition in many of the actions taken in the 1970s to improve programs in the schools.

ASHA Action

ASHA responded in the 1970s to an expressed need for leadership from its members in assisting schools to provide optimal services to children with communication disorders. Working through its Committee on Language, Speech and Hearing Services in the Schools, the organization undertook a major project to devise a national set of standards and guidelines for school programs. Over 4,000 professionals participated in this effort. Several task forces were charged with a variety of responsibilities in developing these guidelines. One was a Task Force on Supervision in the Schools, which prepared detailed guidelines for programs in the areas of administration, consultation, and program development. It made recommendations for ratios of supervisors to clinicians and supportive personnel, and formulated guidelines for preparing supervisors, for supervising supportive personnel, and for the school practicum (ASHA, 1972). In addition, the Task Force encouraged universities and colleges to develop preparation programs for supervisors, urged ASHA to work toward establishing special supervisor certificates in each state, and proposed that states reimburse school districts for supervision.

The final result of the described project was the document, *Standards and Guidelines for Comprehensive Language, Speech, and Hearing Programs in the Schools* (ASHA, 1973–1974), which included a section on administration of speech-language and hearing programs in the schools and a section on program supervision.

A further action of the Committee on Services in the Schools was a recommendation to the Executive Board that a standing committee on supervision be appointed by the organization. The Committee on Supervision in Speech Pathology and Audiology was appointed in 1974. The charge to that committee was as follows:

1. Promote and disseminate current information about supervision in speech-language pathology and audiology.
2. Promote research on the supervisory process.
3. Identify significant issues in supervision in training programs, the Clinical Fellowship Year, and in various employment settings.
4. Recommend standards and guidelines for the roles and responsibilities of supervisors in the settings listed in Item 3.
5. Develop strategies for encouraging the employment of supervisory personnel.
6. Recommend standards and guidelines for training programs in supervision.

In 1978, after extensive study of the issues surrounding the implementation of the supervisory process within the profession, the Committee on Supervision developed a status statement in which nine major issues in supervision were identified and discussed at length:

1. Need for data to validate the supervisory process.
2. Need for role definition for supervisors specific to the context of the various settings in which they work.
3. Need for more supervisors.
4. Need for better quality in the supervision currently being provided.
5. Need for special standards for supervisors, other than the Certificate of Clinical Competence of the American Speech and Hearing Association.
6. Need for training for supervisors.
7. Need for investigation of the status of supervisors, particularly within the academic system.
8. Need for investigation of the ambiguities and problems which exist in the supervision of the Clinical Fellowship Year.
9. Need for accountability systems for supervisor. (ASHA, 1978a)

On the basis of these issues, recommendations were made in two categories: one for ASHA as an organization, consisting of twelve items; another for the committee itself, which included six items.

Organization of Supervisors

Parallel to the ASHA-sponsored activities and the individual efforts at research and writing during this period, another special interest group of supervisors was formed. The College and University Supervisors of School Practicum was organized in November, 1970. Its purpose was to bring together those members of college and university faculties who were engaged in the supervision of the school practicum. In 1974 the organization voted to include supervisors of practicum in clinical training programs and at that time changed its name to the Council of University Supervisors of Practicum in Speech Pathology and Audiology (CUSPSPA). In 1985 the By-Laws of the organization were once again modified to include associate membership. Associate members do not need to hold the ASHA Certificate of Clinical Competence and have no voting privileges. The group meets annually at the time of the ASHA convention and has developed an active interaction among professionals with a common interest in the supervisory process. The organization publishes a quarterly newsletter, *SUPERvision*.

Other Activities

The 1970s saw the real beginning of formal educational programs in the supervisory process. A survey by the Committee on Supervision in the late 1970s, however, revealed that such preparation was still sparse and that its content was not clearly identifiable. Approaches to preparation of supervisors included course work, content in other courses, practicum, internship, and individual study. Further analysis, however, showed that such offerings were often provided only intermittently and those that were available had reached only a limited number of individuals. Much of the education related to supervision still appeared to be offered through the workshop or institute format and often seemed to deal more with the administrative aspects of the supervisory role; that is, *program management* rather than *clinical teaching*, as defined by the Committee on Supervision (ASHA, 1978a).

In 1972, major recognition of the importance of preparation in the supervisory process was shown with the funding by the U.S. Office of Education of a doctoral-level program at Indiana University, the goal of which was to prepare students to teach others how to supervise and to conduct research in the supervisory process (Anderson, 1981).

The Decade of the 1980s

As the profession moved into the 1980s, the interest in supervision continued to increase and extremely important events took place.

The Literature

With the advent of the 1980s, more dissertations were completed (Andersen, 1981; Brasseur, 1980b; Casey, 1980; Farmer, 1984; Kennedy, 1981; Larson, 1982; McCrea, 1980; Nilsen, 1983; Roberts, 1982; Shapiro, 1985; Tihen, 1984; Tufts, 1984). Additional articles were published in *Asha* (Anderson, 1981; Cimorell-Strong & Ensley, 1982; Culatta & Helmick, 1980, 1981; Peaper & Wener, 1984) and one in the *Journal of Speech and Hearing Disorders* in this time period (Pickering, 1984). The most positive move forward in terms of the literature, however, was the publication of the first articles on supervision in the *Journal of Speech and Hearing Research* (Brasseur & Anderson, 1983; Roberts & Naremore, 1983; Roberts & Smith, 1982; Smith & Anderson, 1982a, 1982b). Publication of these articles represented a change in policy of the ASHA Publication Board to permit the publication of research on supervision in journals of the profession other than *Asha*. This change was the result of major effort—by individuals, the Committee on Supervision, and, eventually, action of the Legislative Council. Researchers also published in several journals other than those of their own organization—the *Journal of Communication Disorders* (Dowling, 1983b; Dowling & Bliss, 1984; Dowling, Sbaschnig, & Williams, 1982; Dowling & Shank, 1981; Dowling & Wittkopp, 1982; Irwin, 1981a, 1981b; Oratio, Sugarman, & Prass, 1981), the *Journal of the National Student Speech Language-Hearing Association*, (Dowling, 1981; Shapiro, 1986), and in a new interdisciplinary journal entitled *The Clinical Supervisor* (Blodgett, Schmitt, & Scudder, 1987; Dowling, 1983a, 1984, 1985, 1986; Farmer, 1985-1986, 1987; Peaper, 1984; Runyan & Seal, 1985; Sleight, 1984, 1985).

Two books have been published during the 1980s. The first dealt with the school practicum (Monnin & Peters, 1981) and the other, *Supervision in Human Communication Disorders: Perspectives on a Process*, edited by M. Crago and M. Pickering (1987), covers a variety of topics. In addition, Lemme (1986) has contributed a chapter on supervision in a textbook on intervention in aphasia.

Three conferences held during the 1980s focused on the supervisory process. The topic of the first conference was the preparation of supervisors. The second was the annual conference of the Council of Graduate Programs in Communication Sciences and Disorders, at which a series of presentations was made on the topic of clinical supervision in the university setting. Both conferences resulted in published proceedings (Anderson, 1980; Bernthal, 1985). The third conference was sponsored by CUSPSPA and will be cited later.

Additionally, a perusal of ASHA convention programs reveals numerous presentations during this period on the supervisory process. These offerings at ASHA conventions, still seldom published, are not only increasing in quantity but in quality. Recent papers have demonstrated an identification of issues and a focus in the research that indicates a clearer direction in the study of the process.

ASHA Activities

Several activities of ASHA during the early 1980s have been directed toward certain of the recommendations made by the early Committee on Supervision (ASHA, 1978a), specifically the development of role definitions, guidelines, and qualification standards for supervisors, and investigation of preparation of supervisors. Foremost among these was the adoption by the Legislative Council, upon recommendation of the Committee on Supervision, of a detailed list of tasks and competencies for supervisors (ASHA, 1985b). Implications of this document are discussed in the chapter on preparation of supervisors. Specific competencies are referred to where appropriate in other chapters. Although not validated, this listing of competencies offers a base for future exploration into the intricacies of this most important activity called supervision. Another historical perspective has been presented by Ulrich (1987), which details more specifically the role of AHSA in on-going development of standards which have been relevant to supervisors.

The Committee on Supervision continues to pursue implementation of the recommendations made by the original committee. Current major activity is a document which presents preparation models in the supervisory process.

Organizations

The Council of University Supervisors of Practicum in Speech-Language Pathology and Audiology (CUSPSPA) has grown and strengthened. A national research network, *SuperNet*, has been established to bring supervisors together in their research efforts. CUSPSPA continues to work with the ASHA Committee on Supervision. Its major contribution, however, has been the organization of a national conference on supervision in 1987, the proceedings of which will be published (Farmer, 1987).

Other Activities

There appears to be a continuation of in-service offerings and course work, although this fact cannot be documented at this time. More information should be available soon on educational offerings as a result of efforts of CUSPSPA, which has been attempting to collect such information.

SUMMARY

This overall review makes it obvious that interest in the study of the supervisory process in speech-language pathology and audiology has progressed slowly but steadily, with a recent intensification of efforts. Each decade has brought developments. The increase in the literature, convention presentations, and conferences, and the work of ASHA and other organizations can be documented. What is more difficult to portray is the enthusiasm and vigor of the individuals who have made this happen. Supervisors have developed a network that is strong and operative. There is more to be done, but it seems safe to say that at last certain segments of the profession are taking more seriously than ever before the needs of supervisors, their importance to the profession, and the necessity of studying the process. More important, supervisors are beginning to answer their own questions and solve their own problems through networking, research, teaching, and political action.

Styles of Supervision

Each of us has his own strengths and weaknesses. Therefore, we would hesitate to insist that all of us should supervise in the same way.

Van Riper, (1965)

One of the things known about supervision in speech-language pathology is that, despite the obvious wisdom of the above quotation, most supervisors *do* supervise in the same way. There is now a fairly large body of information about the supervisory conference from many sources. These studies have identified a definite pattern found in supervisory conferences. The details of the studies will be given later as appropriate; but if the data from these studies are combined and the reader conjectures about a typical supervisory conference in speech-language pathology (there are no specific data about audiology conferences), the description of a typical conference would be something like this:

> The conference is brief—probably less than 30 minutes. The supervisor assumes a dominant role, doing most of the talking, initiating and structuring most of the discussion, thereby setting the tone for the entire conference. Topics change frequently. Much of the content of the conference consists of the supervisee providing information about what happened in the therapy session and the supervisor making suggestions about strategies to be used in the future. It is not clear how much of this information is data based or analyzed, but it appears to be a "rehash" or recounting of what happened in the therapy session. Supervisors give a great deal of information, make a great many suggestions, and do not spend much time asking the supervisee for suggestions about future action. Supervisors use praise or other supportive behaviors to create a positive social-emotional climate which probably is perceived by supervisees as reinforcement for certain behaviors. Very little explanation, justification, clarifying, elaborating, or summarizing of statements (all behaviors that enhance communication) are given by either supervisor or supervisee. Discussion probably deals with maintenance or procedural topics with discussion of anxieties, defensiveness, or other affective issues being avoided. Supervisors in different settings (university, off-campus practicum, service delivery settings) may operate differently in some

aspects of supervision, although there are not really enough data to sub-
stantiate this. Emphasis in the discussion is on the teaching-therapy process or the client, not on the supervisee or supervisor. The supervisory
process is seldom discussed. Very few evaluative statements are made
about the supervisee, perhaps because supervisors assume that supervisees can utilize the discussion of the client to learn about their own
behavior. Supervisor style will be much the same from one conference
to another, regardless of the supervisee's experience, expertise, or expectations. In general, the discussion is cognitive, not affective.

Supervisees are usually passive participants in the conference, seldom ask questions, initiate a topic, or ask for justification of supervisory statements. Instead, they react and respond to the supervisors. Their
responses tend to be short, most likely agreeing with the supervisor.
Supervisees' needs for indirect behavior from the supervisor and for their
own participation are probably not met. As with supervisors, supervisees utilize simple utterances without justification or rationalization
and they do not provide reinforcement for the supervisor. (Blumberg,
1980; Culatta & Seltzer, 1976, 1977; Culatta et al., 1975; Dowling &
Shank, 1981; Hatten, 1966; Irwin, 1975, 1976, 1981b; McCrea, 1980;
Pickering, 1979, 1981, 1982, 1984; Roberts & Smith, 1982; Russell, 1976;
Schubert & Nelson 1976; Shapiro, 1985; Smith, 1978; Smith & Anderson,
1982b; Tufts, 1984; Underwood, 1973; Weller, 1971).

Because there is such overwhelming evidence that this is what happens in
conferences, this type of interaction will be referred to from now on as *traditional*
supervision.

It has also been determined that, although supervisors can identify certain
differences in the supervisory behaviors of others (Brasseur & Anderson, 1983)
they are not so accurate in their perceptions of their own behavior (Smith &
Anderson, 1982b). Regardless of different self-perceptions, supervisory behavior
patterns are similar. Self-analysis does not facilitate change even when supervisors
perceive change in their own behavior. Rather, they tend to rationalize the patterns
they perceive (Culatta et al., 1975; Culatta & Seltzer, 1976, 1977).

ASSUMPTIONS ABOUT SUPERVISORY BEHAVIOR

Perhaps the most reliable fact about supervision in speech-language
pathology and audiology is that the vast majority of supervisors are operating
without preparation for the supervisory process and that they have expressed
the need for knowing more about how to supervise (Anderson, 1973, 1974, 1980;
ASHA, 1978a; Schubert & Aitchison, 1975; Stace & Drexler, 1969). Therefore,
it seems reasonable to assume that current supervisory styles have been derived
in a variety of ways, not necessarily based on a conceptual or theoretical
foundation, and possibly not thoughtfully planned or rationally decided.

The speech-language pathology and audiology profession, along with many
other professions, has operated on many assumptions about supervision that
have certainly not been challenged, possibly not even recognized. First, it has

been assumed that supervision is necessary and beneficial, yet there is virtually no documentation that it makes any difference at all in the behavior of the supervisee, either in the educational program or in the service delivery setting, or in the behavior of clients, which is, after all, the ultimate goal of both the clinical and the supervisory interaction. Second, it has been assumed that supervisors are "super-clinicians," and therefore have the ultimate answers about what should happen in the clinical session when they become supervisors. Third, it has been assumed that all supervisors are attempting to produce self-directing, independent, problem-solving clinicians. Fourth, it has often been assumed that the major role of the supervisor is *evaluation*. Fifth, it has been assumed that formal education is not necessary for engaging in the supervisory process—that education and experience as clinicians are sufficient to prepare professionals for the role of supervisor.

IS THERE *A* METHODOLOGY?

The search for *a* methodology for supervision is a will-o-the-wisp, as elusive as *a* methodology for clinical interaction. Clients are different; clinicians have divergent needs; supervisors vary. Validation data on effectiveness of supervision methods are sparse in any field, nonexistent in speech-language pathology and audiology.

Butler (1976), in a discussion of competencies in speech- language pathology and audiology as related to supervision, said:

> Interaction between client and clinician in the therapeutic process reflects an almost kaleidoscopic matrix of events. . . such interactions must take into account the nature and degree of the client's speech, language or hearing disorder, the age and sex of the client, the age and sex of the clinician, the degree of sophistication and experience of both client and clinician in the therapeutic process, certain identifiable teaching-learning behaviors, and certainly, the professional persuasion of the supervising clinician. If you have been a supervisor in a college or university clinic, you know of the perils and the problems of quantifying such a complex matrix. (p. 2)

The supervisor of a service delivery program is no less vulnerable to these complexities. Fisher (1982) addressed the issues in supervising professional personnel in the schools and stated, "This responsibility requires a multitude of skills in human interaction, motivation, and leadership of developing professionals. The role of a supervisor is vastly different from the role of a speech-language pathologist or an audiologist in this respect. In essence, when a person becomes a supervisor, this person changes professions" (p. 54).

Gouran (1980) recognized the fact that supervision remains something of an art and said, "Hence, recommendations related to the practice of supervision should be viewed in probabilistic terms" (p. 87). He further noted that there would be a number of exceptions for any set of recommendations and, thus, it would not be prudent to develop or implement standard operating procedures for all situations. Weller (1971) asserted that a single methodological approach is impossible; rather, supervisory functions related to problems should be identified and methodologies appropriate for each should be proposed.

DEVELOPMENT OF SUPERVISORY BEHAVIORS

In the presence of so many situational variables and so little "how-to-supervise" information, what, then, forms the basis for the actions of professionals when they become supervisors? How do supervisory behaviors or styles develop? Obviously, past experiences in human interactions influence behaviors toward people in all situations. A major factor in the way supervisors interact with those in less dominant positions in the supervisor/supervisee relationship may be the way in which they have been dealt with by others who have held dominant positions over them—parents, teachers, siblings, or others. "The way the important people in our lives treat us largely determines our self-perception" (Gazda, Asbury, Balzer, Childers, & Walters, 1977, p. 2). Much of the perception of the role of the supervisor and the behaviors of persons who find themselves in that role probably have come from their interactions with their own supervisors, modeled directly from their behaviors. They may reflect the style of a significant supervisor, their style may have become a potpourri of behaviors from many supervisors, or they may have learned "what not to do" from those supervisors with whom they have not related so well. A colleague recently told of the student in a class on supervision who, in a role-playing exercise, was challenged on a certain behavior. Her rationale for the behavior was related to what *she* had expected from *her* supervisors while she was in training. Therefore, she felt that her response was appropriate. This type of modeling may be a major source of supervisory style for many supervisors.

Stereotypes of Supervisors

In addition to these personal interactions which shape behavior, the world is filled with stereotypes, many negative, of the "person in charge"—in literature, on the television screen, and in the movies. Most individuals have heard since childhood about their mother's boss, their father's department manager, and they have observed their teachers' principals. They have viewed on various screens the sergeant directing the troops, the business executive managing the employees, the department store manager lurking in the aisles, the newspaper editor shouting orders to reporters, or the boss whose only communication with his or her secretary is "Take a letter." They have heard the words "snoopervision" and "stupidvisor." Occasionally, they have seen a kindly, maternalistic or paternalistic portrayal of the role and, probably less often, an example of a positive, cooperative interaction between superior and subordinate. From all of this they have absorbed certain attitudes about supervision which may be reflected in their own expectations and behaviors.

Other Sources of Supervisory Styles

Some supervisors have read books and articles from other fields about leadership and management and have tried to apply the contents to their own situations—possibly with mixed results. They also may have read much about leadership in the popular literature, that is, books, magazines, or paperbacks. Bookstores now have an abundance of "how-to" books on this topic and, in the current climate of self-improvement-through-reading, they may have searched there for ways to advance themselves or, more likely, what to do once they have *been* advanced!

There are many parallels between the clinical process and the supervisory process. Their education and their competencies as clinicians are probably important influences on the supervisory behavior of most supervisors. This is not to imply that a competent clinician is automatically a competent supervisor. It does seem reasonable to assume, however, that the emphasis in clinical process preparation on such aspects as thorough description of behaviors, meeting individual needs of clients, one-to-one interaction, and productive interpersonal relationships probably contributes more than is realized to competencies in the supervisory process. This hypothesis remains untested, however.

Policies or organizational structure also may influence the way in which supervisors develop a style. Work-load assignments, organizational philosophy, operating policies, delegation of responsibility, and other organizational variables directly affect the way in which supervisors perceive and carry out their roles.

Last, each supervisor's personal characteristics and interpersonal relationship style will determine to a great extent the kind of supervisory interaction that each person adopts. Each person's style reflects his or her approach to dealing with people in any setting. Supervisory styles may be only an extension of life styles. To paraphrase a well-known saying, it is probably true that "You may take the supervisor out of the person but you can't take the person out of the supervisor."

Generally speaking, then, individual styles of supervisors have probably "grown like Topsy"—developed as a result of a variety of experiences rather than as a result of a study of the supervisory process, examination of one's personal philosophy, self-study of one's behaviors as a supervisor, or the application of theoretical models and research findings.

LITERATURE FROM OTHER DISCIPLINES

Perhaps the picture painted is too bleak or too simplistic. Perhaps it is patronizing to the many supervisors who have been influenced by the large and varied body of literature that exists in other disciplines. Perhaps supervisors have been influenced more than is realized by their education from other disciplines—education, psychology, business management, sociology, and others. Certainly the writer's thinking about the supervisory process has been influenced to a major extent by the study of the literature on leadership, learning, communication, and many other subjects. Leddick and Barnard (1980) quote Myers (1971) to support their point that while the study of supervision is made more complex because of its existence in so many arenas, there is an overlap among the helping professions which makes it important to understand the contributions of each.

Attempting to provide a comprehensive review of the literature in relevant areas would be roughly comparable to summarizing the literature on communicative disorders in a few pages. It seems important, however, to trace, albeit sketchily, the evolution of certain ideas or approaches that have, sometimes unknowingly, sometimes directly, influenced supervisors in speech-language pathology and audiology and the organizations in which they work. Therefore, this chapter will contain, not a review, but a brief commentary on literature from such areas as business management, education, counseling, and social work. The serious student of the supervisory process will want to go to original sources to supplement the information given here.

Leadership and Supervision in Business Management

A search for information about supervision naturally takes one to the literature on leadership and supervision from business management or organizational behavior where researchers and writers have been absorbed for many years with the question of how to work with other people—how to lead and how to follow. Much of the literature appears to be applicable to supervision in speech-language pathology and audiology, if not directly, at least in ways which encourage some very pointed questions about the discipline. According to Gouran (1980), "If leadership consists of acts having functional utility in the achievement of shared goals, then it would appear to follow that the supervisor/supervisee relationship represents the kind of social configuration in which a knowledge of leadership principles and practices should have instrumental value" (p. 92).

Scientific Management

Taylor (1911) proposed a theory of leadership called *scientific management*, which was characterized by efficiency, standardization of work behaviors, and a definite hierarchical, bureaucratic system. The objective was to determine the best method to do every job. The manager/supervisor was an authoritarian figure whose responsibility was to see that workers performed the job according to that one best method so that they would produce and meet the objectives of the system. Focus was on the organization, not the individuals within it. Through finding the "right way" to perform every activity, production was expected to increase. This classical approach to management still influences some organizations.

Human Relations

The human factor in the work setting was not considered seriously until after the Hawthorne studies (Mayo, 1933). These well-known studies marked a turning point in the treatment of workers and in the role of the leader/supervisor by clearly demonstrating the importance of the personal interaction within the work setting. Thus began what came to be known as the *human relations movement* in management, which has produced extensive research about the significance of the interactions among people in the work setting, job satisfaction, and the personal relationship of the leader to the led (Hampton, Summer, & Webber, 1982; Hersey & Blanchard, 1982; Kelly, 1980; Pascale & Athos, 1981; Peters & Waterman, 1982; Reitz, 1981; Tannenbaum, 1966).

Differences in leadership styles have been based on assumptions made about humans and the kind of power or authority that must be used on the basis of those assumptions. The classic categorization of leadership behavior as authoritarian (concern for task), democratic (concern for people), or *laissez-faire* (no formal leadership) (Lewin, Lippett & White, 1939) became the foundation for extensive research in psychology, sociology, education, management, and other disciplines concerned with interactions between people.

Early research in leadership was also strongly influenced by the work of Maslow (1954), who classified human needs common to all people as physiological, safety, social, self-esteem, and self-actualization. Maslow contended, and others have built upon the idea, that humans attempt to satisfy these needs in the order in which they are presented—physiological needs first. When these are met, the next level is activated. Although there are many complexities in applying this hierarchy to specific conditions, it is useful background for the study of supervisory behavior. Recognizing needs for self-actualization in supervisees and helping them attain it may be one of the most significant qualities of a supervisor.

McGregor (1960) offered two assumptions about human behavior in the work setting—Theory X and Theory Y. Theory X assumed that most people are innately lazy, unreliable, not interested in assuming responsibility, and want to be told what to do. Theory Y assumed the opposite—people are not innately lazy, irresponsible, and unreliable and, if motivated properly, can be basically self-directed and creative. The theory did not lead to the conclusion that one form of behavior is good, the other bad; rather, that Theory X and Y are attitudes toward people which govern the way in which leaders interact with their followers. Based on the assumption that most people have the potential to be motivated and self-actualizing, McGregor suggested (1) decentralization and delegation, (2) job enrichment, and (3) performance appraisal as activities of leaders which he considered consistent with Theory Y. McGregor also assumed that management must assume the onus of developing employment conditions in which people would feel free to exploit their self-fulfillment needs. The way to do this, according to McGregor, was through participative management.

Argyris (1962) maintained that, despite what had been learned about the advantages of the democratic, humanistic approach to leadership, most organizations operated under authoritarian leadership. Argyris described two types of value systems. In his *bureaucratic/pyramidal* system, the emphasis was on the organization's objectives, where the effectiveness of human relationships increases with clearly communicated direction, authority, and control, and with appropriate rewards and penalties for achievement of the objectives. In the *humanistic/democratic* value system, human relationships are not only related to the objectives of the organization, but to the internal working of the organization. Argyris assumed that human relations are most effective when, in addition to direction, authority, and control, they incorporate authentic relationships, internal commitment, psychological success, and the process of confirmation.

Argyris believed that the humanistic or democratic values he listed would, if utilized in the work environment, result in increased interpersonal competence, group cooperation, and effectiveness in the organization. When people are treated as human beings there is benefit for both the worker and the organization. Argyris also proposed an "immaturity-maturity" continuum in which he listed seven changes that should take place in the personality of individuals if they develop into mature people over time. He further maintained that people are often kept from maturing by the organization (leaders) because they are encouraged to be dependent and subordinate and to fit into the goals of the organization, and that this happens because the power and authority come from the top of the organization. Rather than this, Argyris proposed that management should make it possible for workers to grow and mature by allowing them opportunity for self-direction and creativity. This is an important concept in relation to the supervisory process as it will be presented later.

In *Megatrends* (1982), Naisbitt maintained that new management styles, such as those proposed by Argyris, have "flourished mostly in the business literature. Very few made it to the office or the shop floor." Nevertheless, he believed that the pyramid style by which people have organized and managed themselves for centuries, is being "smashed" and replaced by "networking" where people talk to each other, share information and resources quickly and openly (p. 212). This is a movement that is relevant to those engaged in supervision, as seen in the previous chapter in the formation of special interest groups of supervisors, their own newsletters, and the national research network.

Traits of Leaders

Traits of leaders have been the topic of investigation for approximately 60 years. Efforts have been made to find common traits or personal qualities that would identify leaders who could, presumably, be effective in any situation. "In 50 years of research in what is known as the *trait theory* of leadership—that is, looking for traits which are characteristic of leaders of all kinds—we have failed to unveil one single personality trait or set of traits that distinguish leaders from non-leaders. We no longer believe that a leader can be identified by giving him a test or looking at him or measuring him or weighing him" (Reitz, 1970, p. 21).

This long search for characteristics of leaders led to the identification by many researchers of two dimensions of behaviors at opposite ends of the continuum. Tannenbaum (1966) called these dimensions of behavior *task-oriented* (authoritarian) leader behavior at one end of the continuum, *relationships-oriented* (democratic) at the other. Other writers have identified similar concepts and used other terminology. Researchers at the Survey Research Center at the University of Michigan (Katz, Macoby, & Morse, 1950) called the two different concepts *employee orientation* and *production-orientation*, again parallels to the authoritarian and democratic styles. Studies at Ohio State University described leadership behavior as *initiating-structure* and *consideration* (Stogdill & Coons, 1957). Behavior called task-oriented, production-oriented, or initiating is at the authoritarian end of the continuum, with the leaders using their power to influence the followers and emphasize production and the technical aspects of the job. Leaders initiate the action and develop the procedures and see employees as tools to accomplish the goals of the organization. The employee-oriented, consideration, and relationships-oriented leader is seen as one who is group-oriented, gives the followers freedom in their work, feels that all employees are important, and takes interest in them, accepting their individuality and personal needs. Such a leader provides encouragement, enhances communication, and maintains good relationships (Hersey & Blanchard, 1982). The leader who implements this type of leadership style, according to Cartwright and Zander (1960) provides encouragement, stimulates self-direction, keeps interpersonal relations pleasant, and increases the interdependence among the group members as opposed to the other style, in which the manager initiates the action and sees that the group members meet the goals.

Management by Objectives

Management by objectives (MBO) was another popular development in the management literature of the 1970s which has had its influence on supervision, particularly on the program management or administrative aspects. The concept is based on participative management in reaching the goals of an organization. It assumes joint establishment of goals based on the finding that goals formulated jointly achieve more acceptance than do those imposed by a person in authority (Hersey & Blanchard, 1982; Reitz, 1981).

This concept has been applied to speech-language pathology and audiology programming in the schools (ASHA, 1973; Healey, 1982), as well as in other organizations.

Situational Leadership

Another development, which questioned the idea of a best style of leadership, was the concept of adaptive leadership behavior or *situational leadership*—not one best style but the most effective style for a particular situation (Gouran, 1980; Hersey & Blanchard, 1982; Reitz, 1981). The "leadership contingency model" developed by Fiedler (1967) stated that, although there are more or less effective styles of leadership, they are not effective in every situation. The three major situational variables identified by Fiedler in determining the appropriateness of a style of leadership were (1) leader-member relations, (2) degree of structure in the task, and (3) the power and authority their position provides.

Gouran (1980) suggested that too many people who have supervisory responsibility function "within narrowly and stereotypically conceived notions of what constitutes 'good supervision'." He maintained that practices based on this erroneous conception are "injurious to the task of clinical supervision" (p. 93). He presented the work of Farris (1974), who identified four supervisory styles, labeled *collaboration, domination, delegation,* and *abdication.* The appropriateness of each style is dictated by the relative capabilities of the supervisor and supervisee to deal independently with a specific kind of demand.

Gouran further stated several principles that are applications of Farris's ideas about the relationship between supervisory style and circumstantial influences: (1) No one style of supervision is best. (2) A supervisor must be prepared to deal differently with different supervisees. (3) Within any given supervisor/supervisee relationship, circumstances may require periodic changes in style. (4) Adoption of an inappropriate style in relation to a particular situational demand will reduce the chances for achieving the supervisor and supervisee's mutually shared goals. (5) The measure of success in effective supervision is not the extent of the supervisor's influence on the supervisee, but the extent to which their interaction contributes to the achievement of specified objectives.

Hersey and Blanchard (1982) proposed a "situational leadership theory" utilizing the terms *task behavior* and *relationship behavior* to describe leadership style. Any leadership style is made up of some combination of task or relationship behaviors. Task behavior is defined as the extent to which the leader provides direction, organizes roles and activities, and specifies how they are to be achieved; relationship behavior is the extent to which the leader establishes and maintains personal relationships with the follower(s) that is supporting and facilitating. It is the interaction of style and environment that makes leadership effective or ineffective; therefore, no style is appropriate to all situations. Hersey and Blanchard further proposed that the level of maturity (Argyris, 1962) of the follower is a variable that must be considered in relation to the task. Maturity is defined by Hersey and Blanchard as the ability to set high but attainable goals, ability and willingness to take responsibility, and education and/or experience of either an individual or a group. Since maturity will vary within any one person or group, the leaders therefore must know the level of maturity in determining the appropriate style.

Hersey and Blanchard's model includes four behavioral styles and presents an important parallel to the continuum proposed in this book.

- *Telling* (high task/low relationship)—leader defines roles and tasks
- *Selling* (high task/high relationship)—direction is still provided but it is accompanied by more two-way communication and socioemotional support to encourage participation

■ *Participating* (high relationship/low task)—facilitative, sharing in decision-making
■ *Delegating* (low relationship/low task)—follower "runs own show")

Thus, they proposed that when the follower is immature in relation to a task, the appropriate style will be High Task-Low Relationship, that is, the leader will be more involved in organizing and directing in relation to the task. "As the individual or group begins to move into an above average level of maturity, it becomes appropriate for leaders to decrease not only task behavior but also relationship behavior" (p. 163). In other words, the follower works more independently, socioemotional support is not so necessary, and there is less direction and more delegation by the leader. Style, then, changes as followers become more able to set goals and accomplish the task independently.

LEADERSHIP AND SUPERVISION IN EDUCATION

At the time that this research on leadership and supervision was developing in the management area, a parallel stream of supervision theory and research was emerging in education. Often borrowing from the management literature, but frequently more related to the teaching aspect of supervision, this parallel development has probably had an even stronger impact on supervision in speech-language pathology and audiology than that of the business literature.

Early Approaches

The first approach to supervision in education in the early days of the United States was authoritarian and autocratic. It was related mainly to inspection of schools by lay persons for the purpose of evaluating facilities and pupils, thereby, it was assumed, documenting and evaluating the effectiveness of the teacher. As life became increasingly complex, the responsibilities became too great for lay persons to continue this method of evaluation; thus, professional educators became involved in regulatory and inspection tasks. As schools increased in size, more teachers were employed and the position of building principal began to emerge as an administrative and managerial position (Alfonso, Firth, & Neville, 1975; Owens, 1970). Later, special teachers and supervisors became a part of the total school structure.

Education was not untouched by the scientific management movement espoused by Taylor (1911). This approach, as adapted to education, called for defining educational objectives, finding the "best" methods for teaching, and forcing teachers to use these methods—this was the job of the supervisor.

Human Relations Movement

Again, in the late 1920s, leadership in education paralleled the human relations movement in business management. The roles of teachers with their students and of supervisors with their teachers began to change. "The human relations movement emphasized the human and interpersonal factors for administering the affairs of organizations. Supervisors in particular drew heavily on human relations concepts, placing stress on such notions as 'democratic' procedures, 'involvement', motivational techniques and the sociometry of leadership" (Owens, 1970, p. 10). There began to be an emphasis on participation by teachers in the improvement of instruction similar to the participation of employees in other settings. According to Wiles (1950), the 1930s were characterized by democratic supervision (the kind treatment of teachers), which evolved into a cooperative group decision-making endeavor in the 1940s. In the 1950s the concept of the supervisor as a "change agent" was introduced.

From later research studies, it became clear that teachers wanted "supportive and nonthreatening services that are relevant to the improvement of their performance" (Lovell & Wiles, 1983).

Participative Supervision

The contemporary view of supervision in education requires that supervisors guide teachers within the context of a participating relationship. Teachers are seen as identifying problems and implementing their solutions. This participation of teachers does not diminish the supervisor's leadership position but, rather, directs it toward melding human resources in the organization. The team approach, then, is seen as the current climate for supervision in the schools (Alfonso et al., 1975).

However, Alfonso and colleagues (1975) warn that such actions are valid only when they contribute to the study and the improvement of teaching, which is the only reason for supervision. Supervisors must study formal organization, role theory, communication theory, decision making, personality theory, the change process, and other areas. The mere offering of pronouncements about the power of the group and of the need for "working together" does not represent a supervision program.

Studying the Behavior of Supervisors

Until the early 1970s, the bulk of the writing on supervision in education was related to curriculum development, instruction, in-service, parent and community relations, and similar issues pertinent to the total operation of the educational system, not to the critical elements of supervisory behavior. Underscoring the lack of evidence about effectiveness of supervision in education, Alfonso and colleagues (1975) stated, "Much attention has been directed toward the tasks that supervisors perform; little has been directed at the critical element of supervisory behavior. Few professional roles in education have had as little intelligent study done" (p. 32).

The decade of the 1970s, however, found a few educators seemingly more concerned than previous writers about the relationships between supervisors and supervisees in the supervisory process. Some of the recent literature has been directed toward the specifics of supervisors' *behavior* in their interaction with supervisees. Research on behavior of teachers in the classroom influenced attitudes toward the study of supervision. Flanders (1967, 1969) was among the first to maintain that direct behavioral styles are less productive in problem-solving activities in the classroom than indirect styles. Generally, Flanders maintained from his various studies that children learned better from teachers who did not dominate but who were flexible in their behaviors, who could be direct or indirect, as indicated by a particular situation.

Studies of Direct and Indirect Behaviors

The direct/indirect concept was applied to the study of the supervisory process by Blumberg (1968a), Blumberg and Amidon (1965), Blumberg, Amidon, and Weber (1967), Blumberg and Cusick (1970), and Blumberg and Weber (1968). Influenced by Flanders (1967) and Bales (1950, 1951), Blumberg and his associates maintained that the exclusive use of direct behaviors in supervision increased defensiveness on the part of supervisees. Blumberg (1974, 1980) also recognized that most texts on supervision did not address what happens between supervisor and supervisee in the supervisory interaction. He and his associates conducted extensive inquiries about the human relationships aspect of supervision, particularly the direct and indirect dimensions of the supervisor's behavior. Blumberg's investigations were based on the work of Gibb (1969) on defensive communication, in which he identified six bipolar communication behaviors which were either *support-inducing* or *defense-inducing*. Behavior that was support-inducing, Gibb said, was oriented toward problem solving, spontaneity, equality, provisionalism, empathy, and description. Behavior that was defense-inducing was oriented toward control, strategy, superiority, certainty, neutrality, and evaluation.

Blumberg (1974, 1980) equated Gibb's defense-inducing behaviors with *direct* supervisory behaviors, including such behaviors as telling, giving opinions and suggestions, directing, criticizing, suggesting change, and evaluating. Support-inducing behaviors were equated with *indirect* supervisory behavior and were considered to be such behaviors as accepting and clarifying the teachers' questions, praising teacher behavior, asking teachers for their own opinions and suggestions, involving them in problem solving, accepting their ideas, and discussing teachers' feelings about the relationship between the supervisor and the supervisee. In other words, Blumberg contends that these direct/indirect styles communicate a totally different attitude toward the teacher/supervisee. Direct behaviors communicate that the supervisor wishes to control the teacher, excludes the teacher from problem solving, sees evaluation by the supervisor as the main function of the observation, and does not value the worth of the teacher in the teaching role. Indirect behaviors communicate a concern for the teacher as a person, a desire for collaborative problem solving, and a recognition of the teacher's personal and professional growth.

Using these categories of direct and indirect behaviors, Blumberg and Amidon (1965) investigated whether or not teachers could discriminate between specific types of behavior of their supervisors. Results of this study made it clear that a one-dimensional approach to supervisory behavior was too simplistic. From this study, the authors developed the following set of four supervisory styles which Blumberg and his colleagues used in subsequent studies:

- Style A—High Direct, High Indirect (supervisors are perceived by teachers as emphasizing both direct and indirect behavior, telling and criticizing but also asking and listening)
- Style B—High Direct, Low Indirect (supervisors are perceived by teachers as doing a great deal of telling and criticizing but very little asking or listening)
- Style C—Low Direct, High Indirect (supervisors are perceived by teachers as rarely telling or criticizing but emphasizing the asking of questions, listening, and reflecting back the teacher's ideas and feelings)
- Style D—Low Direct, Low Indirect (supervisors are perceived as passive and not doing much within the interaction)

Blumberg and his associates also found that perception of these supervisory styles made a difference in the way teachers viewed their interaction with their supervisors. The results present support for a mix of the two styles of behavior, but with a strong tendency to prefer high amounts of indirect behavior, and are an important base for the study of supervisory methodologies. Teachers in these studies perceived more positive interpersonal relationships with their supervisors under the two styles containing the most indirect behavior (Styles A and C). Teachers gave positive evaluations of their interpersonal relationships with their supervisors when they perceived the interaction to consist of telling, suggesting, and criticizing as well as reflecting, asking for information, and opinions (Style A) or when there is little telling and much reflecting and asking (Style C). Negative attitudes resulted from perceptions of supervisory behavior as predominantly telling, with little reflecting or asking (Style B), or when the supervisor was perceived as passive (Style D).

Teachers in these studies also indicated that they were able to obtain more insight about themselves, both as teachers and as persons, if supervisors used high amounts of indirect behavior with some direct (again a combination of styles A and C). Thus, Blumberg (1980) stated, "This finding suggests that hearing about oneself is probably most productive, not only when the supervisor (or other helping agent) questions, listens, and reflects back what he hears, but also when he does a bit of telling and gives feedback" (p. 67). Behavioral Styles D (Low Direct, High Indirect) and B (High Direct, Low Indirect) were not seen by teachers as contributing to learning about themselves. According to Blumberg, even Style B, which does include indirect behavior, was not seen as contributing to insight, perhaps because the presence of the direct was *so* potent that, not only did it not enhance the teachers' feelings of worth and acceptance, it made it more difficult for them to accept the indirect.

When supervisors were perceived to use Style B (High Direct, Low Indirect), the teachers understandably perceived their supervisors to be more oriented toward control than problem solving. Teachers under this treatment felt the need to be more strategy oriented and less spontaneous, and they felt that supervisors were more oriented toward superiority than equality, more oriented toward certainty than provisionalism. Also, teachers felt their interaction more dominated by evaluation of their behavior than toward description of that behavior. All of these behaviors are equated with the defense-inducing behaviors of Gibb (1969).

At the same time, teachers whose supervisors were seen to operate under Style C (Low Direct, High Indirect) perceived the highest degree of empathy and productivity and the least degree of the defense-producing behaviors. "Thus," said Blumberg (1980), "our unspoken expectations that Style C would result in communicative freedom and high productivity while Style B would reflect defensiveness and low productivity were met" (p. 69).

Other similar findings by Blumberg and Cusick (1970) present support for the use of both direct and indirect behaviors, together with the first definitive discussion of behaviors and data to dispute the value of the direct style. Their findings support the need to look carefully at the effects of the direct and indirect styles and the probable need to analyze one's supervisory behavior on the basis of these styles. Despite methodological problems in the studies, they provide an interesting parallel to some of the management literature and pose many questions about supervisory style. They have been discussed in depth here because of their significance for the proposal to be made later about supervision of speech-language pathology and audiology.

Interpersonal Approach

Meanwhile, at Teachers College, Columbia University, Dussault (1970) proposed a middle-range theory of supervision in the education of student teachers which was based on Carl Rogers's theory of therapy and personality change. Dussault discussed the relationships that exist between therapy and the teaching function of supervision and developed a theory that parallels Rogers's writings and, in brief, states that if facilitative interpersonal conditions exist during the supervisory conference then certain changes will be observed in the supervisee.

Dussault differentiated clearly between the *evaluative* function of supervision and the *teaching* function. Evaluation, he said, is the process of assessment or judgment about the person's readiness to assume professional responsibilities. The teaching function, on the other hand, is the process of helping the student acquire the competencies necessary to fulfull those professional responsibilities. Thus, he made a distinction between evaluation as feedback and guide and evaluation as judgmental assessment. This concept departs from the negative perception of supervisors verbalized by Cogan (1973) as "someone paid to ferret out weaknesses" (p. 78) or specialists "charged with filling cavities" (p. 78).

More discussion of the interpersonal aspects of supervision was presented by Mosher and Purpel (1972), who attended to the psychological factors experienced by students/supervisees during the student teaching experience. They suggested a method of supervision, based on ego-counseling, which focuses on the personal condition with regard to certain roles or situations. Ego-counseling "*does not* deal with unconscious material" but with "the full range of *conscious* personal response to teaching—both intellectual and emotional" (p. 128–129). This type of supervision takes preparation but, Mosher and Purpel maintain, preparation is necessary for any type of supervision.

Clinical Supervision

Two other authors at about the same time began advocating a style of supervision called *clinical supervision* (Cogan, 1973; Goldhammer, 1969). Their approach to supervision, though not supported with data, was decidedly more specific and more related to the analysis of actual supervisor behavior than any previous writers. The methodology employs shared interaction between supervisor and supervisee, based on objective data collected and analyzed by both supervisor and supervisee. *Clinical*, a term rarely found in the education literature up to that time, was used by both writers to describe supervision as not referring to the pathological, but to "supervision up close" (Goldhammer, 1969, p. 54)—the one-to-one relationships between supervisor and teacher. There is a strong emphasis on the desirability of teachers and supervisors to "be supportive and empathic; to perfect technical behaviors and the concepts from which they are generated; to increase the efficiencies and pleasure of learning and becoming; to treat one another decently and responsibly and with affection; to engage with one another in productive and rewarding encounters; and to move toward our own destinies and toward one another's, honestly" (Goldhammer, 1969, pp. 55–56).

Cogan (1973) described the genesis of the clinical supervision methodology with students in the Master of Arts in Teaching program at Harvard in the late 1950s and indicated that it grew out of the dissatisfaction of many students about the supervision of their student teaching internship. Cogan also defended the use of the word *clinical* and said "It was selected precisely to draw attention to the emphasis placed on classroom observation, analysis of the in-class events, and the focus on teachers' and students' in-class behavior" (pp. 8–9). Cogan formulated eight phases in his cycle of supervision:

- *Phase 1*: Establishing the teacher-supervisor relationship
- *Phase 2*: Planning with the teacher
- *Phase 3*: Planning the strategy of the observation
- *Phase 4*: Observing instruction.
- *Phase 5*: Analyzing the teaching-learning processes
- *Phase 6*: Planning the strategy of the conference
- *Phase 7*: The conference
- *Phase 8*: Renewed planning

Goldhammer (1969) proposed five similar stages for the clinical supervisory process: (1) pre-observation conference, (2) observation, (3) analysis and strategy, (4) supervision conference, and (5) post-conference analysis (nicknamed the "post-mortem"). Both Cogan's and Goldhammer's methodologies definitely mandate recognition of the contribution of both supervisor and supervisee to the supervisory process.

In a revision of Goldhammer's earlier work, Goldhammer, Anderson, and Krajewski (1980) called clinical supervision "that phase of instructional supervision which draws its data from first-hand observation of actual teaching events, and involves face-to-face (and other associated) interaction between the supervisor and teacher in the analysis of teaching behaviors and activities for instructional improvement" (pp. 19–20).

The writings of Blumberg, Cogan, Goldhammer, and Goldhammer, Anderson, and Krajewski have exerted a strong influence on the writer of this book. Although the proposal for supervision presented here is different from that proposed by them, it draws heavily from their writings for illustration and support. The brief review of their work given here should not be considered sufficient to understand their methodologies. Readers are encouraged to read the original texts carefully.

SUPERVISION IN OTHER HELPING PROFESSIONS

There have been additional influences from other helping professions which utilize the supervisory process in training and monitoring the delivery of services to their clients, and they merit brief attention here.

One of these sources has been the counseling literature. Leddick and Barnard (1980) traced the history of supervision in counseling "from a polarized state to its current trend toward collaboration" (p. 186). Supervision began, they felt, with the acceptance of psychoanalysis and evolved as the helping professions of counseling, psychology, and social work were evolving and establishing their identities. The practice of supervision has followed the growth of the professions from the authoritativeness of psychoanalytic thought to the nondirective client-centered approach. The task of the supervisor came to be modeling the behavior of the facilitative, nondirective counselor to provide an example for students. Rogers's (1957) model was refined and came to include didactic teaching and group therapy. At the same time, behavioral approaches were developing and by 1966 the field of supervision had "three major models: dynamic, facilitative and behavioral" (Leddick and Barnard, 1980, p. 190). "The 1970s. . . have been characterized by models rather than theories" (p. 194) and the profession has now reached a position of eclecticism regarding supervisory approaches.

Three models proposed by Hart (1982)—skill development, personal growth, and integration—were differentiated on the basis of the relationship between supervisor and supervisee, the hierarchical distance between them, and the focus of the session. Boyd (1978) provided a comprehensive coverage of counselor supervision wherein he presented many topics familiar to any student of the supervisory process in any discipline—the lack of theory, the need for accountability, the lack of empirical evidence. The work of these authors and others to which they refer offer a profitable source of study for the student of the supervisory process in all professions.

Supervision in the preparation of physicians, according to Kutzik (1977a), exists only during their educational programs and is characterized by a superior-subordinate relationship, the function of which is to educate the student, "not improve services to patients" (p. 6). Once the student becomes a practicing physician, the model becomes that of consultation where the consultee "voluntarily seeks the advice of a consultant. . .and decides whether or not to take the advice" (p. 5).

The history of supervision in social work goes back to the 1800s and takes place in both educational and employment settings (Kadushin, 1976; Kutzik, 1977b; Munson, 1983). The first social work supervision was of agencies and institutions, not social workers as individuals. This emphasis was the result of the "consequence of indiscriminate almsgiving" (Kadushin, 1976, p. 4), yet Kadushin stated that even then the current principle functions of supervision were found in the literature. As a body of information about casework was accumulated, course work was offered in universities and the education of professionals began. Once considered a status achievement, supervision is no longer a "move up the ladder"; now social workers are being prepared in schools of social work "to graduate as supervisors and consultants" (Vargus, 1977, p. 153). The field has moved through the master-apprentice model, group supervision, and peer supervision to a teacher or administration function. Supervision seems to have been important to social work throughout most of its history and its functions identified as administrative, educational, and supportive as early as the 1920s (Kadushin, 1976). Educational supervision was rationalized on the basis of inadequacy of preparation, but as education improved, the supportive function increased, providing a rationale for continuous supervision. Later, social work supervision moved toward consultation (Kutzik, 1977b). Currently, "While consultation has become the norm for experienced professional staff, supervision has remained the norm for semi- or nonprofessionals" (Vargus, 1977, p. 179). Vargus also suggested "teaming" as a method whereby a team "works on the resolution of the problem" and concluded, "But whatever model is used and whatever the title—facilitator, consultant, enabler, or team leader—the effectiveness of the supervision task will greatly depend on a conscious recognition of the supervisor's values, philosophies, and ability in that role" (p. 179).

Psychiatric education also utilizes supervision (Brammer & Wassmer, 1977; Kagan & Werner, 1977), as does the somewhat newer discipline of family therapy (Kaslow, 1977). The literature from this discipline reveals a recognition of the importance of supervision and a concern about its effectiveness.

Whatever the profession, however, the literature shares certain common themes—lack of theory, limited or no validation of a wide variety of models and practices, lack of accountability, confusion of roles, the multidimensionality of the process, the extensive gap between research and actual practice, the need for research, lack of validation of methodologies for preparing supervisors, effects of personal variables of participants in the supervisory process—and the list goes on and on. According to Hart (1982), supervision has been "feared as a practice and, until recently, neglected as a field of study" (p. 5).

Kagan and Werner (1977) have stated: "Supervisory processes need to be validated through studies on the impact of supervision on patient outcome; these same processes need to be defined so that they can be reliably implemented in other settings. Reliability may be as difficult to achieve as has been the validation of effective practice" (p. 36). Brammer and Wassmer (1977) have also noted: "We suspect that supervision will continue to be a highly individual, sometimes rigorous, sometimes haphazard, always unregulated, 'sometime' thing, which no amount of descriptive research will substantially improve. . . . Our lack of knowledge of the nature and conditions of supervision, our lack of outcome criteria, and our lack of knowledge of the comparative effectiveness of various supervisory strategies all demand a moratorium on further speculation and a redoubled effort toward descriptive, evaluative, and experimental research" (p. 82). Though written about psychiatric supervision and counseling, respectively, these statements characterize the status of supervision in all the disciplines where it exists. Yet, parts of the literature from these other areas have, without doubt, influenced the thinking of supervisors in speech-language pathology and audiology in much the same way as the literature from education and business management which have been reviewed in somewhat greater depth.

SUPERVISORY APPROACHES IN SPEECH-LANGUAGE PATHOLOGY AND AUDIOLOGY

Although less extensive and covering a shorter period of history than supervision in the disciplines just reviewed, the speech-language pathology and audiology field has produced a number of suggested approaches to the supervisory process. Most will reveal the influence of work from the other disciplines.

Probably the first in-depth look at the complexities of preparing clinical personnel came twenty-some years ago in two thoughtful articles by Ward and Webster (1965a, 1965b). Perhaps not so well known except to those specifically interested in the study of supervision and the preparation of speech-language pathologists and audiologists, these articles should be required reading for everyone in the profession. Ward and Webster discussed issues that have not yet been resolved. They probed "the nature of the human encounter" (1965a, p. 39) and stressed the importance of providing proper conditions for growth and change for students, as is done for clients, and for developing "concepts of training in which students may gain repeated experience in exploring and exercising their own humanness in the series of human encounters which constitute their training programs" (1965a, p. 39). Their definition of clinical supervision is "an interactive process between student and supervisor in which both are working together to find the most productive ways of effecting the diagnostic or therapeutic relationship" (1965b, p. 104). Supervisors, they believe, must be willing to examine their own attitudes and relationships—the first mention in the literature that both supervisor and clinician behaviors need the same kind of focus given to client behaviors.

A Rogerian orientation to the relationship between supervisor and supervisee was proposed by Caracciolo and colleagues (1978a). Based on Carl Rogers's (1961, 1962) work on client-centered therapy and the proposal for a theory of supervision by Dussault (1970), the authors suggested that the same facilitating interpersonal conditions that most speech-language pathologists or audiologists would agree are important to facilitate change in client behavior are also relevant to the supervisory process. These facilitating behaviors, if offered to the supervisee by the supervisor, will "provide a psychosocial environment which enables the student to develop into a competent, secure, and independent professional clinician" (p. 286). Further discussion of this approach by Caracciolo and colleagues suggests that the supervisor in speech-language pathology, while needing to utilize the nondirective, facilitative orientation to establish a relationship conducive to growth, must also play another role. That role is a more directive one, "when the supervisor must be more directive with respect to giving information to the student, making judgments of the student's behaviors, and establishing requirements and standards for lesson planning, report writing, and so on" (p. 288).

Oratio's (1977) Molar Model of Clinical Supervision encompasses two primary objectives: changing clinician behavior and developing professional independence and clinical autonomy in the clinician. The model employs didactic teaching, clinical practice, demonstration, conferencing, observation, analysis, and microtherapy to meet those objectives.

An approach to supervision in audiology by Rassi (1978) utilizes a framework of competency-based instruction that includes skills in testing, writing, and interpersonal and decision-making areas. Her definition of supervision is clinical teaching in which the student is taught "in a one-to-one situation how to apply his academic knowledge in a practical clinical setting as he functions in that setting. The ultimate goal is to transform the student into an independent clinician" (p. 9).

Later, Rassi (1985, 1987) provided arguments for differences between supervision of audiology and of speech-language pathology. These are related to the greater proportion of the diagnosis-evaluation component in audiology of the and factors within that component which Rassi believes dictate a different approach to supervision. This approach, she says, requires a competency-based type of instruction.

Schubert (1978) suggested an approach to supervision based on the use of an interaction analysis system, the *Analysis of Behavior of Clinicians*. This system will be discussed in the chapters on Observation and Analysis. *The Integrative Task Maturity Model of Supervision* (ITMMS), discussed by Mawdsley (1985a) at an ASHA convention, is an ingenious combination of the Hersey and Blanchard *Situation Leadership Model* (1982), the *Wisconsin Procedure for Appraisal of Clinical Competence* (Shriberg et al., 1975), and the clinical supervision model of Cogan (1973). It includes a system for identifying appropriate supervisory styles and specific techniques to be utilized at different levels of maturity. This model appears to have good possibilities as it is further developed.

A recent valuable addition to the literature in speech-language pathology and audiology has been a book edited by Crago and Pickering (1987). Although presenting several facets of the supervisory process, major emphasis is on the interpersonal aspects.

Most pertinent to the remainder of this book, however, is the application of the clinical supervision model of Cogan (1973) and Goldhammer (1969) by the writer (Anderson, 1981). In discussing previously a developing approach to preparation of supervisors the writer stated:

> The pervading belief underlying the program is that supervision at any level is teaching—a very special kind of teaching—and that, like all teaching, it requires the involvement of the learner. Therefore, the supervisee is not an apprentice to be molded into a model of the supervisor, is not "slave labor," and, although often but not always "less knowing," is not *subordinate* to the supervisor. The model that is developing and being tested through self-study and research is one of joint problem solving by supervisor and supervisee related to client or program needs. It includes maximal use of objective data collection and self-analysis techniques by both supervisor and supervisee. It assumes a dual role for the clinician—that of clinician to the client, and supervisee to the supervisor. Each of these roles demands a different set of behaviors that can and must be identified, observed, quantified, analyzed, and if necessary, modified. The model utilizes an analytical approach to behavior in the supervisory conference and assumes that interaction between supervisor and supervisee is as important to the total learning process and as measurable as the interaction between clinician and client. It also assumes that supervisors, as well as supervisees, can and must grow and develop and improve their own skills as they participate in the supervisory process. (p. 79)

It is this approach that forms the foundation of this book.

SUMMARY

Philosophy and procedures in supervision in speech-language pathology and audiology have been built, to a great extent, on the literature from other disciplines as well as the experiences of the profession itself. It is important for students of the supervisory process to have a broad view of the accumulated knowledge about supervision so that they can build upon, rather than repeat, the events of the past. Further, many speech-language pathologists and audiologists are often supervised by individuals from other professions. Knowledge about the models of supervision generally utilized in the preparation of these people who supervise or administer their programs may increase understanding of the dynamics of their own situations.

A Continuum of Supervision

A leader is best
When people barely know he exists
Not so good
When people obey and acclaim him
Worse when they despise him.
But of a good leader who talks little
When his work is done
His aim fulfilled
They will say
"We did it ourselves."

Lao-tse (c. 565 B.C.)

The definition and description of the supervisory process given in Chapter 1 specifies a goal of professional growth for both supervisor and supervisee. Expansion of that idea leads to the concept of the supervisor's role as assisting the supervisee in reaching a level of independence where their relationship is one of peer-consultation rather than dependency. To create a situation where supervisees can say, "We did it ourselves" seems the ultimate in the supervisory relationship.

This chapter will discuss a continuum of supervision in which the goal is just that type of relationship. It consists of three stages: Evaluation-Feedback, Transitional, and Self-Supervision. The appropriate supervisory styles for use along the continuum will then be presented.

A CONTINUUM OF SUPERVISION

Aware of all the variables that prohibit simplistic answers to the question, "How should we supervise?" and influenced by experience and a study of the literature from many areas, the writer makes the following proposal: that supervision exists on a continuum which spans a professional career and that there are *styles* of interaction which are appropriate to each stage of the continuum. This continuum probably already exists within the nervous system of most supervisors, consciously or unconsciously. At least it is verbalized frequently. It is offered here, not as a new concept, but as a framework for discussion and study of seemingly obvious components of supervision. It offers a structure for supervisors and supervisees to examine their own philosophies about supervision, identify their own behaviors, and determine what changes they wish to make, if any. It is also presented as a base for clarifying some of the many questions that must be answered if the profession is to validate any of the supervisory activities in which personnel have been and are currently spending so many hours. A further tenet of the proposal is that supervisors and supervisees must engage in a study of the supervisory process itself—self-study by those engaged in the interaction, as well as research directed toward determining appropriate methodologies.

STAGES OF THE CONTINUUM

The continuum of supervision is based on the assumption that professionals will be involved in some supervisory or consultative experience for the duration of their professional career and that the expectations and needs of supervisees change throughout this time period. The stages of this continuum of professional growth are shown in Figure 4–1.

Evaluation- Feedback Stage	Transitional Stage	Self- Supervision Stage

FIGURE 4-1. *STAGES OF THE CONTINUUM OF SUPERVISION*

The continuum mandates a change over time in the amount and type of involvement of both supervisor and supervisee in the supervisory process. As the degree of dominance of the supervisor decreases, participation by the supervisee increases across the continuum. As they move into the Self-Supervision Stage, the balance changes to the more equal interaction of peers. Each stage and its appropriate style will be discussed briefly here. More detailed discussion will follow in later chapters.

A most significant feature of the continuum which must be understood is that *none of the stages should be seen as time-bound.* Any individual supervisee may be found at any point on the continuum throughout his or her career, depending upon personal and situational variables. Some may never reach the Self-Supervision Stage, others may begin well beyond the Evaluation-Feedback Stage, as demonstrated by the arrows in Figure 4–2.

It is assumed that this continuum applies to both speech-language pathology and audiology. In fact, Rassi (1978), in discussing the composition of supervision in audiology, presented a similar continuum when she listed eight possible levels of supervision beginning with detailed explanation accompanied by

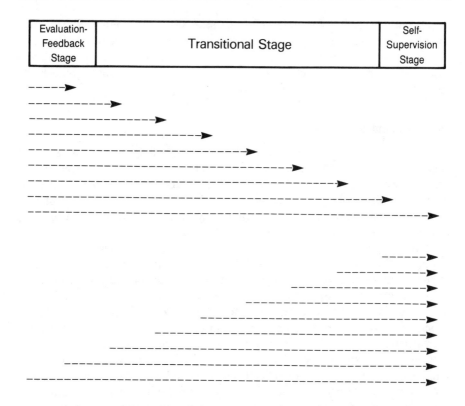

Evaluation-Feedback Stage	Transitional Stage	Self-Supervision Stage

FIGURE 4-2. *PROGRESSION ALONG THE CONTINUUM OF SUPERVISION*

demonstration to a final level where the student is working independently with monitoring and suggestions provided by the supervisor only when necessary. Rassi stated, "Each succeeding level requires less active participation by the supervisor while, at the same time, the student's direct involvement and attendant responsibilities increase" (p. 15). Indeed, it may also be assumed that within each level there will be shifts in the supervisor-supervisee balance over time.

Evaluation-Feedback Stage

In the Evaluation-Feedback Stage the supervisor is dominant. This is where the beginning supervisee may be found, or the supervisee who is working with a new type of client, or the one who has just entered a new setting. The supervisee who is unknowledgeable or clinically inept, often called the "marginal student," may perseverate at this stage. Unprepared for the clinical interaction, unable to problem-solve, overwhelmed by the dynamics of the situation, or accustomed to being told what to do, the supervisee at this stage assumes a very passive role. Additionally, the supervisory dyad may be found at this stage because of the supervisor who does not perceive that the supervisee has the ability to participate or whose only view of the supervisor's role is that of instructor or evaluator. This stage is consistent with the first quadrant of the Hersey and Blanchard model discussed in the previous chapter. The aim of both participants should be to move out of this stage as soon as possible to a point further along the continuum.

Transitional Stage

The Transitional Stage follows the Evaluation-Feedback Stage. It is perceived as the place where the supervisee has reached a level of competency and knowledge and the supervisor has achieved an attitude that results in participation by both, joint problem-solving, and peer interaction—a process of shared deliberation. The supervisee is not yet able to operate independently but is moving along the continuum in that direction.

At this stage, supervisees are able to participate to varying degrees in decision making. They are learning to analyze their clinical action and plan future strategies on the basis of that analysis, to make modifications during their clinical sessions, to problem-solve and collaborate within the supervisory conference. The supervisor is able to allow the supervisee to assume responsibility. As the supervisory dyad moves along the continuum, the interaction becomes increasingly closer to peer interaction or colleagueship (Cogan, 1973) with the ever-present goal of independence or self-supervision. Supervisees may move back and forth within the Transitional Stage, as shown in Figure 4–2, depending upon many variables. Supervisees may have skills that enable them to begin their supervisory experience at any point in the Transitional Stage. Some may have had many hours of experience with articulation and language clients and be able to work independently with them, but when assigned to a laryngectomized client, may find it necessary to move back to the Evaluation-Feedback Stage and receive more input from the supervisor. Such situations may occur in either the educational setting or the service-delivery setting.

Self-Supervision Stage

Self-Supervision is defined as a stage where supervisees have the ability to self-analyze their clinical behavior accurately and to alter it, based on that analysis. It denotes a level of independence in problem solving in which supervisees are no longer dependent upon supervisors for observation, analysis, and feedback about their clinical work. Nevertheless, persons at this level still desire peer interaction or a consultative type of interaction.

Some professionals may never reach a total level of independence. Probably few persons perceive that they have totally reached this stage—that they do not need some kind of peer interaction for continued professional growth and development or consultation on specific problems. Some, on the other hand, may feel a self-confidence not compatible with their actual performance. However, it seems logical that persons who have moved through the Transitional

Stage with a continuous increase in their ability to assume responsibility will come closer to the Self-Supervision Stage than someone who attempts to move directly from Evaluation-Feedback to Self-Supervision.

IMPLICATIONS OF THE CONTINUUM

This continuum has important implications in terms of expectations for professionals during their educational program and after they leave it. Some supervisees may not reach the independence of the Self-Supervision Stage with any type of client during the educational program, despite all efforts. This, then, becomes a question of accountability for the educational program which will be discussed in a later chapter. If the supervisee enters the off-campus practicum, the Clinical Fellowship Year (CFY), or the work force at a point on the continuum below the Self-Supervision Stage, the supervisor in those situations must then maintain a style relevant to that point. In other words, supervisors in all situations must be aware of the continuum as they determine the appropriate style for each supervisee. Additionally, they must possess the flexibility that will enable them to adjust their behaviors as they move back and forth on the continuum with their supervisees. The task of identifying the place at which the supervisor and supervisee should be operating and the behaviors that make up the appropriate style will be the focus of the remaining chapters of this book.

APPROPRIATE STYLES FOR EACH STAGE

The appropriate supervision style for each stage of the continuum is determined by the skill level of the supervisee and the nature of the task as related to the client. The supervisor's flexibility in adapting to these variables also affects the appropriateness of the interaction.

Direct-Active Style

The style for the Evaluation-Feedback Stage is Direct-Active for supervisors, and Passive for supervisees. It is the style that was described earlier as traditional supervision, and is used predominantly, as indicated in Chapter 3. In this style, the supervisor is in a controlling, superior position; the supervisee in a passive, subordinate position. A broad interpretation of the style is shown in Figure 4–3.

This style at its extreme embodies maximum control and responsibility in the supervisor's role; dependence and minimal participation in the supervisee's role. The script for this style in its most extreme version, as illustrated in Figure 4–3, is as follows: The supervisee performs clinical work. The supervisor observes and communicates to the supervisee, in one way or another, "No, that is not the way to do it. Do it this way," probably providing the strategy the supervisor would have used if she or he had been conducting the therapy. This "way I would have done it" is portrayed by the square box at the right of the diagram. In subsequent efforts, the supervisee tries repeatedly to match the supervisor's

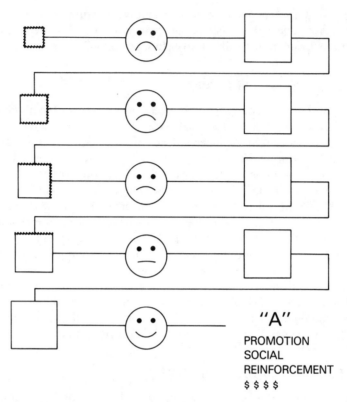

FIGURE 4–3. *DIRECT-ACTIVE STYLE USED IN EVALUATION-FEEDBACK STAGE*

square box, or "right way," finally achieves this objective, to the supervisor's satisfaction at least, and receives whatever the reward system provides for that particular situation—grades, promotion, social reinforcement, or a raise. This "square box" of the supervisor comes from his or her experiences, biases, prejudices, anxieties, fears, interpretations, inferences, perceptions, and disciplined intuition as discussed by Cogan (1973).

This is the High Direct-Low Indirect style of Blumberg (1980), the Domination style of Farris (1974), and the style of choice of many supervisors. It is comparable to the High Task/Low Relationship Stage of the Hersey and Blanchard (1982) model. It may be appropriate, depending upon the needs of the supervisee in relation to the client. The frequency with which it is used may depend upon the perceptions that both supervisor and supervisee have of their role in the supervisory process. Some supervisors may hold a firm conviction that direct behavior produces greater change in supervisees and, therefore, prefer this style.

Available time is perceived by some as a variable that influences the use of this style by the supervisor (Irwin, 1976). Those who use this reasoning say that joint problem solving, which is a characteristic of the Collaborative or Consultative Style, takes time that most supervisors do not have. Supervisors may feel it is necessary to be more directive with supervisees in the interest of the client when time is limited. This assumption has not been tested, however, and the ramifications of time in the supervisory process are unknown.

Although it seems clear that there are situations in which the supervisee is at the Evaluation-Feedback Stage and the direct style is appropriate, especially with the inexperienced or incompetent, the decision to use this Direct-Active Style must be made carefully. The first question to be asked is, By whose judgment is the supervisee declared inexperienced or incompetent? On what basis has the judgment been made that the supervisee is at the Evaluation-Feedback Stage? On the basis of objective data? Or is it merely the result of the subjective appraisal of the supervisor, biased by his or her own experiences and prejudices? Is the supervisor's judgment nothing more than his or her "square box?" Is it the supervisor's style with all supervisees? Or has it been objectively and rationally decided that the direct approach is necessary and appropriate for this particular supervisee?

This style used exclusively has certain hazards. Current research and theoretical writings on leadership and human interaction clearly negate the use of any single style for all situations because of differences in supervisee, supervisor, and situation (Gouran, 1980). One outcome of the exclusive use of this style is the phenomenon of modeling. Although a certain amount of directing, suggesting, and modeling by supervisors may be necessary, appropriate, and desirable at some times, it may also be a deterrent to growth and development of the supervisee. The constant shaping of the supervisee's behavior to match that of the supervisor's behavior or the supervisor's "square box," probably based on what his or her own performance would have been in a similar situation, has the potential for the outcome of the supervisory process to be the creation only of mirror images of the supervisor. This possibility creates potential problems for a profession. If each new generation of professionals does no more than model the behaviors of its supervisors, it does not bode well for the ongoing development of systems for delivering services, nor for the welfare of clients. *The purpose of supervision is not cloning.*

Although supervisors do have experiential and academic information to share with their supervisees (if they didn't, they should not be supervising), no supervisor can possibly have all the final answers to every clinician-client transaction. Certainly, with the proliferation of knowledge from which speech-language pathologists and audiologists draw, each generation of professionals should proceed beyond the level of the last. The objective of supervisors should be not only to impart from their own experience but to encourage their supervisees to go beyond them. The Direct-Active Style as a pervasive style would not seem to do that.

Confusion About Direct-Indirect

Those who have studied the supervisory process in recent years have been introduced to the Direct-Indirect concept and certain misconceptions have grown up around it. Its characteristics have often been distorted from the original description by Blumberg (1974) and its use has been subject to a variety of interpretations. Additionally, a value judgment has been placed on the two styles in some instances—direct supervisory behavior is wrong, indirect right. This "good" and "bad" dichotomy could not be further from the concept that came from Blumberg's research.

Furthermore, the idea that direct supervision is "bad" and indirect is "good" is very guilt-producing for the supervisor who has intellectually espoused an indirect style but actually uses direct behavior at times. Every direct behavior then brings on a "guilt attack."

It is simplistic to discuss any style of human behavior restrictively. Blumberg himself made it clear that he and his associates perceived at least four combinations of direct and indirect supervisory behavior and that teachers perceived a combination of both types of behaviors to be more effective than either one alone. In reality, supervisors probably do exhibit varying degrees of both behaviors; supervisees will also be both active and passive within any one interaction. What becomes important in terms of the continuum is the balance of these behaviors and the appropriateness of that balance to the situation.

Some supervisors also have not interpreted the behavioral components of these styles accurately. Some assume that the mere asking of questions makes the interaction indirect, however, there are many ways of framing questions. 'Do you think the client would benefit from. . ." from the supervisor may appear just as direct to the supervisee as "Have him do. . . next time."

The clinical supervision approach (Cogan, 1973; Goldhammer, 1969), which has influenced much of the thinking about supervision in recent years, makes no allowances for the appropriateness of direct behavior. Cogan rejected the superior/subordinate relationship between supervisors and supervisees as incompatible with his approach; Goldhammer insisted on cooperative, shared interactions. They, however, were writing about the professionally employed teacher. It is the opinion of the writer that, particularly in an educational program, supervisors must allow for the fact that some supervisees will need varying amounts of direct assistance in learning how to begin their work as professionals, and that there are times when supervisors will legitimately need to provide specific directions or to demonstrate techniques. It is only when that direct behavior persists throughout the interaction or with all supervisees and inhibits their opportunities for problem solving that it should be viewed negatively. There should be a rationale for whatever behaviors are used. It is the *balance* of the two types of behaviors that must be carefully orchestrated. This balance will be discussed in the section on the Collaborative Style. The model presented by Hersey and Blanchard (1982) may be more appropriate in terms of that balance than the clinical supervision model.

Is the Terminology Accurate?

The terms *direct* and *indirect* have become a part of the language of supervision in recent years. The salient behaviors of each have been identified earlier—direct supervisory behavior is characterized by initiating, criticizing, telling, directing; indirect by listening, supporting, asking for opinions and suggestions, and other behaviors that encourage activity by the supervisee. These terms do not seem to be adequate, however, for describing all aspects of behavior in the supervisory process. For example, indirect might be interpreted as inactive or may imply less participation by the supervisor, yet the behaviors previously listed are certainly active and purposeful. Some supervisors may be operating in the adbication style of Farris (1974) or the Low Direct, Low Indirect style of Blumberg (1980), where very little is happening between supervisor and supervisee, and none of the descriptors for indirect or direct are applicable. The terms also do not adequately describe the behaviors of supervisees, a fact supported by Smith (1978), who identified a passive clinician factor in ratings of conferences.

Therefore, it is suggested that the terms *active* and *passive* be incorporated where necessary to more precisely and accurately describe the behavior of both participants. Thus, a supervisor's behavior may be direct-active, characterized by the descriptors for direct behavior; indirect-active, characterized by purposeful behaviors that encourage problem solving such as asking for opinions and suggestions, accepting and expanding supervisees' ideas, or asking for rationale or justification of supervisee statements; indirect-passsive, characterized by listening, waiting for supervisees to process ideas and problem-solve; or passive, characterized by not listening, providing little or no input, or not responding to supervisee input. These terms are more descriptive of the complexities of the interaction than simply *direct* and *indirect*.

The use of the terms *active* and *passive* are particularly important in describing supervisee behavior. An active supervisee would be participating by collecting and analyzing data, initiating, problem solving, questioning, suggesting, giving opinions, and requesting rationale and justification for supervisor statements. A passive supervisee would be listening, accepting, asking for suggestions and guidance, seeking strategies, and waiting for information from the supervisor.

Collaborative Style

The appropriate style for moving away from the Evaluation-Feedback Stage, through the Transitional Stage to Self-Supervision is the Collaborative Style (Figure 4–4). This style is a dynamic, problem-solving process wherein supervisor and supervisee work together to achieve optimum service for clients as well as the professional growth and development of both participants. The supervisor's role is less direct but not inactive. Both participants assume responsibility and provide input in varying degrees at different times about both the clinical and the supervisory process. Objectives are established jointly. The supervisor provides feedback but also encourages input from the supervisee, accepts the supervisee's ideas, problem-solves with the supervisee, analyzes clinical behavior, encourages self-analysis and further planning by the supervisee, and recognizes

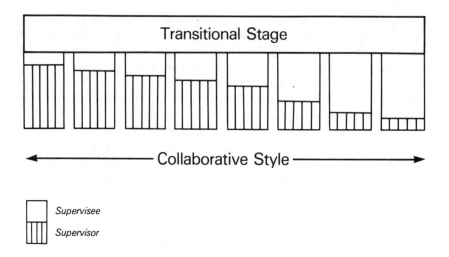

FIGURE 4-4. COLLABORATIVE STYLE USED DURING THE TRANSITIONAL STAGE

and respects the worth of the supervisee as a professional and as a person. The supervisee, in turn, accepts responsibility for participation in the clinical and supervisory process, provides input, accepts suggestions, questions the supervisor, requests rationale and justification for supervisor statements, engages in self-analysis and problem solving, and works toward independence. The supervisor, though responsible for structuring and facilitating the interaction, is *not* the responsible individual within the interaction, does not make all decisions, or provide all the information. Rather, supervision is seen as a joint process where the supervisor and supervisee share responsibilities and interact as professionals to meet common objectives. As progression continues along the continuum, the amount of participation from each is altered as shown in Figure 4-4. This becomes what Kurpius and colleagues (1977) termed "increased ownership" by the trainee in the joint experience of supervision. Furthermore, the interactions between supervisor and supervisee are subjected to study to increase the learning that results from participation in the supervisory process. Based on clinical supervision as presented by Cogan (1973) and Goldhammer (1969), this style is seen as necessary to move from the Evaluation-Feedback Stage to the ultimate objective of Self-Supervision.

Some supervisors resist the Collaborative Style because they assume it means a compromising of the supervisor's position or that it is impossible to obtain appropriate input from supervisees. Some do not realize that it employs a mix of behaviors. This is definitely a misinterpretation of the style. The supervisor using the Collaborative Style may employ both direct, indirect, active, or passive behaviors in any combination, depending upon the situation. None of the styles will be seen in a pure form. Only at the Evaluation-Feedback Stage does the supervisor come close to a totality of direct behavior, and even then there will be a mix of behaviors. The aim of the Collaborative Style is to move away from direct supervisor and passive supervisee behavior as rapidly as possible to involve the supervisee in decision making. Supervisors should have input however. They must share their experience and expertise—but not to the exclusion of meaningful participation by the supervisee.

Munson (1983) described supervision in social work in terms that are similar to the Collaborative Style proposed here:

> If we enter supervision viewing it as the place where supervisors give answers, check up on the practitioner's work, and find solutions for the therapist, we will have started off on the wrong foot and will stumble. Supervision should be a mutual sharing of questions, concerns, observations, speculations, and selection of alternative techniques to apply in practice. I call this process the *congruence of perceptions* in supervision. Practitioners should, and want to, participate in supervision rather than be recipients in it. (p. 4)

Caracciolo and colleagues (1978a) described this mix of behaviors when they said that the supervisor plays two roles—a nondirective one that enables the student to express ideas without fearing judgment or penalty, and a directive one of giving information where appropriate, establishing standards and guidelines, and judging when necessary. "The speech-language pathology supervisor must, therefore, be sensitive to the continuously changing needs of the student clinician within any given moment of the supervisory conference period and must be able to match the supervisory behavior to the student clinician's needs and expectations" (p. 288).

In certain instances, a supervisor and supervisee may virtually change roles at some points in the Transitional Stage. For example, a student clinician, well-trained and with extensive experience in the clinical program with a specific disorder area, may be working with a supervisor whose background in this area is different, limited, or not current. The supervisee might then assume a more active role in the collaboration, with the supervisor receiving the input about certain techniques or a differing philosophy. This requires openness on the part of the supervisor, and confidence, if not courage, on the part of the supervisee.

As in the Evaluation-Feedback Stage, there may be hazards. If the proper place on the continuum is not identified, supervisors may expect supervisees to operate beyond their level, resulting in frustration for both. The Collaborative Style could easily become more of an *abdication* style if supervisors do not provide the correct amount of input.

Consultative Style

Following the continuum through to its conclusion of Self-Supervision, the burden of responsibility now shifts to the supervisee. Self-Supervision requires a continuing search for professional growth through self-analysis. It suggests a peer relationship between supervisor and supervisee, which is represented in Figure 4–5 by the horizontal lines, signifying the ultimate cooperative interaction between supervisor and supervisee. This interaction has been developing throughout the previous stages of the continuum and the supervisee has now been empowered to make decisions about his or her own needs and proceed to find solutions. The professional who reaches this stage will be able to self-identify strengths or weaknesses, make appropriate behavioral modifications, and seek assistance or further knowledge when appropriate. Although this knowledge may come from other sources—peers, in-service or course offerings, readings, or creative problem solving—the supervisory relationship remains important, even though supervisees now have the major responsibility for initiating consultation, even when it is not automatically made available to them.

Consult is defined as "to seek advice or information" as in "consult a specialist," "to exchange views," or "to give professional advice" (Webster, 1984, p. 303). This is exactly the concept intended in the use of this term as the appropriate style for the Self-Supervision Stage, a style that involves a more voluntary nature of interaction between peers than the previous styles. "*Consultation* is a helping process which emerges out of a need to solve a problem. The consultant and consultee engage in a voluntary relationship which focuses on change (i.e., solving a problem) in a client or client system within a given environment (i.e., behaviors, structures, system, and/or situations). In the work-related process of consultation, the consultant helps the consultee use his/her knowledge, skills, and expertise to solve a problem" (Brasseur, 1978, p. 2).

As with the other stages, Self-Supervision is *not time bound* and, therefore, the Consultative Style may be utilized at appropriate times in the educational program, the off-campus or Clinical Fellowship Year experience, or the

Consultative Style

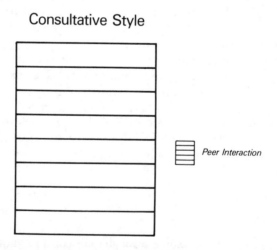

Peer Interaction

FIGURE 4–5. *CONSULTATIVE STYLE USED DURING THE SELF-SUPERVISION STAGE*

employment setting. The supervisor may serve in this capacity when the supervisee no longer needs continuous monitoring. This style may be used when supervisees are working with certain types of clients with which they have developed expertise while, at the same time, the supervisor may be utilizing a Direct-Active Style with the same supervisee while working with another client. In the employment setting where supervisors are probably less available, supervisees may find it necessary to be specific in their requests for help. If a true consultative style is to be a reality here, both participants must enter the interaction with a clear concept of their roles, the problems to be solved, and the procedures to be followed. As with the other stages, differences in perceptions and unmet expectations can create negative reactions, leading to a variety of negative results.

Supervisor behaviors used in the Consultative Style will be mainly listening, supporting, problem solving, and, where appropriate, direct suggestions. If a true peer relationship exists, these suggestions may be accepted, rejected, or built upon by the supervisee. The two will be relating as peers in a productive interaction. It is critical, therefore, that the supervisor recognizes and accepts the supervisee's options, especially that of rejecting suggestions.

Striving to reach the Self-Supervision Stage is important in speech-language pathology and audiology since so many professionals work alone or without supervision or consultation from persons trained in their own profession. Working alone is not necessarily synonymous with self-supervision. When working in such situations, the responsibility for professional growth lies with the individual. Some professionals are able to continue their self-analysis and professional growth to a greater extent than others. Supervision in the service delivery setting will be discussed in greater depth in a subsequent chapter, but it should be said here that the lack of supervision or consultation in the employment setting by trained persons is a serious issue in terms of continuing professional growth. It is also a fact that increases the need for educational programs to produce self-analytical students.

PLACE ON THE CONTINUUM

A composite of the stages of the continuum and their appropriate styles is seen in Figure 4–6. Determining at which level the supervisor and supervisee are functioning, and therefore, the appropriate style to use, is a decision that requires insight and analysis on the part of both participants. It is somewhat analogous to the diagnostic process used to determine the needs of clients. This process will be discussed in detail in the chapter on planning.

Attitudes Toward the Continuum

Most supervisors would probably say that this continuum is what they actually are following, that they *do* treat supervisees differently, that they *do* change their style depending upon the level of expertise of the supervisee, and that their style *is* a collaborative one. In reality, as has been discussed, data on

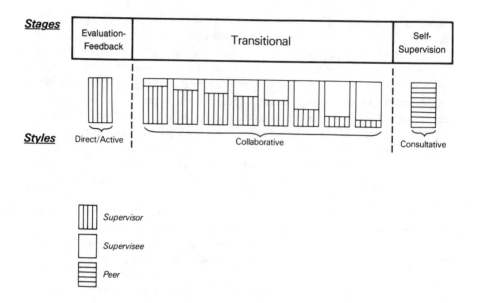

FIGURE 4-6. *COMPOSITE OF STAGES OF SUPERVISION AND THE APPROPRIATE STYLES FOR EACH STAGE*

the supervisory conference indicate that not only is the Direct-Active Style the most frequently used style, but that supervisors do not change their styles over a period of time, even when they perceive that they do. Supervisors appear to have one style that they use consistently with all supervisees. Some supervisors, accustomed to the Direct-Active role, may be unwilling or unable to change their style; some supervisees may prefer to remain dependent and passive. Nevertheless, the continuum is presented as a vehicle for professional growth and development.

SUMMARY

Supervision exists on a continuum along which supervisors and supervisees progress throughout individual supervisory interactions as well as their total careers. Although individuals may enter the continuum at any point or may move back and forth on it, depending upon situational variables, it is the continuous *movement* along the continuum toward the ultimate objective of independence that is critical. The Collaborative Style is seen as a means to facilitate this movement.

Components of the Supervisory Process

Supervision, as a field of study, is filled with myths, unclear definitions and distinctions, and untrained supervisors who operate with good intentions as their main resource.

Hart (1982, p. 5)

What are supervisors and supervisees talking about when they talk about supervision? Where do they begin in studying such a complex process? What do they mean when they say they are supervising? What is involved in carrying out the tasks they assume as supervisors? In the preface to a book on counselor supervision, Boyd (1978) stated that there is a generally accurate perception of what people do when they are counseling but "when counselor supervisors say they are supervising, one must guess what kind of procedure or activity is being performed" (p. xiv).

The same can be said of supervision in speech-language pathology and audiology. Student clinicians have been carefully prepared in observation and analysis of the clinical process. They have been taught to isolate the components of the clinical process with informal supervisor-developed methodologies or by the use of highly structured behavior recording systems such as those described by Boone and Prescott (1972) and Schubert, Miner, and Till (1973). Supervisors have discussed with their supervisees reinforcement or modeling or other behaviors that make up the total clinical act. If they are to understand the supervisory process in the same way they need to attend to its various parts. Supervisors and their supervisees need to be provided with a way to dissect and examine those components that make up the total process.

The continuum proposed in the previous chapter consists of three stages: Evaluation-Feedback, Transitional, and Self-Supervision. A Collaborative Style is seen to be the appropriate supervisory style to facilitate movement of supervisees along the continuum. This style consists of certain components: (I) Understanding the Supervisory Process, (II) Planning, (III) Observing,

(IV) Analyzing, and (V) Integrating. The point on the continuum at which supervisor and supervisee are operating will dictate the quantity of time spent on each component, the amount of input from supervisor and supervisee in each component, and the operational specifics of each supervisory interaction.

Each component will be treated in a separate chapter. A brief overview of all components is presented here.

COMPONENT I—UNDERSTANDING THE SUPERVISORY PROCESS

One of the premises of this book is that supervisors need to be prepared for their roles. Another premise is the need for collaboration between supervisor and supervisee in the process. If these are both valid assumptions, does it not follow that supervisees also need preparation for their roles? For some supervisees, this preparation is nonexistent. For others, it may consist of academic consideration of the supervisory process as an entity which differs from the clinical process and which can be broken down into manageable components for discussion. Whatever the previous preparation, it is proposed here that the supervisory process should be a topic of discussion between supervisors and supervisees at the beginning of every new supervisory experience and throughout the relationship.

Each person brings to the total supervisory experience his or her own needs, expectations, concerns, and objectives. Because of the variety of stereotypes brought into the supervisory experience and because supervisors and supervisees have different perceptions of the same supervisory interaction (Blumberg, 1980; Culatta et al., 1975; Smith & Anderson, 1982b), it is important for the two participants to discuss the supervisory process throughout the entire interaction. If there is a lack of congruence about objectives and procedures at this point, attempts can be made to resolve it. If not resolved, differences can, at least, be raised to a level of consciousness or compromise.

For example, supervisors who believe that the "best" supervisory style is the Collaborative Style may incorporate into their behavior such activities as broad questioning, listening, using supervisee's ideas, and supportive responses to supervisee's ideas with strong attention to encouraging problem solving by the supervisee. If supervisees, however, perceive that the supervisor's role is to evaluate, tell them what they did right or wrong and help them to "do better," there will be an incongruency which may disrupt the supervisory relationship and the learning that should take place (Larson, 1982). A period of discussion about the process into which the supervisor and supervisee are about to embark, preparation of the supervisee for his or her part in the experience, and sharing expectations and objectives should alleviate problems which might arise from such differences in perceptions.

This activity is perceived as being more than just an introductory phase, however. It is important that such discussions of the supervisory process be on-going as needs and objectives are altered, levels of expertise change, and new insights or new problems arise.

COMPONENT II—PLANNING

Speech-language pathologists and audiologists have spent a great deal of time planning for the client and supervisors have spent time educating their students in the planning process. This client-centered approach is certainly necessary and important, but other planning is needed. If the continuum proposed here is to be followed, it will require joint planning as follows:

■ *Planning for the Clinical Process*
   A. Planning for the client
   B. Planning for the clinician
■ *Planning for the Supervisory Process*
   A. Planning for the supervisee
   B. Planning for the supervisor

Planning for the client is not new. Planning for the clinician may not be new for many; planning for the supervisory process itself may be an activity that will necessitate some change of behavior for most supervisors and supervisees.

COMPONENT III—OBSERVING

Traditionally, the script for observation has probably been as follows: Supervisor enters observation room, pencil in hand. Observes clinician at work. Takes notes continuously or intermittently. Notes consist mainly of evaluations of supervisee's behavior. Supervisor leaves observation room. Evaluations are communicated to supervisee in a variety of ways (written notes, check lists, or verbally).

Observation is not to be considered as the time when evaluation takes place. Rather, it is seen as the place where real objectivity begins in the supervisory process, where data are collected and recorded by both supervisor and supervisee for further analysis and interpretation which then lead to the evaluation. Cogan (1973) defined observation as "those operations by which individuals make careful, systematic scrutiny of the events and interactions occurring during classroom instruction. The term also applies to the records made of these events and interactions" (p. 134). Substitute clinical or supervisory sessions for classroom interaction and it becomes a definition that is applicable to the thrust of the proposal made here.

COMPONENT IV—ANALYZING

The analysis stage of the supervisory process is a bridge between observation and evaluation. The objective data collected during the observation really mean little by themselves. It is in the analysis component that the supervisor and supervisee begin to make sense of the data (Cogan, 1973; Goldhammer, 1969). The data are examined, categorized, and interpreted in relation to the change, or lack of change, in the client or clinician. Analysis comes naturally from the planning and observation stages, for if planning is well done both supervisor and supervisee will have determined exactly what data will be collected and what is to be done with it.

An important facet of the analysis stage is the joint responsibility for analysis or interpretation of the data. This is where supervisees, to whatever extent possible, begin to self-analyze, to problem-solve about their own behavior, and to look for the relationships between their behaviors and those of the client.

COMPONENT V—INTEGRATING

At various points throughout each supervisory experience the contents of the components must be integrated. This is ordinarily done in a conference between supervisor and supervisee, individually or in groups, although there are other procedures that contribute to integration.

SUMMARY

The complexities of the supervisory process will be better understood if they can be isolated into specific components for discussion and study. Thus, this chapter has presented five components: Understanding, Planning, Observing, Analyzing, and Integrating, which make up the content of supervision. Each will be discussed thoroughly in subsequent chapters.

Understanding the Supervisory Process

Both (teacher and supervisor) must learn a great deal about each other and about their roles in clinical supervision before they can begin the processes of planning, teaching, observation, analysis, etc., in the cycle of supervision.

Cogan (1973, p. 78).

Regardless of their place on the continuum, supervisors and supervisees in all settings must at some time engage in a special type of interpersonal interaction to accomplish their objectives. This interaction is so important in the supervisory process that it deserves all the effort and attention that can be brought to it to make it a satisfying and rewarding learning experience for all participants.

There are many ways to teach people to swim. One is to toss them into the water and hope that they will suddenly acquire the necessary techniques to reach the edge of the pool. At one time, some clinicians were introduced to the clinical process in much the same way—sink or swim! This practice has been addressed and modified in recent years as a result of ASHA requirements for observations by students preceding clinical practicum and more specific requirements for supervision of the practicum. College and university programs also include in their curricula certain clinical courses and experiences which prepare and then gradually introduce the neophyte clinician to the intricacies of the clinical process. The introduction to the supervisory process, however, still appears to be "sink or swim," as few educational programs appear to teach about the supervisory process and as there is little discussion of the supervisory process in supervisory conferences at any experience level.

PURPOSE OF THE COMPONENT

This chapter will present ways to (1) prepare supervisees for meaningful participation in the supervisory process, and (2) communicate about the process throughout the entire period of interaction between supervisor and supervisee.

The premise for such preparation is that mutual understanding of the various components of the supervisory process will enrich the supervisory experience and enable both supervisors and supervisees to better use that process to strengthen clinical behavior and promote professional growth. Further, the interaction will be most effective when all participants are able to observe, discuss, and analyze the process so that the experience can be modified to meet their needs. This mutual understanding will come from (1) a basic knowledge about the supervisory process, (2) the preliminary investigation of the expectations and needs of both participants, and (3) discussion of the dynamics of the ongoing interaction between the participants. It is maintained that this continuous dialogue about what is happening in the supervisory interaction will increase the value of the experience and the opportunities for professional growth for both supervisor and supervisee and will ultimately result in better service to clients.

This first component of the continuum consists of several facets—an awareness of the possible roles of participants, the importance of supervisors and supervisees knowing and understanding each other's expectations as they enter the activity, the anxieties that supervisees (and perhaps supervisors) bring to the process, and the importance of self-knowledge. What will be presented is a rationale and a method for preparation of both supervisor and supervisee for an interaction that will best address the needs of all participants in the clinical and supervisory process—client, clinician, supervisee, supervisor. What insights, knowledge, and strategies are needed to ensure optimum results from this learning process called supervision?

The Name of the Game

This Understanding component of the supervisory process relates to learning about the basic principles of supervision, but should not be assumed to be relevant only to the beginning of the process. The understanding of such a complex set of behaviors as supervision is developmental. There is no one word that is quite adequate to capture the totality of this component. It might be called "orientation to the supervisory process," but orientation seems too narrow if it is interpreted as "adjustment or adaptation to a new environment, situation, or belief" or "introductory instruction concerning a new situation" (Webster, 1984, p. 829). Cogan (1973) called it an induction phase. However, it is more than an introduction or induction. It is applicable to more than a new situation. It is ongoing and applies across the continuum.

Interpreting is also not totally satisfactory as a descriptor. Such definitions of interpret as "to explain," "to expound," "to represent or delineate the meaning" (Webster, 1984, p. 638) are not inclusive enough. Further, they seem to be unidirectional rather than multidirectional; that is, they might be considered as information coming exclusively from the supervisor, a concept that is inconsistent with the theme of this book. *Rapport* is a term that is used frequently in describing the relationship between clinician and client. It is certainly a desirable objective in the supervisory process; however, what is being discussed here requires a deeper understanding of each other than the usual concept of rapport. The understanding component is a composite of all of these definitions, and refers to an in-depth understanding, not only of the process, but of the thoughts and feelings of the partners in the relationship.

CURRENT TREATMENT OF THE SUPERVISORY PROCESS IN CONFERENCES

Data obtained from analysis of supervisory conferences in speech-language pathology make it clear that conferences, as now conducted, do not include much discussion of the supervisory process or of the needs and behaviors of the supervisees or supervisors who are participating in these conferences (Culatta et al., 1975; Culatta & Seltzer, 1977; Pickering, 1984; Roberts & Smith, 1982; Shapiro, 1985; Smith & Anderson, 1982b; Tufts, 1984). One can make certain assumptions about that fact. Such discussion may not be perceived as an important component of the interaction by either supervisor or supervisee; therefore, it is intentionally omitted from the conference. It may be that the classic view of the supervisory process as evaluation or as a supervisor-dominated activity is so strong and so accepted that it is assumed there is no need for discussion of the process. It may be that supervisors, who generally control the direction of the conference, do not have an understanding of the components of supervision, and feel inadequate to deal with the topic. Additionally, supervisees have probably not been prepared for supervision in such a way that they are able to either initiate or participate in meaningful discussion of the process. Whatever the reason, the data consistently indicate that the focus of the conference is on the clinical process, mainly the client and not the clinician; certainly not on the supervisee or supervisor and the supervisory process. Supervisors seem to plunge into discussion of client needs without attending to the needs or concerns of the supervisee except as related directly to the client.

Appropriateness of Current Practice

It would be ludicrous to argue against the importance of discussing client needs. The intent here is not to eliminate the focus on the client. Rather, the intent is to encourage interpretation and discussion of the supervisory process, in addition to the clinical process, as a means of contributing to the growth and development of the supervisee and supervisor, thus enriching the clinical process.

Speech-language pathologists and audiologists have always been concerned about the ability of the client for carryover or generalization of behaviors acquired during the clinical session. Of equal concern should be the generalization of behaviors acquired by clinicians through the supervision process. However, it appears that supervisees are expected to extrapolate from discussion of the client's behavior to their own to determine the changes that they should make in their own clinical performance. Such an approach is probably limiting in its contribution to the total professional growth of the clinician.

Two strategies for altering this traditional approach to supervision seem possible. The first and most obvious is to move beyond individual client behavior and beyond clinician behavior as it relates to one client, or even one disorder, and to look for patterns of clinical behavior that can be generalized across the clinical process. Unable to resist the restatement of a well-worn bit of advice, the author finds here an analogy in the statement "Give me a fish and I eat for a day. Teach me to fish and I eat for a lifetime."

The next possibility is to attend to the behavior of clinicians as supervisees to try to determine if their participation is such that they obtain maximum benefits from the supervisory process, enabling them to learn problem-solving techniques they can utilize in other situations. It is hoped that these two strategies will move supervisor and supervisee beyond extrapolation from discussion of the client. This point of view was supported by Munson (1983) in the social work literature when he directed his discussion away from "what to learn and how to learn" about social work toward the supervisory process as a learning experience.

UNDERSTANDING THE ROLES IN THE SUPERVISORY PROCESS

Role is usually considered to be a set of expectations about the behavior of persons who occupy certain positions in social units or as actions that are perceived as appropriate to certain positions. It is a set of prescriptions for behavior that are shaped by the rules and sanctions of others and by each person's conception of what his or her behavior should be in a certain situation (Biddle & Thomas, 1966).

The sources of preconceived stereotypes about supervisors and supervision have been discussed in earlier chapters, together with the many roles that supervisors and supervisees have available to them and the fact that they may be performing several roles at one time. If communication is to be open, objectives are to be met and professional growth is to take place as a result of the supervisory process, that is, if supervision is to be productive, participants should be aware of the role perceptions they have for themselves and each other and the expectations they bring into the supervisory interaction.

Perceived Roles for Supervisors

Supervisors are viewed as assuming a variety of roles, among them that of teacher, overseer, controller, evaluator, and counselor (Hatten, 1966) and decision maker (Schubert, 1978). In education, Cogan (1973) listed six types of relationships between supervisor and supervisee, all of which would demand very different roles for each of the participants—the superior-subordinate relationship, the teacher-student relationship, the counselor-client relationship, the supervisor as evaluator or rater, the helping relationship, and the colleagueship relationship. Weller (1971), in discussing the three functions of "counselor, teacher, and trainer," made an important point when he said, "Supervisors can rarely expect to be equally competent in all three functions, yet neither can they afford to be ignorant of any one" (p. 8).

The concept of supervision as a temporary, miniature social system in which one role holder is the control figure (Blumberg, 1980; Dussault, 1970) is of interest and importance in understanding many of the variables in the supervisory process. In a review of supervision in several helping professions, Kurpius and colleagues (1977) suggest that the traditional role of the supervisor in the educational process has generally been that of an autonomous figure who tends to answer to his or her own goals and philosophies rather than to an authority or to a model of supervision. Other concepts of the role of supervisor are inherent in the purposes of supervision as discussed in Chapter 1. In reality, each supervisor probably plays several roles in any one supervisory relationship, as does each supervisee.

Importance of Shared Expectations

Expectations are the perceptions of appropriate behavior for one's own role or the role of others and, as such, are a potent influence on the individual's behavior as well as on how he or she believes others should behave. To speak of *shared expectations* implies that each individual perceives his or her own and others' roles similarly (Biddle & Thomas, 1966). This is considered an important prerequisite to communication and to meeting objectives, especially in the supervisory relationship. "Leaders must either change their style to coincide with followers' expectations or change follower expectations" (Hersey & Blanchard, 1982, p. 132). If supervisors and supervisees operate from different sets of assumptions about what should take place between them, then communication barriers are raised even before the interaction begins (Blumberg et al., 1967).

Discrepancies between expectations and perceptions of what actually happened lead to confusion and conflict. Individuals expressing such role conflict have been found to be less effective than others, suggesting that the consequence of role conflict may be not only ineffectiveness for the institution within which they work, but frustration for the individual (Cooper & Good, 1983; Getzel & Guba, 1954; Trow, 1960).

Tihen (1984), after an extensive review of the literature on expectations of education students regarding the student teaching experience, stated, "It is apparent from the reviewed literature that the realization or lack of realization of the supervisee's expectations of his/her supervisor will have a significant effect upon the supervisory process and clinical practicum. If there is a discrepancy between the supervisee's expectations and the supervisor's actual behavior, both the performance of the supervisee, and the satisfaction which he or she derives from the supervisory process may be negatively affected. Conversely, if the supervisor's behaviors are congruent with the supervisee's expectations, both the supervisee's performance and satisfaction may be positively affected" (p. 7). Hersey and Blanchard (1982) stated that what is important is how leadership is perceived by their followers, not how the leaders think they behave. "Thus, leaders have to learn how they are coming across to others" (p. 129). This position was supported by Smith and Anderson (1982b), who recommended periodic checking of perceptions of conference behavior.

Without clarification of roles, expectations, and needs, the supervisory experience may be characterized, for either of its participants, by uncertainty, confusion, lack of direction, frustration, and stress. In fact, sharing of goals and objectives, the defining of needs and expectations, and the clarification of the differences and similarities in perceptions of roles may well be one of the most important components of the entire supervisory interaction, probably forming the pattern for the entire relationship. It also is reasonable to assume that needs, expectations, and perceptions are not static, and are altered by maturity, experience, and the influence of the many variables within each situation. Therefore, there is a need for *continuing* exploration of perceived role, as well as expectations and needs, in every supervisory relationship as it progresses through a semester, a year, or an ongoing situation such as an employment setting.

EXPECTATIONS FOR SUPERVISION

Studies from Other Disciplines

The literature from other disciplines contains many studies that identify expectations and needs of supervisees and the extent to which they are met. Much of this literature is overlapping, contradictory, and equivocal; some is trivial. A few themes stand out, however, as important, and provide insights about the wide variety of expectations that may be present in any situation.

Many writers have related the meeting of expectations or needs to motivation, effectiveness, productivity, and attitudes toward the situation in which the supervision took place (Delaney & Moore, 1966; Gross & Herriot, 1965; Hersey & Blanchard, 1982; Kelly, 1980; Likert, 1961, 1967; Reitz, 1981; Shapiro & Shapiro, 1971; Smith, 1978; Wernimont, 1966). Some have speculated that a criterion for effectiveness of supervision should be a measure of how well supervisees' needs are fulfilled (Bowers & Scofield, 1959). Some have strongly suggested that supervisees' satisfaction with the supervisory process and their subsequent evaluation of the experience are related to the degree of discrepancy between supervisees' expectations and their perceived realization of those expectations (House, Filley, & Gujarati, 1971; Likert, 1961; Stuntebeck, 1974). Others have identified specific areas where discrepancies exist between what supervisors and supervisees believed was good supervision (Worthington & Roehlke, 1979). Some studies have indicated that supervisees' expectations change over time—within a short period of time such as a practicum experience, for example, or between the educational setting and the employment setting (Gyshers & Johnson, 1965; Hansen, 1965). Training, experience, personality traits, and situational variables have been investigated relative to expectations and needs (Vander Kolk, 1974).

Expectations Related to Direct/Indirect Styles

Apropos to the discussion of expectancies are certain investigations of preferences of supervisees for direct and indirect supervisory behavior. This dichotomy of styles has been of particular interest to researchers in education, although the findings have been mixed. Blumberg and Amidon (1965) were among the first to study this dimension and found that supervisors of teachers who utilized a high amount of indirect behavior (listening, questioning, reflecting back teacher's ideas and feelings) more nearly met teachers' expectations.

Copeland and Atkinson (1978) studied students who had completed elementary student teaching and found that their subjects clearly preferred directive (authoritarian style) to nondirective (interrogatory and reflective style) supervisory behavior. The authors related this finding to the inexperience and insecurities of students that lead them to desire concrete and immediate solutions to their problems or to their dependence on the supervisor for a grade.

In another study of male and female secondary student teachers, Copeland (1980) again found a preference for the directive over the nondirective. He cautioned that the results cannot be used to support an argument for one supervisory approach over the other, but said, "It seems logical, however, that a relationship between a supervisor and a teacher is more likely to continue and to be productive if the teacher perceives the supervisor's approach as being appropriate" (p. 41).

Other Variables in Expectations

While the literature has investigated many variables related to expectations of supervisees, one area that does not appear to have been a subject for much research is the influence of such factors as gender, race, or age on expectations or role perceptions for supervision. Copeland (1980) found a strong preference of female subjects for male supervisors and a slight preference of male subjects for female supervisors. Although Copeland stated that these findings must be interpreted carefully, he confirmed that they are consistent with other research which has shown preferences for counselors of the opposite sex and which show opposite sex experimenters as more potent reinforcers. Vander Kolk (1974) found that black graduate counseling students differed from white graduate counseling students in their anticipation of the supervisory relationship, black students anticipating a destructive or less than facilitating relationship with the supervisor. These and others may be extremely important variables in relation to expectations for supervision and they deserve careful investigation. For example, are expectations of supervisees different for older supervisors than they are for those who may be near-contemporaries of the supervisee? Are they different for males or females, Ph.D. academic professors, or master's degree supervisors? Are there other such factors that influence expectations? In the face of the lack of much information about these issues, they at least deserve to be raised to a level of consciousness on an individual level.

Expectations of Supervisors

The expectations or needs of supervisors appear not to have gained as much attention as those of supervisees. If differences between role perceptions and expectations exist and if they result in lack of satisfaction or interfere with communication and effectiveness for supervisees, they must also affect supervisors. Munson (1983) reported on a study in social work which showed that, although supervisees had a high level of satisfaction with their supervisory experiences, the factors that provided high levels of satisfaction and met the needs of supervisees produced little satisfaction for supervisors. He further raised an important question when he asked, "At what price to the supervisor are these supervisee satisfactions being met?" (p. 20). Investigation of supervisors' expectations and needs and their satisfaction with the supervisory interaction may be an important key, not only to affective components of the relationship, but to overall effectiveness. If supervisors' expectations for their role are not being met, it may relate to the finding that supervisors' behavior remains static over time, not adapting to supervisee variables (Culatta & Seltzer, 1977; McCrea, 1980; Roberts & Smith, 1982; Tufts, 1984). This may be important as either the cause or the result of a lack of satisfaction with their job, if it exists. Anyone not achieving satisfaction from work activities may slip into stereotypical, repetitive responses to the demands of the job. Conversely, in a "Catch-22" script, lack of variation in activities may quickly cause boredom. Supervisor expectations and satisfactions with their job are a fertile area of study.

Studies from Speech-Language Pathology and Audiology

Students of the supervisory process in speech-language pathology and audiology have also investigated and/or made suggestions about what supervisees see as important in their supervisors, about perceived needs and expectations that supervisors and supervisees have for each other, and the discrepancies that may exist.

Some insight about what supervisees consider important can be gleaned from a study by Russell (1976), in which she asked student supervisees to indicate their perception of the importance of 65 different supervisor competencies or behaviors and also to indicate what behaviors were actually exhibited by their supervisors. Her subjects listed the following ten most valued competencies (i.e., competencies supervisors should exhibit):

- Being fair and impartial in the evaluation of the clinician.
- Treating the clinician in a fair and impartial manner.
- Encouraging the clinician to question, disagree, and express ideas.
- Guiding the clinician to make clinical decisions.
- Being flexible and adaptable.
- Providing the clinician with constructive evaluative information.
- Being responsive to the clinician's feedback and evaluation.
- Perceiving the clinician's feedback and evaluation.

The ten least valued competencies were:

- Guiding the clinician to provide written feedback to the client.
- Providing specific academic coursework concurrent with clinical training in the disorder(s) of concern.
- Being procedure-oriented.
- Guiding the clinician to provide the client with feedback at designated intervals.
- Providing the clinician with indirect feedback and evaluation.
- Providing specific academic coursework prior to clinical training in the disorder of concern.
- Guiding the clinician to provide indirect feedback to the client.
- Providing the clinician with written feedback and evaluation.
- Guiding the clinician to be procedure-oriented.
- Guiding the clinician to foster decision making on the part of the client.

Interestingly enough, when Russell's supervisees were asked what supervisors *do* most frequently, the ten items were different from those listed as most valued. The only item that appeared in both the actual and the most valued categories was "treating the clinician in a fair and impartial manner." Of the other nine items listed as behaviors that actually occurred, all were specifically related to client behavior or the clinical process. Discrepancies between expectations and reality were greatest in terms of supervisor's attention to clinician needs, feelings, and problems and to evaluation.

Some researchers have looked at needs or expectations of speech-language pathology students at different experience levels. Myers (1980) found that, although student supervisees perceived that their needs for demonstration and discussion of theoretical bases and rationale underlying therapy approaches decreased over time, affective needs were continuous throughout the educational program. Similar changes in needs of students were identified by Russell and Engle (1977), who found students changing from concern about therapy procedures to concern about their client and the clinical *process*.

Russell and Engle (1977) also found some differences between expectations of audiology and speech-language pathology students. Audiology students, more than speech-language pathology students, perceived that it was important for supervisors to guide them in being nonthreatening to their clients, developing a clinical atmosphere, and helping them to be procedure-oriented and to provide oral feedback to the client. Audiology students placed great importance on receiving help when encountering difficulty. Speech-language pathology students valued flexibility and adaptability in their supervisors as well as guidance in developing clients' understanding of goals, providing feedback, and utilizing resources. These differences in expectations would seem to reflect the difference between the one-time diagnostic interaction and precise requirements of audiology and the on-going and variable nature of the therapeutic interaction in speech-language pathology.

Dowling and Wittkopp (1982) found differences in perceived supervisory needs between experienced and less experienced students in six different universities. Assistance in writing lesson plans and the need for frequent observations were given greater value by the less-experienced clinicians, whereas the more-experienced clinicians wished to assume more responsibility for the client. The authors suggested, on the basis of certain of their findings, that students do not have preconceived notions about what supervision is or what it should be, thus lending support to the need for preparation of supervisees for the experience.

Inconsistencies between student clinicians' perceptions of the supervisory process and the role of the supervisor and the clinician's own willingness to assume responsibilities were reported by Wollman and Conover (1979). Although students felt that their supervisor's biases and opinions were imposed upon them, limiting their opportunities to incorporate their own procedures, they also indicated a desire for direct supervisory intervention in improving their therapy and suggesting the "best" therapy techniques. Students in this study also indicated that to avoid criticism from the supervisor, they would prefer going to colleagues for advice, thereby avoiding supervisor confrontation. The authors drew some negative conclusions from their findings about the willingness of students to assume responsibilities in the supervisory process. It may be, however, that these findings illustrate the confusion supervisees may have about role and responsibility and lend support to the importance of a basic understanding of expectations.

Larson (1982) looked at both needs and expectations of supervisees. Although she found similar expectations for supervision both from inexperienced (no clinical hours) and experienced (over 150 hours) supervisees—to ask questions, to participate in the conference, to express their opinions and have their ideas used, for supervisors to be supportive—the inexperienced students had slightly higher expectations for supervision and expressed stronger needs than the experienced, as might be expected. Inexperienced clinicians expressed a high expectation that supervisors would tell them about their clinical weaknesses.

In terms of their needs, both groups felt a strong need to be allowed to express their opinions, for supervisors not to assume a superior role but to be supportive and pay attention to what supervisees say—in other words, they felt that their point of view should be considered. Both groups expressed a strong need to have supervisors exhibit supportive communication behavior as well as to function in instructional roles as teachers, by helping them with client goals and therapy strategies.

In another study in speech-language pathology, Tihen (1984) studied the importance that three different levels of student clinicians attached to each of five categories of expectations and whether they perceived their supervisors attaching similar or dissimilar importance to the same categories. Tihen found, as did other investigators, that inexperienced clinicians expected more direction from supervisors than the more experienced groups. They also did not differentiate as much as more experienced clinicians did between the importance they attached to their expectations and the importance they felt their supervisors attached to the same expectations. As clinicians gained experience, they placed greater value on the expectations related to their own responsibility in the supervisory process. Tihen suggested that this means that clinicians enter the supervisory process without priorities for their expectations of their supervisors and that their priorities develop as a function of the supervised practicum. He further proposed that knowledge of the expectation profile of each supervisee would assist supervisors and supervisees in planning supervisory programs that would be compatible with supervisee needs.

These findings suggest that supervisees do change in terms of their perception of need and the expectations for supervision as they move along the continuum. This is perhaps not surprising, but the question that supervisors must ask themselves is whether or not their supervisory approaches are compatible with these changes. As has been stated, the literature suggests that supervisory styles do not adjust to changing expectations of supervisees.

ANXIETY IN THE SUPERVISORY PROCESS

The role of the emotions in the communication process and in the learning process is significant and should be considered in any study of the supervisory process. Gazda (1974), in discussing the emotional tone of the classroom, stated that, while it is true that students who are emotionally involved learn best, it is the specific emotion and its intensity that may "either facilitate, distract from, or inhibit learning" (p. 10). He then quoted Mouly (1960), who wrote, "A certain amount of emotional tension (e.g., motivation) is beneficial if the individual utilizes the energy which is generated to further the attainment of his goals. However, when the tension is too great. . .the individual becomes so concerned with the tension itself that he is no longer able to devote himself to dealing with the problem confronting him" (Gazda, 1974, pp. 139–140).

Anxiety of Supervisees

Weller (1971) said that the initial years of teaching produce great stress, especially for persons who set high standards for themselves. One contributing factor is that the feedback about failures is often more obvious and persistent than feedback about successes. "This may be the first instance of failure for the novice who has had an academic history of success, and such perceptions of failure are frequently taken in an intensely personal way" (Weller, 1971, p. 8). This is probably just as much of a certainty in speech-language pathology and audiology. In fact, the first practicum will probably be the first time the supervisee has had his or her behavior subjected to the type of scrutiny it receives during the observation and conference.

Small wonder, then, that supervisees approach the experience with a broad range of emotions. Anyone who has overheard a conversation between students prior to their first practicum will be aware of the "jitters" which accompany this "rite of passage." All professionals probably remember the great amount of anxiety, as well as time, that accompanied the preparation of lesson plans in the early days of their own practicum experience. They also may remember the threat of the unseen, but nevertheless acknowledged, observer on the opposite side of the observation room window. Or they may remember the even worse, ever-present possibility of an unplanned interruption of the therapy session by some supervisors. For some, the anxiety produced by observations diminishes only slightly, even with experience.

Very possible sources of anxiety for supervisees during their educational program, including off-campus experiences, no matter how good the interpersonal interaction may be, are such factors as evaluations, grades, recommendations for graduate school, or job placement. In the employment setting, anxiety over evaluations that relate to retention, promotions, or recommendations for other jobs are realistic. Additionally, in the work setting, anxieties are often created for speech-language pathologists or audiologists by the fact that they may be supervised by individuals trained or experienced in another discipline. This may also be true in the school practicum where the university supervisor may be a representative of the university's general education faculty (Anderson, 1973a).

Openness and the ability to communicate freely will certainly be affected by feelings of anxiety. Such feelings may result in hostility, an inability to think clearly or to be flexible, and will probably increase the amount of "selective listening." People hear what they want to hear or what their emotional state allows them to hear. Some may focus only on the negative; others may hear only the positive. Supervisors need to do what they can to decrease the anxiety of supervisees (Lovell & Wiles, 1983).

Munson (1983) believes that supervisee anxiety grows out of lack of mechanisms to cope with problems encountered in practice. He considers the authority of the supervisory position to be a factor in the creation of anxiety. It is true that, even with the best of intentions on the part of supervisors, the reality is that they do hold a position of power. All the factors mentioned previously—grades, evaluations, job recommendations—provide a very real threat.

The anxiety factor is discussed at length in relation to the colleagueship aspect of the clinical supervisor model which Cogan (1973) proposed. In discussing teachers in the field, he said that they perceive supervisors as a threat for a variety of reasons. They often perceive the supervisor as someone who is looking only for their weaknesses, a perception that may be accurate in some cases. They endorse supervision in principle but not in practice. Further, Cogan attributed most of the teacher's anxiety to the "one-shot, hit-and-run" supervision that may be common in the schools, to a lack of trust by teachers, to capricious behavior by supervisors, to the fact that supervisors' criteria for good performance are often unknown to teachers, to supervisors' personal approach to supervisees, to the effect of supervisors on the classroom as they visit, and to their estimation of the supervisor's competencies. Although Cogan was addressing the issue of the classroom teacher, there is food for thought here for supervisors in any situation.

Stress and anxiety are created in the student teaching situation by the gap between the requirements of the job, the student's self-expectancies, and his actual performance based on his immediate capacity to deal with the situation, according to Mosher and Purpel (1972). They listed the possible reactions of the supervisee—intellectualization, reaction formation, suppression or denial, rationalization, projection, regression, or dependence. Such discussions of anxiety are all relevant to supervisors and supervisees in speech-language pathology and audiology. Energy dissipated through excessive anxiety is energy lost to the task at hand.

Kadushin (1968), in an article inspired by Berne's (1964) theory of gamesmanship, noted the anxieties of supervisees that may be generated by the need for change of behavior and, perhaps, personality, the threat to autonomy and sense of adequacy, the return to a relationship similar to the parent-child relationship, and the threat of evaluation and confrontation. Kadushin said that supervisees have developed some clearly identifiable games as a result of these anxieties and suggested, among others, the following games: "Be Nice to Me Because I am Nice to You," "Protect the Sick and the Infirm," "Treat Me, Don't Beat Me," "Evaluation is Not for Friends," and the wonderful avoidance devices that may be familiar to supervisors—"I Have a Little List" which is, in turn, related to "Heading Them Off at the Pass." Sleight (1984) has suggested similar games for supervisees in speech-language pathology and audiology. Although the games concept tends to be a simplistic approach to the complexities of supervision, as indeed it is to life in general, supervisors will find amusing and insightful glimpses of themselves and their supervisees in these articles.

Studies of Anxiety in Speech-Language Pathology and Audiology

In the speech-language pathology and audiology literature there is also reference to the anxieties of supervisees. Rassi (1978) included in her qualifications for the supervisor in audiology a practical knowledge of human behavior and the ability to deal with supervisees regarding their uncertainty about the future and other concerns. Ward and Webster (1965a) said that a student may find clinical practice "fraught with terrors of which he has little understanding" (p. 39). Oratio (1977), on the basis of informal interviews with students, related fear and anxiety experienced by students entering clinical practicum to three sources: anxiety about their inability to attain supervisory standards, the responsibility for the welfare of the client, and the fear that they will be unable to put academic knowledge into practice.

The *Sleight Clinician Anxiety Test* (SCAT) was developed to rate fears and anxieties of new practicum students (Sleight, 1985). The 40-item scale describes four areas of fears: (1) living up to supervisory standards and relationships between supervisors and supervisees, (2) responsibility for clients, (3) transferring theory into practice, and (4) general feelings about the practicum. On the basis of a study in which this test was used with students, Sleight said that during the practicum, students decreased their anxieties and increased their confidence regarding supervisor/clinician interactions and general fears but not regarding client well-being or putting theory into practice. At no time did any group show decreases in anxiety about responsibility to clients. This seems to be a continuing source of anxiety, as perhaps it should be. Feelings of anxiety or confidence did not change in Sleight's study with repeated clinical experience in the same clinical setting. When the test was given following completion of the school practicum, however, the students showed an increase in confidence in the areas of transferring theory to practice and general functioning in the practicum. The author stated, "It appears that additional experience in the same setting does not affect a student's confidence, but additional experience in a different setting increases confidence in some areas" (p. 41). It may also be the usually intensive nature of the school practicum that "wears down" the anxiety. Sleight further stressed the importance of supervisors recognizing students' anxieties about the practicum. The SCAT provides an instrument which supervisors might find useful for exploration of the anxieties of individual supervisees.

Anxieties of Supervisors

One cannot assume that all the anxiety and apprehensions brought into the supervisory experience are brought there by supervisees. Most supervisors have not been prepared for the tasks they must perform as supervisors. Their perceptions of their roles have come from as many different sources as have those of their supervisees. Perhaps they bring even more stereotypes or preconceived ideas for they, at least, have been supervised, even if they have not supervised.

Supervisors, in speech-language pathology and audiology at least, do not usually plan to be supervisors—their preparation, their career objectives, their self-perception as professionals, is as that of a clinician—and often one who works with children. To be suddenly thrust into the new role of supervisor of professional adults, without preparation, may result in a difficult and stressful transition which requires the development of a new and different self-concept. Additionally, supervisors may begin work with little or no organizational assistance or support, that is, job descriptions, models, or opportunity for in-service education to help them learn new skills or define their new role. Indeed, the importance of the role of supervisor may be downgraded by the casual way in which supervisors are selected and the lack of guidance they receive. Off-campus supervisors, for example, may be provided with very little in the way of guidelines or support from the university for whom they are supervising. University supervisors or supervisors in a service delivery setting may receive no input about their responsibilities and, thus, may operate autonomously. These are only a few of the sources of anxieties for supervisors.

Most supervisors recognize the importance of their tasks along with their lack of preparation. Most are conscientious about fulfilling their roles. Some supervisors' perception of their role is of a professional who must have the answer to every possible clinical question, who must be able to solve every problem or issue that arises. That "heavy" self-perception, along with the inner knowledge that one does not really have that kind of information, skill, or power will surely produce anxiety. This self-concept—that supervisors must have all the answers—has serious consequences in the development of the Collaborative Style.

Sometimes the dispelling of this myth comes as a great surprise and a great relief. Every supervisor has the right—and the responsibility—to say "I don't know."

This initial anxiety about role may continue. There are very few data in any of the areas where supervision is utilized that supports any particular methodology that will bring results. Supervisors who want to find hard and fast answers about what they should be doing will search without much result. Cogan (1973) addressed this in relation to supervisors in education when he stated that professional uncertainties have existed for a long time and will probably persist for a long time. 'Supervisors," he said, "need to be prepared to live with partial knowledge" (p. 52). Until they can accept the fact that they must make decisions without a clear-cut rationale or that they must be satisfied with less than a "yes" or "no" answer they will work under extreme "psychological and ethical strains." Cogan continued on to say that many professionals establish a satisfactory adjustment to these unknowns. The process of achieving this status, however, may be extremely stressful for conscientious professionals.

Some supervisors experience difficulties in using the various types of authority inherent in their positions—administrative, evaluative, educational, and consultative. The attempt to deal with these difficulties may lead to two categories of games—games of abdication and games of power, neither of which resolves the problem. According to Hawthorne (1975), supervisors must examine their own feelings and needs concerning the authority of their professional role. Ward and Webster (1965b) also discussed problems of authority and relationships for both supervisor and supervisee.

Supervisors, in their role as evaluators, often have to make or participate in "life-altering" decisions—retention or dismissal from an educational program, recommendations for a job, for promotions, or for tenure. If dealt with seriously and responsibly, these are awesome responsibilities that understandably create tension and anxiety.

What are the effects, then, of supervisor anxiety and what is its relationship to supervision at this stage of the continuum? Why insert it at this point in the discussion? If supervisors are, indeed, responsible for structuring the supervisory experience, they should have, in addition to information, some sense of comfort in the role. Excessive anxiety or uncertainty on the part of the supervisor will surely be communicated to the supervisee through various means—aggression, neglect of duties, uncertainty, erratic behavior. On the other hand, too much complacency about the role is not desirable.

Very little is known about the feelings of supervisors. Pickering (1984; Pickering & McCready, 1983) touched upon it in their studies, especially when they wrote about the use of journal writing by supervisors, as did McCready, Shapiro, and Kennedy (1987). Like most other aspects of the process at the present time, supervisor anxiety must be considered as thoughtfully as possible, without the benefit of a great many definitive answers. It is speculated that perhaps the judicial use of a modicum of self-disclosure might contribute to collegiality, encourage better communication—and possibly diminish anxieties of both supervisor and supervisee. The image of the supervisor who knows all is difficult to maintain; more reasonable is the image of the supervisor who knows how to problem-solve and is willing to enter into this type of activity with the supervisee.

IMPLICATIONS FOR PARTICIPANTS IN THE SUPERVISORY PROCESS

What does all this mean to the supervisor and the supervisee facing each other across the conference table for the first time? Or the twenty-first time? In implementing the Understanding component of the supervisory process as presented here, supervisors are dealing with two distinct entities. The first is an interpersonal factor; the second a teaching factor, that is, teaching about supervision.

It has already been stated that the interpersonal components of the supervisory process will not be dealt with in great detail here other than to point out the wealth of information on this topic that is available from other sources and the importance of an in-depth knowledge of the interpersonal aspects of human relations. However, this component is one of the places where an understanding of the dynamics of interpersonal interaction is not only relevant but essential.

The very essence of this component is mutual understanding, not only of the mechanics of the process, but of the other person in the interaction. Therefore, supervisors will need to bring to bear all their knowledge, insight, and skills about interpersonal interactions to successfully accomplish the goals of this component. Supervisors have learned and have taught clinicians to apply these interpersonal skills to their clients; can they not apply the same principles to their supervisees? This does not necessitate perceiving or dealing with them as "clients," but as humans. Ward and Webster (1965a), in one of their significant articles on preparing clinical personnel, stated it thus:

> It seems of critical importance, if only to the advancement of our pro-
> fession, that we apply these concepts about human beings to our clinical
> students, too. These are the people who will tend to view others as they
> have been viewed, to treat others as they have been treated. They can
> use knowledge with compassion and meaningfulness or they can apply
> techniques mechanically. They can feel challenged to advance knowledge
> of speech and hearing disorders and their treatment from their creative
> understanding of themselves and others, or they can avoid the risk of
> seeking new knowledge. They probably cannot go beyond their own
> level of growth to help their clients grow and change. (p. 39)

Role Discrepancies

Literature on the importance of shared expectations has been reviewed earlier. Its application is an important issue. A lack of congruency about role expectations may be one of the major sources of breakdown in communication that makes interpersonal interaction less than successful. The possible scenarios for situations where there is a lack of congruence regarding role expectations are many. Consider, for example, supervisees who have had little opportunity in previous family or educational experiences to participate in problem solving and decision making and who have learned to expect authority figures—parent, teacher, employer, and others—to tell them what to do and then to provide evaluative feedback. Such supervisees will probably expect supervisors to assume the same role. They may have a difficult time with supervisors who perceive their own role as facilitators in a joint problem-solving situation where supervisees are expected to assume decision-making responsibilities.

The *immediate* needs of such supervisees will probably be met by supervisors whose perception of their role is an authoritarian one in which evaluative feedback is given and followed by information and suggestion or direction. One may question the long-range results of such interaction, however. Conversely, supervisees who perceive themselves as able to work independently and who perceive the supervisor's role as that of a facilitator, matched with supervisors who see their role as authoritarian, will probably experience frustration, if not bitterness and disillusionment with the supervisory process, and possibly even with the clinical process. Kavanagh (1975) stated "An employee who expects to be treated as a 'person' by his supervisor would be upset if he were treated as just another 'cog in the wheel' " (p. 28).

Supervisors, too, may be frustrated if they assume a facilitative role and find that the expectation for independent behavior from the supervisee is unrealistic. Caracciolo and colleagues (1978a) discussed the importance of the student clinician's understanding of the supervisor's expectations and stated, "It is quite conceivable that some student clinicians may welcome and readily adjust to the non-directive supervisory experience while others may be unable to cope with it; that is, some student clinicians may prefer direct tutorial supervision" (p. 289). Supervisor frustration may be alleviated somewhat by a knowledge of these expectations and abilities.

Learning About Discrepancies

If supervisors are to know about the discrepancies that exist between themselves and their supervisees or between expectations and reality, they must take the lead in talking about the supervisory process itself. If they are to do this, they must first raise to a conscious level what it is that *they* believe about or expect from supervision. They also need to assist their supervisees in developing an ability to discuss their feelings, concerns, and expectations.

Further, supervisors must recognize the individuality of their supervisees. Each person is unique—novice clinicians who bring their anxiety, blatantly obvious in a variety of reactions or covered by false self-confidence, bravado, or hostility, into the conference; slightly more experienced, but nevertheless anxious, clinicians; supervisees who have been supervised often and frequently by supervisors with divergent styles and philosophies; the mature, competent supervisee—all have different needs, different expectations. Supervisors must learn all they can about each one—while still dealing with their own anxieties.

Dealing with Discrepancies

Possible mismatches of expectations can be dealt with in several ways. One possibility is supervisory assignments made to avoid such situations. This alternative can be discarded almost immediately. Such variables as experience, ability, training needs, and organizational constraints make scheduling difficult enough in most settings as it is. Time, requirements for clinical hours, and availability of clients often dictate scheduling in educational programs. In most off-campus assignments, there are only limited numbers of supervisors in each setting and, in the service delivery setting, there is usually only one supervisor available, often for many supervisees. Furthermore, information is not available for making the "perfect" match for the most effective supervision even if it were logistically possible. More important, if supervisees are to grow professionally and move from the evaluation feedback position to the self-supervisory and consultation stage discussed previously, one can assume that the nature of the supervisory experience should not be determined by the supervisee's preference or expectations alone. In other words, the supervisee who prefers or feels a need for guidance and direction from authority figures would not necessarily profit from being matched with a supervisor who will meet that need—very little growth is apt to take place. What supervisees perceive as their needs may not be what is best for their professional growth. Supervisees' preferences for supervisor behavior are not necessarily related to the effectiveness of supervision (Copeland & Atkinson, 1978). Children like and want candy, but it may, after all, produce dental cavities, hyperactivity, and weight gain. What is more consistent with the proposal made here is that both participants in the process become aware of the other's role perceptions or expectations, that communication take place about the incongruencies that exist and the changes that may be necessary for both supervisor and supervisee if communication is to be enhanced and professional growth is to take place throughout the entire experience. Accommodations must be made where there are discrepancies if the interaction is to be successful (Hersey & Blanchard, 1982).

PREPARING FOR SUPERVISION

It has already been stated several times that supervisors, by and large, have not studied the supervisory process. Basic to the approach presented here, however, is some understanding of the dynamics of the process, whether from this book or other material. The first step is for supervisors to prepare themselves for the encounter, learning about themselves as well as the process. This not only will increase their understanding but will perhaps allay some of their anxieties.

Study of the Process by Supervisors

Although it is true that formal coursework has not been or may not now be available to many supervisors, there are ways for them to become more knowledgeable about the process once they have assumed the role of supervisor.

The listing of tasks and competencies adopted by ASHA (1985b) may be the best starting place for study, and there are other sources. The position paper that lists those competencies also makes suggestions about ways for supervisors to become more knowledgeable about the process (see Chapter 12). The implication seems to be that there is no justification for a lack of information about supervision if one seeks it out.

Speech-language pathologists and audiologists seem to be earnest in their desire for continuing education regarding their clinical expertise, as evidenced in attendance at conferences, conventions, and other continuing education activities. Supervisors need to recognize that they have the same kind of professional obligation in relation to the supervisory responsibilities they have assumed. Clinicians who would not attempt to deal with a client with an unfamiliar disorder without study or consultation may take on the job of supervisor with neither.

It is recommended, then, that supervisors avail themselves of some of the many opportunities for making themselves more knowledgeable about the supervision process. Reading, coursework, conferences, and presentations at professional meetings are ways to begin. In many organizations or areas, supervisees have formed discussion groups. Additionally, self-study, which will be discussed at length in another chapter, is a valuable tool for supervisors who wish to monitor their skills.

Supervisor Self-Knowledge

The admonition to "know thyself" is as important in the approach to the supervisory process as it is in the many other situations in which it is wisely offered as a guideline. Self-knowledge in several categories is critical. Supervisors first must define, or raise to a conscious level, their basic philosophy of what supervision really is. They need to define the purpose of supervision and the principles upon which they determine their supervisory techniques. They must be honest about what they really believe about the supervisory process and the values they bring to it.

In a recent discussion of supervisory techniques, a supervisor described her own use of indirect behaviors such as questioning and asking supervisees for ideas. The techniques were consistent with the clinical supervision model, but then she said, "The supervisee came up with a good idea, so I could go along with it. I don't know what I would have done if I hadn't been comfortable with it." Obviously, there were some discrepancies between what the supervisor *really* believed and what she perceived she was doing.

Supervisors need to understand their self-perception of their own roles. They need to analyze their own behavior to determine if it is consistent with their basic philosophy, and must have a rationale for their behaviors. They must recognize the complexity of the supervisory process and determine if they see it as teaching, evaluation, modeling, collaboration, or any of the many other available models. They need to examine their belief in a scientific approach to observation, data collection, and analysis and their own dedication to maintaining a scientific approach. The number of questions that supervisors must ask themselves is infinite, but they must honestly analyze their own philosophical foundation for the practices in which they engage before they can expect to discuss the process with their supervisees.

A further area of self-knowledge is that of personal motivations in relation to supervision. Why do individuals become supervisors? Many would answer the question with lofty statements about the professional growth and development of young professionals and the obligations of passing on that which they have learned through education and experience to new generations of clinicians, thereby contributing to their profession. Those are certainly valid reasons and, for the most part, sincere and honest motivations. The reality is, however, that most supervisors became such by accident. Rather than planning to be supervisors, they were in the right place at the right time and, lo!—they became a supervisor. As they continue in this role, however, there is always the specter of the seductiveness of power and authority lurking in the background. Brammer (1985) suggested that many people who are involved in the helping process do so "to meet their own unrecognized needs" (p. 3). This can also be true of supervisors. Other writers have suggested that the helping process may be destructive rather than facilitative (Carkhuff, 1969a,b; Carkhuff & Berensen, 1967). Supervisors need to be aware of their basic attitude toward people and their worth. If, in their role of supervisor/helper they are going to step back and *permit* their supervisees to grow, then they must value them as autonomous individuals, believe fully in their ability to think and learn, and recognize these abilities when they are present. If they believe that role includes assuming all responsibility for the supervisee's growth and development, if they do not believe that individuals can function independently in problem solving and move toward growth, they may become manipulative and self-serving in their roles. They may perceive themselves as "rescuers" and the kinds of satisfactions they obtain from this so-called helping relationship may not be healthy ones. Supervisors can determine these values and attitudes only after considerable soul-searching, but it is important as a preliminary to assuming the role of supervisor.

TEACHING SUPERVISEES ABOUT THE SUPERVISORY PROCESS

Introducing the student to the supervisory process may take several forms, organizationally or individually based, between supervisor and supervisee. The approach is analogous to the first experiences students have in observing therapy. Without guidance, many students may look at live or taped clinical sessions globally, unable to identify individual behaviors or patterns of behavior, much less understand their significance. The same possibility exists for the supervisory process.

In teaching about the clinical process, various methods are used by different programs. In addition to a great amount of coursework related to normal and abnormal speech and language development, the student is introduced to the clinical process through discussion of clinical issues in academic courses, and clinical process courses (i.e., Introduction to the Clinical Process, Introduction to Therapy, Methods of Clinical Practice, and so forth). Students are gradually introduced to therapy through observation and participation prior to their first experience in supervised therapy. This is considered an important component of the educational program for all students, as substantiated by ASHA requirements.

Certain techniques are used to teach about clinical behaviors in the early observations before the student clinician enters the clinical world—joint observations, guided observations, check lists, interaction analysis systems, followed by reports and analysis of observed behaviors. Once the practicum is begun, the focus is on the clinical process in a wide variety of ways.

If students or employed professionals are to be successful as supervisees, it is just as important that they be introduced to the supervisory process in a similar manner. Munson (1983) said that supervisees have a more difficult time establishing the supervisory relationship than supervisors because supervisors have a certain power by virtue of their position (p. 118). Yet, because educational programs have not assumed responsibility for providing access to this type of study to their students and because in-service offerings on the topic are limited, there is a rather common lack of information about the process in all settings.

Tihen (1984) suggested that the interaction of expectations, satisfaction, and performance make it essential that the identification of supervisee's expectations of the supervisor become an integral part of the supervisory process. He further suggested that preparation for supervision relative to expectations should involve: (1) an identification of the student clinician's expectations, (2) determination of possible supervisor/supervisee role behaviors that may facilitate or impede the realization of expectations, (3) a process for identifying and addressing expectation discrepancies throughout the supervisory process, and (4) a determination as to whether or not expectations are realistic or unrealistic and/or productive or counterproductive.

It has been suggested (Dowling & Wittkopp, 1982; Myers, 1980; Tihen, 1984) that supervisees, particularly beginning clinicians, do not differentiate clearly between the various components of the supervisory process. This is not surprising. Supervisees who have not given much thought to the supervisory process can scarcely be expected to analyze its components and state their own needs in relation to the process in a clear manner. These and other findings point to the conclusion that instruction should be given about the supervisory process. If supervision is a joint process, as suggested repeatedly, then supervisee as well as supervisor must be prepared for the experience.

Responsibility of Supervisors

Supervisors must take the lead in this endeavor. Although the stated goal of supervision is to create a self-supervising clinician through joint problem solving in which the supervisee plays a collaborative role with the supervisor, the supervisor still has the responsibility for setting the stage and directing the supervisory interaction. As the person who is responsible, and presumably more knowledgeable, about supervision, the supervisor will be accountable for preparing the supervisee to participate. In discussing the colleagueship relationship of the clinical supervision model, Cogan (1973) maintained that the supervisor is responsible for structuring the framework of discussion but not the total content of the interaction. Supervisors must get the study of the process started while still making it clear that the supervisee has equal responsibility in the relationship.

Such an approach to supervision requires a certain amount and type of information on the part of the supervisor. The remainder of this book will discuss the components of supervision from one point of view—the reader is reminded that there are also others (Acheson & Gall, 1980; Carraciola et al., 1978a; Cogan, 1973; Dussault, 1970; Goldhammer et al., 1980; Harris, 1975; Mosher & Purpel, 1972; Oratio, 1977; Rassi, 1978).

Introducing the Supervisory Process

Responsibility for this phase of supervision may be assumed by the organization or by individual supervisors. Organizational responsibility is evidenced in a variety of ways. Some educational programs include academic study of the supervisory process in connection with the study of the clinical process. It is considered to be another level of the clinical process and there is discussion of the objectives of supervision, the role of the supervisor and supervisee, and the components of the process. This activity will be discussed further in the chapter on preparation.

In the employment setting, this same introductory component is appropriate, though perhaps at a different level. Understanding of mutual needs and expectations is important at all stages. Cogan (1973) considered this preparation so important that he recommended introduction of his clinical supervision approach in the schools through workshops for all teachers at the beginning of the year. Tanck (1980) demonstrated that the clinical supervision model can be incorporated into a school system through in-service offerings and an administrative structure that supports it.

Although some educational programs provide such an introduction to the supervisory process, probably more do not. Whether the process is treated in coursework or workshops or not at all, *each supervisor should take time at the beginning and throughout each interaction* to talk about supervision as the situation dictates. Topics for discussion at the beginning of the experience might include any of the following and not necessarily in the order given:

1. Components of the supervisory process. This discussion will reflect a content approach to supervision based on the components in this book or on some other approach. It should include not only supervisors' philosophies about supervision but should allow for some input from supervisees about their general impressions of the supervisory process.

2. Perceptions of supervisees about supervision. Information about perceptions of roles are shared here. Supervisors will want to know what

supervisees' role expectations are for them. They need to know if supervisees think that supervisors are there to provide all information or if they see supervisors as authority figures only. They need to know if supervisors' role is perceived as that of evaluator—someone to tell them what they did right or wrong, point out their weaknesses, and then tell them the "right" way to do it again. They need to know if supervisors are perceived as helpers, teachers, counselors; and, if so, what these titles mean to supervisees.

Supervisees' perceptions of their own roles must also be discussed. Do they perceive themselves as passive participants in the process? As helpless pawns? Do they have insight about their responsibilities in problem solving? Can they verbalize about the supervisory process as differentiated from the clinical process? Do they have confidence in their own ability to make decisions about objectives for clients and methods for reaching those objectives? Do they have major anxieties to be diffused?

3. Goals and objectives for supervision. The setting of specific goals and objectives for the supervisory process will be studied in the chapter on planning. At this stage, supervisees need to know that there are goals to be set, not just for clients, but for themselves as supervisees and clinicians, and that goals are also set for supervisors.

4. Prior experiences in supervision. Supervisors and supervisees need to discuss supervisees' past experiences in supervision, the types of interactions they have had with supervisors, their feelings about supervision, and what they have learned about the process.

5. Preferences for supervisory styles. Supervisors will want to know if supervisees can differentiate supervisor behaviors. They need to discuss with supervisees their preferences for styles of supervisory behavior and their reasons for these preferences. They must also discuss the consequences of the preferred style, as related to supervisees' places on the continuum. The kind of feedback they prefer should also be discussed and analyzed for appropriateness. If the views of supervisors about supervision and the expectations of supervisees are not congruent, they need to be resolved at this point.

6. Dealing with anxieties. One major task of supervisors here, especially with an inexperienced clinician or one who is working with a new type of client, is to deal with supervisees' anxieties and uncertainties about the interaction they are about to begin (Cogan, 1973). Identifying anxieties and discussing their source may be enough to diffuse them adequately. For others this will be a longer process of support and positive interactions.

7. The continuum of supervision. This discussion begins to blend in to the planning stage as supervisors introduce the concept of the continuum and the appropriate style of supervision for each place on the continuum, based on supervisee needs, expectations, experience, and the situation. The identification of the location of each supervisee on the continuum is a part of the planning process.

Notice that discussion of the client has not yet been suggested. This is appropriate since this is the time for the supervisee to become aware of his or her own feelings and to share expectations with the supervisor. Once the relationship is established, then supervisor and supervisee can move on to the more traditional planning for the client, as well as for clinician, supervisee, and supervisor.

Operationalizing the Discussion

The discussion described previously may be elicited and enhanced in a variety of ways. The supervisor first must be a good listener. Scattered throughout the literature on expectations of supervisees are several references to the supervisee wanting the supervisor to listen and to take seriously what they say (Larson, 1982; Russell, 1976; Tihen, 1984). The fact that this is stated at all is significant. Have supervisors communicated to supervisees that they are not taking supervisees seriously? That they do not respect their ideas and abilities? The supervisor who takes the time to *hear* what the supervisee expresses about needs and expectations and anxieties will learn some valuable information and probably enhance the relationship immeasurably.

At this point, good communication and interpersonal skills are vital. Acceptance and regard for the supervisee's ideas and feelings are paramount. Good questioning techniques are important. Modeling of a communication style may be of more significance here than what is actually said. Supervisors who proclaim that supervision is a joint problem-solving process or who state their wish to have supervisees involved must show at this initial point that they are willing to listen and accept the supervisee's exploration of ideas and must encourage them if they are not forthcoming. Supervisors cannot afford to play the "Do as as I say, not as I do" game. Responses, both verbal and nonverbal, must be monitored carefully to avoid these behaviors.

Supervisors may wish to give students some reading material about the supervisory process. Dowling (1979b, 1982) has written articles specifically for students, as have Shapiro (1985) and Bernthal & Beukelman (1975).

Getting accurate statements of how supervisees feel at this point may be difficult. They may not know how to express their ideas. The supervisor or the total situation may be so threatening that supervisees' reactions will be inhibited. The supervisor may not be able to resist loaded questions in which the expected answer is obvious. It is sometimes gratifying or easier to hear what one wishes to hear, but it is also not very productive in the effort to learn supervisees' real feelings. Also, supervisees may have learned from the "grape-vine" what each supervisor likes or expects and may play their own little game of "Please the Supervisor—Tell Her What She Wants to Hear." The skill and sensitivity of supervisors in asking questions determines much of the outcome here.

Others may wish to use all or portions of the questionnaires used in Larson's study (1981) as a basis for discussion (Appendix A). A scale developed and validated by Powell (1985) to measure attitudes toward the clinical supervision model of Cogan (1973) could also be used at this stage to learn more about the supervisee's ideas about supervision, thus forming a basis for discussion (Appendix B). Indeed, supervisors who have not yet worked out their own personal beliefs about the supervisory process might also find it useful. The Individual Conference Rating Scale (ICRS) developed by Smith (1978) may also be used to obtain specific information about supervisees' perceptions of individual conferences (Appendix C).

One supervisor known by the writer asks students at the beginning of their interaction to write an informal statement of their feelings at this time about the impending experience. This may be difficult for some students but, as presented by this supervisor, it works well and provides a good basis for future discussion.

Supervisees at this stage frequently need help to see supervision as a larger issue than "What do I do with the client?" One supervisor reported an interesting experience relevant to this point. As she presented to the supervisee the concept of setting objectives for herself as clinician and as supervisee a look of insight flooded the supervisee's face and she said, "I didn't know supervision was for *me*. I thought it was just for the *client*!" It must be added that this was a very capable student who had already had considerable clinical and supervisory experience. Further proof of the fact that the focus is on the client?

Information from supervisors about what to expect from the situation is helpful in allaying anxieties of supervisees. More of this will be discussed in the planning section, but supervisees deserve to know the organizational requirements, as well as those of the individual supervisor, the format under which they will be operating, and the criteria for success in each experience.

ONGOING INTERPRETATION OF THE PROCESS

Once a foundation has been laid for understanding of the process, further discussion can be maintained as the interaction continues. Perceptions must be checked to see that needs are being met as the process develops. Questions posed at the beginning of the interaction may be equally relevant at a later time.

Smith and Anderson (1982b) found that perceptions of effectiveness of conferences varied, depending upon the rater, and stated, "This result suggests that supervisors and supervisees should keep their self-perceptions of the conference at a conscious level, investigating them at frequent intervals to determine if their perceptions are similar. A lack of information regarding the convergence or divergence of perceptions of those involved in conference interactions, if allowed to exist over time, may greatly diminish the effectiveness of the conference" (p. 258).

Much of this ongoing procedure is related to the planning which is discussed in the next chapter. Once objectives have been set for the clinician/supervisee they must be assessed frequently to see if they are being met, and revised if necessary. More than that, however, the supervisee and supervisor must be sure that their perceptions are matching. Attitudes and insights, as well as needs, *do* change.

SUMMARY

The foundation of a productive supervisory relationship is a basic understanding of the supervisory process and effective communication between supervisor and supervisee about philosophies, expectations, perceptions, and objectives. This is more than merely an introduction to the process; it requires ongoing discussion about the continuing interaction.

Planning the Supervisory Process

The planning conference sets the stage for effective communication.

Acheson and Gall (1980, p. 42)

Planning in one form or another has long been a major task of professionals in speech-language pathology and audiology. The main thrust appears to have been planning for the client. However, reflection upon the complexity of the needs and expectations of the clinician/supervisee leads to the conclusion that, if all participants in the supervisory process are to grow and develop professionally, clinical teaching cannot take place haphazardly or spontaneously. Every facet of it must be planned.

FOUR-FOLD PLANNING

Professional growth for all participants comes as a result of careful, systematic four-fold planning: (1) for the client, (2) for the clinician, (3) for the supervisee, and (4) for the supervisor. In other words, it is not enough to plan the clinical process, the process through which the client learns; the supervisory process, through which the supervisee and supervisor learn, must also be planned if maximum growth is to be achieved. This concept is supported in two of the ASHA tasks for supervisors (ASHA, 1985b): Task 2—Assisting the supervisee in developing clinical goals and objectives (p. 58) and Task 8—Interacting with the supervisee in planning, executing, and analyzing supervisory conferences (p. 59). (Program planning will also be the responsibility of many supervisors and supervisees, but only the planning of clinical teaching will be treated here.)

Four-fold planning must be seen as the very foundation of the on-going supervisory process. All future action in the process and its evaluation are based on what is done during the planning component. All activities for all participants are planned—not only clinical activities but also observation, data collection, methods of analysis, participation in conferences, self-analysis, and evaluation. Planning, then, is a continuous process from the first interaction between supervisor and supervisee to the last. It is always integrated with data collection and analysis. Predictions are made on the basis of the data about what will or will not work; the accuracy of these predictions will form the basis for further planning with each set of plans coming out of the data from previously planned activities. Furthermore, this component is considered necessary in all settings where supervision takes place—clinics in educational programs, off-campus practicum sites, and service delivery settings—although the procedures may differ.

IMPORTANCE OF PLANNING

There is little definitive literature in speech-language pathology and audiology to verify the importance of planning, although it has been discussed frequently, often in general terms and mainly in relation to the client (Irwin et al., 1961; Kleffner, 1964; Knight, Hahn, Ervin, & McIsaac, 1961; Miner, 1967). Villareal (1964), in discussing the importance of lesson plans in educational programs, suggested a three-phase sequence in which the supervisor demonstrates during the initial phase, the student and supervisor plan together the patient's clinical program in a second phase, followed by a final phase in which the student assumes primary responsibility for planning and management of the patient's clinical program. This method is perhaps closer to the supervision style used in the Evaluation-Feedback Stage than it is to the Collaborative or Consultative Style of supervision. Too much demonstration at an early point in the practicum may create supervisee dependence, encourage clinicians to become "clones," and set supervisors in the superior role and supervisees in the subordinate role. Once established, these roles are difficult to alter.

Van Riper's (1965) view of planning in the educational program also is client-centered and places final approval with the supervisor. The first responsibility of the supervisor, he said, is to review the client's needs with the student. The student comes to the conference with a plan and then a series of transitional goals for the client are outlined. The plan is discussed and revisions made; the student then submits the revised plan, which he or she is expected to follow. Students are told that they can spend some time in exploration with the client, although further revisions in the plan may be made only after consultation with the supervisor.

Prather (1967) proposed that one of the best supervision tools is the lesson plan for the client where each procedure is evaluated individually. Subsequent planning of therapy then utilizes the data about the past procedures. Schubert (1978) devoted an entire chapter to lesson plans in which he said, "The lesson plan maps out the future work for the clinician and the supervisor" (p. 14). The importance of planning for children's needs and establishing goals for therapy in the supervised school practicum has been discussed also by Flower (1969), Kirtley (1967), Monnin and Peters (1981), and Rees and Smith (1967, 1968).

In actuality, there is very little choice about whether or not to plan for clients (Flower, 1984). 'Not only is it good professional practice to clarify therapy plans as specifically as possible, this clear delineation is an almost universal requirement in any setting where regulations of governmental agencies, accreditation agencies, or third-party payers apply—which is to say, virtually all settings in which speech-language pathology and audiology services are delivered" (p. 105).

This brief review of literature on planning in speech-language pathology and audiology further confirms that the focus has been on the client—not the clinician, supervisee, or supervisor. Certain concepts about planning as a part of the clinical supervision model as defined in education are more relevant to the approach urged in this book and supported by the ASHA tasks quoted earlier in this chapter.

Cogan (1973) talked of joint lesson planning for the teacher and takes a long-range view of planning in which the daily lesson plan is only one element of a continuum of planning. He believes that the daily plan produces episodic, discontinuous supervision and prefers to take a long view while at the same time checking to see that the daily lesson is "in tune" with the larger objectives. Planning for supervision of teachers was presented by Goldhammer and colleagues (1980) as the preobservation conference. They stressed the importance of mutual understanding of the plans and how each participant is to function. This collaborative phase of the process includes goal setting, developing rationales for instruction, and deciding upon instructional methods with an emphasis on teacher behavior.

Planning was so important to Acheson and Gall (1980) that they differentiated between planning conferences and feedback conferences. The planning conference, the first phase of supervision in Acheson and Gall's framework, includes (1) identifying the teacher's concerns about instruction, (2) translating these concerns into observable behaviors, (3) identifying procedures for improving instruction, (4) assisting the teacher in setting self-improvement goals, and (5) arranging the details of the observation (time, observational instruments, behaviors to be recorded, context in which behaviors will be recorded). Although Cogan (1973), Goldhammer and colleagues (1980), and Acheson and Gall (1980) referred to the supervision of teachers who are working in the schools, it will be shown that the ideas are also applicable in speech-language pathology and audiology.

As with so many features of preparation and service delivery in speech-language pathology and audiology, the value of planning has not been validated; rather, it has been assumed that it is important and professionals have developed their own methodologies or assumed those of the institutions in which they work. In reality, there are no data to support existing practices in planning, nor what should be done, despite the requirements cited by Flower (1984). Descriptive data on conferences in speech-language pathology and audiology relevant to planning suggest strongly that so much time is spent on discussion of client behavior in past sessions that little time is left for planning other than for the supervisor to provide the strategies based on the raw data provided by supervisees (Culatta & Seltzer, 1976, 1977; Roberts & Smith, 1982; Tufts, 1984). Supervisors and supervisees probably operate across the spectrum in terms of planning—from detailed scripts in some cases to brief notes, verbal discussion, or to incorporating plans in other record keeping (Flower, 1984) for what will be done subsequently. However, it does not seem debatable that some planning is necessary.

PERCEPTIONS ABOUT PLANNING

Although there are no validation data on planning, there is some literature documenting perceptions about the extent of planning and its value. Two studies have indicated differences in perceptions between supervisors and supervisees about planning. In a survey of participants in school practicum, 88 percent of supervisors ranked the preparation of lesson plans as a highly important activity whereas only 60 percent of their students indicated that their lesson plans were checked and returned by supervising clinicians (Anderson & Milisen, 1965). Culatta and colleagues (1975) reported similar discrepancies between supervisors and students. Sixty-one percent of their supervisors reported that they assigned lesson plans as a major part of preparation for therapy whereas only 44 percent of students recalled that such plans were required. Further, although supervisors complained that students were "too tied to their lesson plans" and not flexible enough in therapy, supervisees reported, contrary to the descriptive data on conferences, that most of their time with supervisors was spent in detailed structuring of lesson plans. Culatta and colleagues then asked some important questions: Is this perceived extensive attention to planning simply the provision of strategies by the supervisors, as reported by the authors? Does it imply to trainees that they should not deviate from those suggestions? Does it imply that they use only the supervisors' suggestions in their plans? Other questions might be asked: Through the process of structuring the plans with the supervisor were the plans so exclusively the product of the supervisor's thinking that the supervisee's learning was stifled and his "ownership" of the plan so negated that he was unable to deviate from the plan? Or was it his perception that he *should not* deviate from what had so generously been provided by the supervisor?

Although the earlier literature talked about *lesson plans*, there has been a recent trend toward other types of planning as shown by Peaper and Wener (1984), who have collected the most extensive data in speech-language pathology about the frequency and perceived value of various types of planning required in educational programs and professional settings. Administering a 55-item questionnaire to 219 clinical supervisors, students, and working professionals, they found that, although 93.7 percent of the students and 80.6 percent of the clinical supervisors reported written lesson plans were required in practicum, only 21.9 percent of the working professionals indicated that they were required in their work settings. Respondents from work settings reported a higher percentage of use of long-term goals or Individual Education Plans (IEPs) than those in educational programs. IEPs were used by all professionals working in schools. Therapy logs were used most frequently in hospitals and rehabilitation centers, with 100 percent of the respondents from those settings indicating they used logs along with long-term goals (87.5 percent) and lesson plans (12 percent).

Peaper and Wener questioned "the value of the considerable time spent in training programs on the lesson plan which is required in only 21.9 percent of professional settings," which "suggests that training programs should direct their efforts more strongly toward the long-term goals process which is more commonly required in professional settings (97.6 percent)" (p. 38). However, respondents in their study strongly indicated a belief that all types of pretherapy planning should be included in educational programs. Students agreed that long-term goals provide direction in the total therapy process and that lesson plans help provide order and direction to daily therapy, although respondents did not perceive that a new lesson plan is necessary for each session. Supervisors strongly agreed with the need to require written long-term goals for each client throughout the practicum experience. Although working professionals perceived written long-term goals to be essential, they also believed that therapy logs are valuable because they provide a basis for therapy progress reports. All groups rejected the use of commercial programs, projected treatment plans, or IEPs as a *substitute* for written lesson plans. Only the presession conference with the supervisor appeared to be an acceptable substitute for such plans. Working professionals, although they reported a low use of written lesson plans for themselves, seemed to view them as a necessary part of the practicum experience. Students and supervisors did not share this view. Working professionals also supported the requirement of therapy logs throughout the practicum.

An interesting finding was that students with the least experience (under 100 hours) did not agree as strongly as more experienced students that a presession conference to discuss goals and procedures was an acceptable substitute for a written lesson plan. Peaper and Wener suggested that this may indicate a recognition of the need to develop written planning skills or a reluctance to propose goals and procedures on a face-to-face basis with the supervisor in a limited conference time. The latter seems a viable hypothesis given the previous discussion of anxiety. It may also be that less-experienced supervisees feel the need for more time to "get their act together" even though they complain about the amount of time spent on lesson plans.

In summarizing these and other data from the study, Peaper and Wener speculated that the results indicate that all types of written planning need to be included in the preparation process, especially written long-term goals, and they suggested an alternative to daily lesson planning: first-year students might be required to write fairly detailed weekly lesson plans to develop skills in identifying short-term goals and accompanying procedures. Second-year students might eliminate the weekly lesson plan after the projected treatment plan has been submitted, with a brief lesson plan being required if goals and procedures are revised. Based on the continuum proposed here, it seems more appropriate to base planning requirements on the individual competencies of supervisees and their place on the continuum. Emphasis should also be placed on projected treatment plans and therapy logs with special attention to writing long-term goals, since so many professional settings require them. Despite what has seemed to be a recent trend toward the writing of long-term programs, this study seems to reflect the opinion held by many supervisors in educational programs, that the detailed writing of lesson plans is a necessary phase of the preparation of students for the future planning they will need to do—a "good experience." If, however, other types of planning are used in service delivery settings, does the emphasis on detailed plans revealed here neglect the preparation of students for other types of planning?

Because this study identified only perceptions of various groups about planning, there are still many unanswered questions. Why are professionals so sure that writing lesson plans in the educational program is important? How can those perceptions be validated? How well were these professionals prepared for any other planning method? Do they support the requirements for plans because this was a part of their preparation and they are comfortable with it? Or could they, if asked, really identify the benefits that have carried over into their own jobs, even though they are now doing a very different type of planning? As with so much of the literature on supervision, this study was dependent upon perceptions and the real effect of the extensive time and effort put into written lesson plans during the educational program is still not known.

PLANNING AS A JOINT PROCESS

The principle that all direction and input in the supervisory process should not come from the supervisor is tested most rigorously in the planning stage. Planning begins as soon as the supervisor, presumably the more knowedgeable of the dyad, has introduced the supervisee to the supervisory process or has provided the opportunity for discussion of the process, as presented in the preceding chapter. The supervisor is responsible for operationalizing the planning process and for involving the supervisee at whatever level of the continuum she or he is able to participate. In addition, it is the major responsibility of the supervisor to help the supervisee increase the amount of participation in planning over time, commensurate with the supervisee's capabilities. The planning component is particularly important in encouraging and assisting supervisees to develop a willingness to participate and to gain a sense of "ownership" of this endeavor in which they are engaged. Most supervisory programs are ineffective because the design of the program does not involve supervisees; therefore, they are not committed to it because it is the supervisor's program, not theirs (Champagne & Morgan, 1978). Perhaps this is what makes supervisees ask their supervisors, "Is this what you want me to do?" Planning, then, should be approached as a joint effort by supervisor and supervisee to determine what is best for the client and for themselves to ensure professional growth.

The early part of the planning component is the place to begin avoiding situations that encourage supervisees' dependence upon the supervisor. It is a time for encouraging and accepting supervisees' ideas, being sensitive to their feelings of insecurity and threat, and fostering their sense of responsibility. Here, as in the previous component, is another place where the supervisor models the communication style that will probably become the standard for subsequent interactions.

Perhaps the *process* is equally, if not more, important than the product at this point. The way in which the planning is carried out lets supervisees know that supervisors really mean it when they talk about supervisees' participation, that supervisors are really planning *with* supervisees, not *for* them (Cogan, 1973). It is a time when supervisors can demonstrate to their supervisees that it *is* possible for them to hold back in the conference and *allow* supervisees to problem-solve and participate.

ASSESSMENT OF SUPERVISEES

References have been made elsewhere to analogies between the clinical and supervisory processes, but nowhere is that analogy clearer than it is in this early stage, which might be thought of as the assessment phase of supervision. Speech-language pathologists and audiologists have been prepared to respect the essential role of thorough assessment in planning treatment procedures that will meet the individual needs of every client. Why, then, when they become supervisors, do they neglect to apply the same principle of assessment to supervisees and assume that one style of supervision can meet the needs of all supervisees?

Part of the planning process, basic to the successful implementation of the supervisory methodology presented here, is the accurate determination of the point on the continuum at which supervisees are capable of functioning and the appropriate supervisory style to be used for each point. Several issues need to be resolved in making this determination:

■ The supervisee's ability to problem-solve
■ The degree of dependency/independency of the supervisee as clinician *and* supervisee
■ The ability of the supervisee to self-observe and self-analyze
■ The supervisor's flexibility in adapting his or her style to supervisee levels

Four-fold planning cannot be accomplished until these issues are resolved. Only then can the supervisor and supervisee break away from the traditional patterns revealed in the data and place themselves properly on the continuum.

This thrust adds a new dimension to what is probably the traditional procedure where the supervisor spends some time at the beginning of the interaction obtaining information about the *clinical* experience of the supervisee. This new dimension makes it necessary for the supervisor to learn what kinds of supervisory experiences the supervisee has had. Discussed also in the previous chapter as a part of the Understanding the Supervisory Process component, it must be recognized that the features of that component may overlap with the Planning component. Some distinction may be made between the two if the first component is thought of as one where information is gathered about perceptions and attitudes; the second component is where actual skills as clinicians *and as supervisees* are identified.

Rockman (1977) supported an assessment approach to the supervisory process when she pointed out the parallels between the clinical and the supervisory processes and emphasized the importance of the assessment of the clinical skills of the supervisee prior to the beginning of the treatment program or supervision. "The most fundamental area in which to begin the comparison between clinician and supervisor is that of initial assessment or diagnostic evaluation. Just as the clinician does not begin a treatment program without an overview of the client's behavior, the supervisory process should be preceded by the supervisor's 'evaluation' or 'assessment' of the students assigned for supervision. The supervisor engages in a diagnostic-like process for each assigned clinician examining the background, experience, and skills that the student clinician brings to the situation" (pp. 2–3).

Rockman continued on to say that the supervisor must rely here on questionnaires, personal interview, and direct observation for this entry level evaluation. She suggested "exploration of academic background, prior clinical experiences, personal experiences, and work history" (p. 3) and stressed the importance of early observation in obtaining information about basic clinical skills. Although directed mainly toward clinical skills, the procedure can be extended to obtain information about the individual as supervisee.

Obtaining Information About Supervisees

Assuming that the supervisor and supervisee have engaged in some preliminary discussion of the supervisory process, then each supervisory interaction will begin with an assessment procedure, as does every clinical interaction.

The following outline is a brief overview, certainly not exhaustive, of information needed *before* the point on the continuum can be determined. Some supervisors will want to explore further in certain situations. As soon as this information is collected, planning can begin.

1. Clinician Information
   a. General clinical experience
   b. Experience with clients with the disorder
   c. Academic background in disorder area
   d. Other experiences relevant to the client or the disorder
   e. Clinician's perception of strengths and needs in terms of the client
   f. Anxieties about this client or disorder
   g. Understanding of the needs of the client
2. Supervisee Information
   a. Type(s) of supervisory interaction experienced previously
   b. Perception of self in terms of dependence/independence in general and with this client
   c. Prior responsibility in data collection and analysis of client behavior
   d. Experience in data collection and analysis of own clinical behavior prior to conferences
   e. Perceptions of responsibility for bringing data and questions to the conference, assisting in problem solving, and decision making
   f. Expectations for learning or modification of clinical skills from the current situation

    g. Perception of need for feedback (amount and type)

3. Supervisor Information

    a. Clinical and supervisory experience (general)

    b. Experience with this type of disorder or client

    c. Theoretical and practical approach to the disorder as compared to that of the supervisee

    d. Preferred or customary supervisory style

    e. Expectations for the supervisee as a clinician and as a supervisee

    f. Expectations for the supervisory interaction

    g. Self-perception of role

Determining Dependence/Independence

Shriberg and colleagues (1974, 1975) have provided a valuable instrument for use at this point. Over a period of several years, Shriberg and several members of the clinical staff at the University of Wisconsin-Madison developed and validated the *Wisconsin Procedure for Appraisal of Clinical Competence* (W-PACC) (Appendix D). This appraisal form will be discussed later under the topic of evaluation, but it is relevant here because of its basic approach. Rather than using client or clinician change as the criterion for effectiveness, this instrument "appraises the extent to which effectiveness is dependent upon continued supervisory input" (1975, p. 160). The instrument provides for clinicians to be designated as operating at one of four levels at the beginning of the supervisory interaction, which might be different in every setting. The criteria for assigning levels, as suggested by Shriberg and colleagues, are hours of experience, number of clients, experience with the disorder area or management approach, and the supervisor's judgment of the supervisee's academic preparation. Although these items are more related to the clinical process than to the items just suggested for the supervisory assessment, the part of the W-PACC relevant to diagnosing the needs or skills of supervisees is the scale used to identify the level of dependence or independence of the supervisee. The scale consists of the following levels of scoring: Score 1—Specific direction from supervisor does not alter unsatisfactory performance and inability to make changes, Scores 2–3–4—Needs specific direction and/or demonstration from supervisor to perform effectively, Scores 5–6–7—Needs general direction from supervisor to perform effectively; and Scores 8–9–10—Demonstrates independence by taking initiative, makes changes when appropriate, and is effective. Each of the 10 Interpersonal Skills and the 28 Professional-Technical Skills that make up the instrument is scored according to this scale.

The listed skills are mainly directed toward the clinician/client interaction but a few are related to the action of the clinician-as-supervisee, for example, Item 6—Listens, asks questions, participates with supervisor in therapy and/or client-related discussions; is not defensive, and Item 7—Requests assistance from supervisor and/or other professionals when appropriate.

This instrument is of value in several ways. It can be used as a diagnostic tool to determine level of dependency. It can be used by supervisees as a self-appraisal of their perception of their own independence and as a means to define their own goals. It can be used by the supervisor and supervisee together, in total or in parts, for the same purpose. The scoring method is appropriate for other items more closely related to the supervisor/supervisee interaction, for example, ability to analyze and report data in the conference. Furthermore, if all supervisors in an organization used this instrument, and could maintain agreement, appraisals from previous semesters could provide a ready basis for determining the stage of dependence/independence. Conceivably, the continued use of this instrument could help both supervisors and supervisees to focus on the general goal of clinician/supervisee independence rather than on individual client behavior. This focus is basic to progress along the continuum of supervision and it must be done with self-knowledge of the clinician. The W-PACC authors have made an invaluable contribution to speech-language pathology and audiology with this instrument, which should be included in the armamentarium of every supervisor, especially in terms of the dependency/independency variable.

COMPETENCIES FOR PLANNING

Clinical competencies specific to planning for the client are not new to speech-language pathologists and audiologists. These competencies have always been a part of the many different evaluation forms used in training programs and service delivery settings. It has also been assumed that teaching those skills and evaluating them is the job of the supervisor.

For example, of the four subdomains that make up the Professional-Technical Skills in the W-PACC, Shriberg and colleagues (1975) included one that deals with planning, entitled Developing and Planning—the Approach to the Task. In this subdomain, they itemized eight skills to be appraised which are related to planning by the clinician for the clinical process (See Appendix D).

Other evaluation instruments include planning competencies. The Pennsylvania State Evaluation Form (Klevans & Volz, 1974) covers planning with the following items: ability to establish appropriate goals, ability to develop lesson plans, and ingenuity in developing original techniques and materials. Dopheide, Thornton, and McCready (1984) validated a clinical practicum evaluation form which contains a component entitled *Planning Skills*: (1) utilizes professional literature and resources in a critical manner, (2) for each session develops sequenced objectives based on client's long-range goals, current levels of performance, and functional communication needs, (3) prepares and utilizes setting to meet needs of client and others, and (4) plans and utilizes appropriate assessment measures and behavioral probes throughout the remedial process.

All supervisors could reach into their files and find one or more such evaluation checklists that include planning competencies for clinicians, and probably more written evaluations than not would discuss such competencies. In summary, then, planning for the client is a clinician competency, the development of which has been seen traditionally as the responsibility of the supervisor.

IMPLEMENTING THE PLANNING COMPONENT

Supervisors must orchestrate all the various aspects of the four-fold planning in collaboration with the supervisee. The four-fold planning expands that basic responsibility to a shared responsibility between supervisor and supervisee to plan for all participants. Methodologies for planning for each will be discussed in this section. Because planning for the client is discussed first, each method will be treated with somewhat greater detail in that section than in following discussions. It should be remembered, however, that any method described for clients can also be applied to planning for other participants. Planning for them should be perceived as an extension of planning for the client. For example, behavioral objectives should be set for *all* participants. Written plans, programs, or contracts should include planning for more than the client.

Planning Strategies

Planning strategies have evolved over the years into several types which vary depending upon site, supervisor, and supervisee—long- and short-term objectives, written lesson plans, presession conferences, contracts, patient records, IEP, programs, logs, and others.

Influence of Behavioral Objectives Movement

Whatever the format, it does seem that nearly all planning has been strongly influenced by a movement which has come from business management, education, and psychology—the setting of behavioral objectives. "A behavioral objective is any educational objective which is stated in terms of behaviors which can be observed and measured" (Mowrer, 1977, p. 146). This approach has been treated generously in the literature in several fields, particularly education, where the value of setting behavioral objectives has been stressed repeatedly (Baker & Popham, 1973; Mager, 1962, 1972; Mager & Pipe, 1970; Popham & Baker, 1970). Mowrer (1977) stated that the behavioral objectives movement "has touched almost every speech clinician" (p. 148).

Such objectives have become standard in planning for clients in speech-language pathology and audiology. Although the principles are often included in clinical coursework, supervisors are usually responsible for implementing their use. Andrews (1971) described their importance to the student in clinical practicum, not only in measuring progress, but in learning to rely on something other than intuition and subjective impression. "Among the advantages," he said, "are that both the student and the supervisor know exactly the purpose of each therapy session and whether or not the purpose has been accomplished" (p. 387). Dublinske (1970), and Dublinske and Grimes (1979), have written about setting behavioral objectives in school programs, as has Healey (1982). Though written about the schools, the basic principles apply in other settings.

It has been assumed that there are advantages in using behavioral objectives—that it makes the session more conducive to learning, that the therapy session is more focused, that it is necessary to state objectives for therapy sessions so that change can be documented and measured and results evaluated, and that it makes it easier to establish appropriate procedures and devise materials for use in therapy sessions.

On a practical level, behavioral objectives keep clinicians directed toward what is to be taught rather than first planning an activity and making what is to be learned fit the activity. It puts the cart and the horse in the correct sequence. If clinicians are unsure of what is to be learned and how to achieve it, writing it in a behavioral objective often helps to clarify it in their minds.

Because the principles and procedures of preparing behavioral objectives have been a part of the clinical education of most supervisors and because the process is discussed so thoroughly and so well in many other publications, the reader who feels the need for further study of this area is referred to the cited materials and the topic will not be given more space here. It will be assumed, however, that the knowledge of how to set behavioral objectives is basic to all planning and that it will be incorporated into all phases of the four-fold planning.

Written Plans

Traditionally, supervisors in speech-language pathology and audiology have worked on the assumption that written plans are important, indeed necessary, for the adequate preparation of students and for appropriately meeting the needs of clients (Peaper & Wener, 1984). Requirements, format, and criteria for such plans have largely been determined by individual supervisors or the organization in which they work, and usually consist of certain categories: objectives, procedures, materials, and assessment.

These written plans frequently become ordeals for the student, sometimes requiring much more time in their preparation than in their execution. After laborious efforts and much time spent writing what they seriously hope will be appropriate objectives and devising procedures and materials to be used to meet those objectives, the plans are usually submitted to supervisors who may make constructive suggestions or who may "mutilate" the plan with red pencil, frequently creating a devastating reaction in the clinician. Some clinicians, after becoming conditioned to supervisor's red pencils, may subsequently begin to write cursory plans because "My supervisor is going to change it anyway." This may be the first point at which the supervisor's "square box" (Figure 4–3) becomes apparent and it may set the tone for future interactions. Certainly no supervisor behavior is more direct than a written note suggesting a different procedure than the one in the supervisee's plan. The appropriateness of such directness is, of course, determined by the place of the supervisee on the continuum. Supervisors should be aware, at a conscious level, of the impact of their choice of feedback on a written plan.

Monitoring and alteration of plans by supervisors are considered by most who use them to be essential to ensure learning by students and clients. Comments by the supervisor may help students to use time more efficiently or to avoid pursuing inappropriate objectives or nonproductive and negative experiences. Such comments may also deprive clinicians of using their own initiative and prevent them from learning through their mistakes. This also assumes, of course, that supervisors have all the skills and information necessary to make such judgments appropriately in every situation. If supervisors do not have these skills or are working from a base of inappropriate perception, their alterations of the plan may make the session no better than it would have been with the original plan. Furthermore, the supervisee will not have had the dubious pleasure of learning through trial and error. Further, if the clinical procedures suggested by the supervisor do not work, the clinician can place the responsibility for the failure on the supervisor's shoulders, a practice not conducive to learning or to the appropriate acceptance of responsibility.

Conversely, the constant responsibility of monitoring individual lesson plans can become a chore to supervisors and may result in cursory attention and stereotyped suggestions. Small wonder, if these negative experiences are regular or frequent occurrences in the educational program, that clinicians develop negative attitudes toward planning which may carry over into the work setting, leading them sometimes to work without adequate planning. Cogan (1973) indicated that teachers sometimes claim that lesson plans are a waste of time, but that "in actual practice, it turns out that a sizable percentage of the teachers who deprecate the written plan actually work from an unwritten plan, often well rehearsed through frequent use" (pp. 110–111). This is not an unknown phenomenon in speech-language pathology and audiology!

The practice of clinicians writing plans that are revised and altered by supervisors also does not encourage the joint participation advocated for all phases of the supervisory process. A more desirable approach would be to allow time for joint planning during the conference where there is input from both supervisor and supervisee based on data collected in previous therapy sessions and analyzed by either or both of the participants. This approach was supported by Peaper and Wener (1984). Verbal planning can be formalized into a written plan if it is needed for the clinician's guidance during the next session. Verbal planning also provides the foundation for the observation and analysis phases. At some point on the continuum it may also lead to the setting of long- and short-term objectives or to the use of other methods instead of a detailed written plan.

Contracts

Joint discussion and joint planning lend themselves to another form of written plan—contracts, which are mentioned frequently in the literature on supervision in other professions. Goldhammer and colleagues (1980) stressed the importance of agreement between supervisor and supervisee on the plans that have been discussed in the preobservation conference and suggested that a supervisory contract is a good way to reach such agreement, assuming that both are willing to modify the contract at a later time if it should become necessary. "In other words," they said, "after certain rules have been decided upon—'This is what you will do, this is what I will do, and here's why' (the contract)" (p. 35), those rules should not be changed in the middle of the game except by mutual agreement and with mutual understanding. The contract, as they perceive it, is an agreement between the teacher and the supervisor which includes the objectives of the lesson and their relationship to the overall learning program, activities to be observed, possible changes to which supervisor and supervisee may agree, feedback desired by the teacher, and methods of evaluation. The contract may be for a specific lesson or a long-term agreement covering a specific period of time. This type of contract can easily be modified to include planning the other three aspects of the four-fold planning.

Contracts based upon goals are termed a powerful tool for supervision in social work by Fox (1983). The contract is an agreement between supervisor and supervisee that includes "purpose, targets issues, clarifies goals and objectives, states procedures and constraints, identifies participant's roles, describes techniques and sets limitations on time. Incorporated directly into the supervisory process, goal oriented contract supervision promotes genuine collaboration in exploring needs and identifying goals between the supervisor and worker" (pp. 37–38). It is performance oriented, and goes beyond "tell me what to do" to mobilize the resources of the worker in self-directed activity, and enlists the worker's cooperation in identifying and determining to a significant degree the shape of supervision. "Furthermore, the goal oriented contract for supervision provides a concrete and objective means for measuring and documenting progress and performance" (p. 37).

One study in speech-language pathology has addressed the effectiveness of written commitments, essentially a form of contract between the supervisor and supervisee (Shapiro, 1985). Shapiro classified commitments into five types: clinical procedures (implementation or changes in techniques), clinical process administration (client-centered planning, analysis, or evaluation), supervisory procedures (changes or implementation of supervisee behaviors, conference interactions, supervisory roles and responsibilities, discussion of clinical or supervisory processes), supervisory process administration (planning, analysis or evaluation of the supervisory process related to clinician/supervisee skills), and academic information/teaching function (gaining academic information). Shapiro's findings about type of commitment support other findings about the content of conferences. The greatest number of commitments involved planning, analysis, and evaluation of the clinical process with particular focus on the behavior of the client (47 percent of total commitments) with the second most frequent being commitments related to specific therapy or diagnostic techniques, again focusing on client behavior (39 percent).

Shapiro used two types of treatment in his study. In one treatment there was discussion of commitments about activities to be carried out by the supervisee in subsequent clinical sessions, but no written agreement, only note-taking by the supervisor; in the other treatment, supervisor and supervisee agreed in writing to the commitments made, in essence, a contract. The documentation also included the specification of the observable behaviors that the supervisee would demonstrate to indicate follow-through of each commitment. Inexperienced clinicians completed more commitments when written agreement was required; experienced clinicians completed more when no written documentation was required. The value of structured written documentation of assignments and commitments with beginning clinicians is supported. The study has provided an important methodology for supervisors to identify and measure the completion of behaviors that are discussed in the conference. This seems to be a reasonable procedure for individual supervisor/supervisee dyads or groups to determine follow-through from the conference to the clinical session, a very necessary step in determining the effectiveness of the supervisory process.

A contract or written commitment between supervisor and supervisee will vary in its content depending upon the situation, but, if approached as a plan that will be followed to help both participants have a clear understanding of their goals and the procedures they will follow to meet those goals, it is a natural way to approach collaborative supervision. The process of agreeing on the specifics of the contract forces discussion. If goals are written and agreed upon by both, there should be much less opportunity for incongruency between supervisor and supervisee expectations. There will also be direction for the supervisory process that may not otherwise exist.

Programs

Another form of planning that first developed in psychology and education is that of programmed instruction. With foundations in the work of Skinner (1954), this form of planning went through a period of evolution before being adapted to speech-language pathology and audiology. Programmed instruction, as defined by Costello (1977), is "a systematically designed remediation plan which specifies *a priori* the teaching and learning behaviors required of both the teacher and the learner" (p. 3). Seen as a means of improving instruction, it consists of materials arranged into a sequence of events and stimuli in which there is immediate feedback about the client's response. Such programmed instructions, or *programs* as they have come to be called, may be written for individual clients, or can be found in published form; computerized instruction is an example of programs, whether obtained commercially or written for a specific client.

Instructional programs were almost unheard of in speech- language pathology before 1960 (Mowrer, 1977). Holland and Mathews (1963) wrote about using a teaching machine to teach discrimination of the /s/ to children with defective articulation, and Garrett (1963) reported on programmed articulation therapy. Clinical projects and research investigations have subsequently appeared in the speech-language pathology literature, demonstrating the validity and clinical usefulness of programmed instruction. (Baker & Ryan, 1971; Connell, Spradlin, & McReynolds, 1977; Costello & Onstine, 1976; Fristoe, 1975; Gray & Ryan, 1973; Holland, 1970; McReynolds, 1974; Sloane & MacAulay, 1968; Van Hattum et al., 1974)

Costello (1977) presented principles and procedures that would enable clinicians and experimenters to produce their own programmed instruction since very few commercial programs were available at the time. Although such commercial programs have proliferated since then, the principles described by Costello are still appropriate and valuable for the supervisor and supervisee who wish to devise a program for their client or to evaluate commercial programs. A more thorough treatment of programmed instruction by Mowrer (1977) is suggested as further reading on this topic; and two detailed manuals are also available (Collins & Cunningham, 1976a,b). Mowrer's book includes a section on evaluation criteria for the selection of such programs which is of importance. His suggestion that clinicians keep abreast of new instructional materials and demand data from field test results is also timely for supervisors who will be participating in decisions about the use or writing of such programs.

The writing of programs has provided an effective method of long-range planning for clients which can also be applied to clinician, supervisee, and supervisor. Techniques for this activity should also be a part of the total training in planning which prepares students for a variety of approaches in the service delivery setting.

Individual Educational Plans

With the passage of the Education for All Handicapped Children Act of 1975 (Public Law 94-142), long-range planning was mandated in the schools through the requirement for Individual Educational Plans (IEPs) for all handicapped children receiving a free and appropriate education under that legislation. This requirement formalized or structured what most speech-language pathologists and audiologists had been taught to do and, in one form or another, were probably already doing for their clients—setting individual behavioral objectives and developing procedures for meeting those objectives. Emphasis in this type of planning is on the client. There is no reason, however, why the same type of planning cannot be employed for other participants in the supervisory interaction. Fantasy runs wild, in fact, when considering the Individual Clinician Plan (ICP), the Individual Supervisee Plan (ISeeP), and the Individual Supervisor Plan (ISorP)! Supervisors in educational programs need to be aware of their responsibility in preparing supervisees for their role in writing IEPs in the future. The role of school program supervisors in developing the IEPs is not clear-cut. It would seem that their involvement would be partially administrative, that is, seeing that the procedures are carried out. Or they may serve in a consultant role to some speech-language pathologist or audiologist for certain cases. Additionally, they may serve as monitor or in a Direct-Active Style for persons who are having difficulty producing such plans. The procedures for writing IEPs have been written about extensively by Dublinske (1978), Dublinske and Healey (1978), Garbee (1982), and Neidecker (1980).

Other Types of Planning

Planning is frequently influenced by the setting in which it takes place and the type of records used in that setting. Hospital records, for example, are very different from those maintained in schools (Flower, 1984). Kent (1977) and Kent and Chabon (1980) have modified a system for medical record keeping and planning (the Problem-Oriented Medical Record [POMR]) for implementation in a small, university-based speech and hearing clinic. The system includes four components: (1) the collection of a data base for each client, (2) identification of specific problems from the data base, (3) design of written plans to favorably affect or resolve each problem, and (4) record of progress in therapy. Each plan describes in telegraphic style the diagnostic, therapeutic, and educational plans for the client. Progress notes provide a complete chronology of case management. The author states advantages to the client, student, supervisor, and the institution. These advantages include the fact that there is little "busy work" of lesson plans and evaluation summaries, therefore, supervisory time can be spent in planning to remediate the client's problem. This point addresses the problem stated earlier that not much supervisory time is spent in planning.

Another plan for client management that is consistent with the recommendation to prepare professionals to write long-term objectives was reported by Lemmer and Drake (1983). Based on the Kent and Chabon (1980) report, the plan is entitled *Student Training Cycle* (STC) and is used in an intensive residential program in a university where students work as a team in diagnostics, treatment, and report writing. After diagnostics, students generate a Problem List which becomes the basis for treatment. Rather than writing a detailed lesson plan, students formulate three objectives for each therapy session. Each objective contains the following information: (1) area of deficits, (2) goals, (3) objective statement, and (4) decreases and increases in difficulty. Data are collected and client performance documented. These notes are submitted in rough draft form to the supervisor until a professional writing style is developed. All student-generated notes for files are read and cosigned by supervisors.

According to the authors, this plan results in improved accountability, better interstaff communication, increased quality of client care, a continuity of service between therapy teams, as well as increased ability in students to draft effective treatment objectives, and development of a professional writing style. Students report a clearer understanding of the therapeutic process and clinical expectations. Here, as in traditional lesson planning, the dependence or independence of the supervisee may determine the supervisor's style of participation, and vice versa.

Other approaches to planning were noted by Flower (1984) and Oyer (1987) and, together with the Peaper and Wener (1984) study, help supervisors in educational programs to recognize the future planning needs of their students. Applicability will vary for the other planning domains.

Planning for the Clinician

The previous discussion of planning objectives and activities for the client is only one component of the planning needed for the four-fold approach to supervision. Similar documentation and planning of objectives and procedures for the clinician are equally important.

Plans for the clinician will include, of course, the planning of the specific clinician behaviors that are to be utilized to modify client behaviors. This statement might seem unnecessary. However, student clinicians often say, "My supervisor never talks about *my* behavior—just the client's." This may be the result of errors in perception, although analyses of conference content have repeatedly established that the *client*, not the *clinician*, is the focus of most of the discussion (Culatta & Seltzer, 1976; McCrea, 1980; Pickering, 1979, 1984; Roberts & Smith, 1982; Shapiro, 1985; Tufts, 1984). Some studies (Blumberg, 1980; Culatta & Seltzer, 1977; Roberts & Smith, 1982; Tufts, 1984) have also indicated that evaluation is not frequently included in the conference. This, too, is probably correctly interpreted as a lack of discussion of clinician behavior.

Lack of specific discussion of clinician behavior probably had its beginning in the traditional concept of planning as reflected in the literature—plans are for the client, not the clinician, and goals are set for clients. This is particularly incongruous when one considers two points: (1) supervisee's expectations for supervision, and (2) the types of evaluation forms used by supervisors.

Planning as Related to Expectations

Expectations of supervisees are usually related to their own needs. Supervisees in Russell's (1976) study, for example, indicated that they wanted fair treatment in terms of *their* evaluation. Such studies have consistently indicated a desire by supervisees not only to learn what to do with the client, but for feedback about their own behavior, that is, to know if they are doing what they should be doing (Larson, 1982; Tihen, 1984). Although these expectations will have been addressed during the first component while interpreting and helping the supervisee to understand the supervisory process, such expectations are important in planning activities. If specific behavioral objectives have been set for clinician activities, if data have been collected and analyzed, clinicians will be able to determine more clearly the progress being made and whether or not their expectations have been met. If the approach to supervision presented here is to become a reality, then specific attention must be given to the behavior, growth, and needs of *clinicians* in the clinical process, as well as clients.

Planning as Related to Evaluation

Although not the topic of this chapter, evaluation must be noted here in terms of the setting of objectives. Evaluation forms, for the most part, consist of lists of clinician, not client, behaviors (Dopheide et al., 1984; Klevans & Volz, 1974; Shriberg et al., 1975). If discussion in the conference is about client behavior but evaluation is based on clinician behavior, where is the bridge between the two? Certainly clinicians should be aware of the criteria for themselves on evaluation forms and, if they are to be used in the total evaluation process, they should be considered in whatever planning is done.

Planning for the clinician must be undergirded by the same rationale used traditionally for establishing clear objectives for clients—to aid in accountability and evaluation of clients. "Unless we know where we are going, how can we know when we arrive?" Stating terminal behaviors for clinicians should be as readily accepted as a necessary part of planning and of evaluating their progress as it has been for clients. This parallel activity of stating terminal behavior for clinicians is apparently not such a common topic for discussion in supervisory conferences.

Again, Rockman (1977) has cited the need for identifying both short- and long-range goals for the student clinician's behavior.

> Objectives may be as specific as improving the accuracy of phoneme judgments or learning to administer a specific test battery, or as general as "ability to plan therapy" or "ability to analyze therapy interaction." Obviously, the more specific the objective, the more easily achievement of that objective can be documented. If the supervisor is as stringent in evaluating her or his objectives for the student as in evaluation of the student's objectives for the client, she or he will have no difficulty in recognizing appropriate behavioral objectives. Basically, we have to ask ourselves the same questions we ask the clinicians. Are the objectives we have selected clear, unambiguous, reasonable, appropriate and capable of being achieved? (p. 4)

The importance of planning the role of the clinician was stressed also by Hunt and Kauzlarich in an ASHA presentation (1979) in which they reaffirmed that the *base* of the supervisory interaction triad is between the supervisor and the clinician rather than the client and the clinician. They also discussed the importance of objectively defining the competencies of clinicians on which they will be evaluated.

Further support for the need to attend to more than client behavior is found also in the task and competency list for clinical supervision (ASHA, 1985b), which places a major focus on assisting the supervisee to develop certain skills and abilities.

This setting of objectives for the clinician is related to subsequent steps in the supervisory process—observation, analysis, further planning and, certainly, to evaluation. These components are more meaningful if based on stated objectives and procedures. Evaluation is more fair and more objective if based on specified behaviors and quantified progress toward goals. If attention continues to be on client behaviors, evaluation of clinicians will continue to be imprecise. Clinician progress can only be measured adequately if clear objectives have been set and behaviors relating to those objectives are quantified.

Long-Term Planning

Generalization of clinician behavior to a variety of situations should receive fully as much attention as does the generalization of client behavior. Generalization is considered by Elbert and Geirut (1986) to be the "hallmark of a 'successful' remediation program" and is defined as the "accurate production and use of trained target sounds in other untrained contexts or environments" (p. 121). Generalization of clinician behavior should be of equal importance in the supervisory process and might be defined as "The appropriate use of trained clinical behaviors in other untrained clinical contexts or environments." This generalization is dependent upon the overall goals of planning for total professional development as independent, analytical, problem-solving, self-evaluating clinicians. Thus, clinicians must (1) set both short- and long-term goals and objectives for themselves; (2) plan procedures for their own performance; and (3) plan the observation, data collection, and analysis that will measure whether or not the objectives have been achieved.

Clients come and go. Even supervisors come and go. Although clients may have similar problems, their responses to treatment may be very different. Activities for one client may have some generalizability to other clients. It would seem, however, that it is clinicians' ability to observe objectively, to analyze their own behavior, to problem-solve and to set objectives for themselves that will enable them to generalize to other situations and to be effective with all their clients. The ability to problem-solve, to devise techniques for each situation, and to determine what may or may not have produced change seems fully as important and probably more far-reaching, in terms of professional development, than assembling a series of techniques that work for individual clients. Specific clinical techniques may never be used again or, more unfortunately, may be used at the wrong time. But self-knowledge is transferable from one situation to another.

Supervisors need to be aware of a broader responsibility than simply session-to-session planning. They should assist clinicians/supervisees in setting objectives for on-going professional growth. Moreover, when general professional development is considered as the overriding purpose of the total supervisory process, short-term objectives must be seen as fitting into this larger perspective of total professional growth. In the educational program, where interaction with any one supervisee may be fragmented because of short-term assignments (for example, one semester with one client and/or supervisor), it is easy to lose sight of general long-term professional development. Supervisors may, for some students, view the trees but not see the forest. Students, too, may not see the relationship between today's events and tomorrow's professional responsibilities unless they see the day-to-day activities against a framework of long-range goals. They need to be helped to understand the importance of their long-term goals and to assume responsibility for them. Long-term goals for clinicians that will apply to all situations may be such behaviors as collecting and analyzing data appropriately, modifying verbal or nonverbal behaviors, sequencing tasks in reaching objectives, and utilizing reinforcement techniques appropriately.

The site where the supervision takes place may have a major impact upon this issue. In all service delivery settings, the first and foremost responsibility is the client. The immediate concerns for delivery of service to clients may make the urgency of the moment seem more important than the growth of the clinician. In the educational program, however, and in off-campus or CFY settings, the supervisor has a dual responsibility— preparation of clinicians and service to clients. This will be discussed further in the chapter on accountability, but for now it should be said that all supervisors must learn to balance the needs of supervisees with the needs of clients. Awareness by both supervisor and supervisee of the supervisee's long-term professional goals will make it easier to coordinate them with client needs. This is best dealt with in all settings during the planning component. Setting long- and short-term goals and objectives for client, clinician/supervisee, and supervisor makes it clear throughout the interaction what each person's responsibility will be.

Perhaps it is in the off-campus or service delivery setting where joint participation in setting long-term objectives for clinicians during the educational program will "pay off." Clinicians who have been involved in the development of their own goals and objectives and who have learned self-analysis and self-evaluation skills should be able to carry their long-term objectives from one client to the next, from one semester to another, from one practicum site to another, and then into the employment setting where professional development continues. If their goals for themselves have been related solely to one client at a time, however, or have been imposed by the supervisor, they may have difficulty in carrying them over into other settings.

In fact, responsibility for carrying their own objectives from one supervisor to another, and from one setting to another may be most important for clinicians in terms of off-campus sites. One of the dilemmas of the university supervisor of the practicum is how much information to give the on-site supervisor about the student clinician, particularly about clinical weaknesses or problem areas. Some off-campus supervisors want information about supervisees, some do not. If university supervisors provide information about a specific problem, they run the risk of biasing the on-site supervisor. If information is not provided, the problem may not be identified by the on-site supervisor until it is too late to begin efforts to modify behaviors as needed. This may be because of the inexperience of the supervisor, the different criteria of supervisors, or the ability of the clinician to avoid exhibiting the problem behavior. It is much better when clinicians, who have been involved in setting their own objectives for professional growth, who know exactly where they stand in relation to meeting them, and are not threatened, can see the off-campus setting as an opportunity to move further toward their long-term objectives rather than feeling that they must hide their weaknesses.

Such planning for the clinician is not a separate and additional activity which necessarily requires more time. It is not a different process, but rather, a change of focus from the customary planning which is solely for the client, to a broader-based type. It is included naturally as the counterpart of the planning for the client. Later it will be seen how supervisee and supervisor planning builds on to this.

Short-Term Planning

Short-term planning for clinicians focuses on current, session-to-session interaction between the clinician and the client. It includes (1) identification of clinician competencies or needs related to specific clinical sessions, the current client, or specific clinical problems, (2) determining how a baseline of clinician behaviors related to these competencies will be obtained, (3) identifying clinician strategies to be used to modify the client's behavior, and (4) planning the observation, including (a) identification of data to be collected on the clinician's behavior by both supervisor and clinician, (b) planning the logistics of the observation, and (c) the identification of data collection methods.

Identification of Clinician Competencies and Needs

In educational programs, supervisors may be familiar with clinicians' skills from previous supervisory situations, from evaluations of previous experiences, or from clinic "grapevines." The ever-present danger here is in the possible bias from other opinions (Andersen, 1981). The emphasis in the Collaborative Style or the Consultative Style would mandate that clinicians assume some responsibility in identifying their own strengths or needs.

Further, it will be noticed that equal emphasis is placed on competencies and needs. This is a more positive approach than the philosophy that directs the supervisor to attend only to weaknesses of the clinician. Cogan (1973) addressed this issue in depth. He suggested that the "weakness strategy" (p. 202) is not very productive, and instead, supervisors should address themselves to the improvement of strengths. This is not to say that weaknesses do not exist or that they should not be dealt with. Rather, the weaknesses must be addressed in situations perceived to be critical, defined by Cogan as situations that essentially prevent students from even "minimally adequate learning" (p. 202). Only then does Cogan believe that weaknesses should be given priority. Many of the decisions made about strengths or weaknesses are subjective. Collection of data and its use is the best way to ensure against the subjectivity of such judgments, although, because they are made by human beings, they can never be totally objective.

How are these competencies or needs identified? Some may be identified during the first conference as the supervisor and clinician progress through the orientation component. The discussion of items from evaluation forms to assist clinicians who are uncertain about their competencies or needs has already been suggested. Not all competencies and needs can be identified prior to beginning the clinical experiences. Others will be identified after clinical work has begun through a process of observation, data collection, and analysis of clinical sessions. As a part of the planning, supervisor and clinician will decide what data will be collected on the clinician. These data will be studied in the analysis phase, and strengths and needs identified.

Determining Baselines of Clinician Behaviors

The same procedures used for determining baselines for clients are relevant for determining baselines for clinicians. The clinician evaluations described previously, clinician-stated needs or preferences, and information obtained from interaction analysis systems (see the chapter on Observation) are all sources of baseline data on behaviors of clinicians that may need modification. Methods of obtaining baselines on clinical behavior described by Brookshire (1967) would be helpful to clinicians and supervisors at this stage.

Identification of Clinician Strategies for Modifying Client Behavior

Clinicians need different amounts of assistance in planning strategies for the clinical session. It is tempting for supervisors, however, to provide too much from their own experience at this point, thus not encouraging creative participation by the clinician in the planning of clinical activities.

This is a crucial point in the process of supervision. It is where the supervisor uses all his or her skills in assisting the clinician to develop clinical strategies, in allowing the clinician to try and to succeed or fail, to assume responsibility, and to be a participant in the conference, not just a receiver of information. Although supervisor input is necessary at this point, it should not dominate unless the supervisee exhibits major inadequacies. Again, the continuum must be kept in mind.

Information needed about clinicians has been identified earlier in this chapter. Methods for obtaining this information will vary widely, but the clinician's competencies in relation to a specific client must be assessed in each new supervisory experience.

Setting Objectives

An example of clinician planning has been contributed by a colleague as follows:

> After my clinicians have completed baseline testing on the client (usually two or three sessions) and three therapy sessions, I require them to complete the W-PACC (Shriberg et al., 1974). This independent self-evaluation enables me to see how they perceive their own strengths and weaknesses. They are also required to write three personal goals on the back of the W-PACC at the same time. During our next conference we discuss and refine these goals to ensure that they are measurable and attainable (that is, reasonable expectations for a semester).
>
> Some typical first-time goals may be (1) to feel more comfortable with my client and not feel nervous in my sessions, (2) to make sure I have enough things to do to keep my client interested and involved for the entire session, (3) to help my client improve, and (4) to be an effective clinician. When I get this type of general goals, we talk so I can identify sources of anxiety and get more specificity. For example, related to the first goal, the comfort factor may involve (a) identifying appropriate long-term/short-term goals, (b) developing and searching for activities that are motivating and productive and that lead to goal attainment, (c) overplanning—trying to ensure that they don't run out of activities, (d) developing branch steps for each step of the program in case the client is unable to perform the planned tasks, and (e) the fear of making mistakes, for example, incorrectly evaluating client responses.

Just as client objectives are planned together, based on baseline data, so are clinician objectives. Based on the general goals previously stated, specific goals may be

1. The clinician will formulate a hierarchy of short-term goals (number is specified) for each semester objective. The appropriateness will be measured by intra- and intersession percentages of correct/incorrect responses.

2. The clinician will incorporate at least x number (usually one or two) new activities or materials into the therapy session weekly.

The clinician will use at least x number of activities for each session goal. Appropriateness will be determined by her subjective evaluation of client interest and objectively by the number of elicited responses (the number to be determined as a part of the planning).

3. The clinician will plan at least x number of activities for each session.

4. The clinician will develop x number of branch steps for each major/primary step. A branch step will be implemented when the client's level of success is below 60 percent in x number of consecutive responses.

5. The clinician will evaluate client responses during 10-minute audio- or videotape segments of each therapy session until she achieves 90 percent or more intrarater agreement in three consecutive sessions. This will be completed for each new target behavior/response.

6. The clinician and supervisor (this, then, becomes a supervisor objective) will independently evaluate and record client responses for selected 10-minute portions of each therapy session until a 90 percent or more point-by-point interrater agreement is achieved for three consecutive sessions. (We mutually decide whether to do this live, via audio- or videotape, or a combination of both. Often one of the clinician's peers assumes my role about mid-semester in evaluating responses.)

Other typical clinician semester goals might be:

1. I will be able to discriminate correct-incorrect-close approximations of _____ phoneme, as measured by intra- and interrater agreements by mid-semester.

2. I will decrease "off-task" behaviors in therapy sessions from _____ percent to _____ percent by the end of the semester as measured by the Boone-Prescott or ABC systems and/or the total number of responses (minimum desired number = 250 in 50-minute session) per session.

3. I will be able to modify a strategy *within* a session (versus planning a modification for subsequent sessions) when the client's behavior indicates he is unable or unwilling to perform at least 50 percent of the time by the end of the semester. (Brasseur, personal communication, 1986)

Planning the Observation

The essential factor in the on-going identification of needs and competencies of clinicians is in the collection of appropriate data and its interpretation. The next chapter will cover the principles and operationalizing of observation, but what must be stated and restated here is *the need to plan the observation.* Traditionally, supervisors have decided what data will be collected, but often this decision is made after the supervisor enters the observation situation. Clinicians, then, have little or no opportunity to participate in the decision making or to have their concerns considered. Bernthal and Beukelman (1975) stressed the importance of providing specific information to clinicians about their own behaviors. The list of behaviors on which data may be recorded is endless— statements of instruction or direction, use of client cues, on-task behaviors, talk behaviors of all types, types of questions.

The important point is that the behaviors to be observed and on which data are to be collected must come out of the stated objectives for the sessions and out of the concerns of both supervisor and supervisee, not just the supervisor's subjective approach, probably based on his or her "square box." This should not be interpreted to mean that observations are so tightly planned that there is no opportunity for the supervisor to record unexpected events.

The logistics of the observation are also included in planning. Will the supervisor be in the room with the clinician and client? Will the clinician collect data on his or her own behavior in addition to data on the client? Will there be audio- or videotape recording? If the supervisor is to enter the room to demonstrate for the clinician, how will this be handled? What means will be used for recording the behaviors?

Basically, then, the purpose of planning the observation is to allow input from the clinician, and to ensure that the observation time is spent profitably and that appropriate data are collected that will make it possible for the subsequent steps to be completed adequately and easily. Such planning should reduce anxieties of supervisees about the observation and its outcome.

Whatever form the planning takes—written plans, contracts, programs—it should include clearly stated objectives for the clinician. In addition to "The clients will _____ ," a portion of the plan should always include such items as "The clinician will _____ ." Such statements give clinicians more direction for self-observation and data collection and for modifying behavior. They are measurable, if written appropriately, by both supervisee and supervisor. Statements based on such measurable objectives should be much more meaningful than a subjective statement from either clinician or supervisor that "Your behavior was much better this time" or "I think I did better than before."

Planning for the Supervisory Process

The Supervisee

This is the point at which clinicians change roles (see Figure 1–1). In terms of a superior/subordinate paradigm, they shift from a superior role with the client, where they are "in charge" to the subordinate role of supervisee, where the supervisor is in charge. This is where the supervisee's role in the process is defined. In the Direct-Active Style of the Evaluation-Feedback Stage, the supervisee will play mainly a passive role and will need assistance in planning an expanded role in the conference. In the Collaborative or Consultative Styles, supervisees will be much more involved. If the first component has been conducted thoroughly and well, supervisees will understand their role in supervision and the purpose of planning their participation in it.

The importance of planning this aspect of the interaction has already been discussed. There seems to be little provision for this type of planning in the speech-language pathology and audiology literature, and probably also in practice.

From the literature in education on supervision, however, comes a range of suggestions for the important concept of planning for the supervisee. Cogan (1973) said, "The lesson planning session is not complete until the teacher has been prepared for the role he will take in the supervisory conference to follow" (p. 130). Maintaining the collegial role, as implied in the clinical supervision model, requires that supervisees understand their role as active participants in the conference, that they are not just passive responders to the supervisor's input, that they do not abdicate responsibility in the joint problem solving that is important in any type of cooperative supervision. The literature indicates that supervisees are not active in conferences; that is, they do not ask questions, and only provide raw data while the supervisor provides strategies and suggestions. One may conjecture about the reason. Perhaps they are burdened with stereotypes of their role as supervisees. Perhaps supervisees do not know how to be active even though it has been indicated in the expectancy studies that they want to be. Perhaps supervisors are too overpowering or do not set the stage properly for them to be active. At any rate, there is a discrepancy between what supervisees say they want to do in the conference and what actually happens (Tihen, 1984). The solution to this may be found in the planning stage.

Planning for the role of supervisee will include (1) setting objectives for the supervisory process; (2) planning the data to be collected from the conference by the supervisee; (3) planning the self-analysis of the conference data by the supervisee; (4) planning what the supervisee will bring into the conference on the basis of those data; and (5) planning the role of each participant in the conference, that is, planning an agenda for the conference.

Planning for the supervisee will become clearer as subsequent chapters are read. For now, examples of overall long-term objectives for supervisees might include: more active participation in planning, data collection and analysis; modifying their own verbal behavior in the conference so that it is clear, specific, and concrete; participating in problem solving about their own clinical performance rather than expecting solutions from the supervisor; and others that will make the supervisory process more productive. The long-term objectives can be broken down and stated behaviorally. There are many others that will apply to the active participation of supervisees in the supervisory process. Such planning for supervisees should help to decrease the domination of the supervisor by stating specifically what it is that supervisees will do as they move along the continuum to independence and self-supervision.

The Supervisor

Planning for the supervisor is the component of the proposal made in this book that is probably farthest from the traditional model of supervision. Such planning is based on the thesis that joint participation by supervisor and supervisee in the process produces not only independence in the clinician but growth and satisfaction in the supervisor. What type of planning is appropriate for the supervisor if this growth is to take place?

First, the supervisor must be aware of his or her own behavior. The fundamental importance of self-knowledge and self-study for supervisors is discussed in other places in this book. Behaviors must be identified which make up patterns in the supervisor's behavior and which may need to be modified or strengthened overall, and in relation to each supervisory interaction. A total plan for the supervisory process, then, should include objectives and procedures for the supervisor, as well as the client and the clinician/supervisee. Because procedures for the supervisor will be fully addressed later, this section will focus only on planning objectives.

Supervisor objectives, like those of other participants in the clinical and supervisory processes, may be long or short term, that is, overall broad objectives related to the supervisors' general patterns of behavior or specific to certain interactions with supervisees. The setting of such objectives assumes some ongoing self-study by supervisors and supervisees of their interactions. This may come as the result of listening to audiotapes or viewing videotapes, from evaluations by supervisees, analysis with their own supervisors or administrators or their peers, and, in the best of all experiences, from open discussion with supervisees about whether or not what is happening is congruent with their perceived needs and expectations or the objectives that have been set. This process of planning objectives is comparable to what is done in the clinical process. The list of tasks and competencies adopted by ASHA (ASHA, 1985b) can provide a focus for both supervisors and supervisees in formulating objectives, especially for those who are just beginning to analyze the supervisory process and are attempting to modify it. Examples of objectives for supervisors might be such general ones as reducing verbal behavior in the conference, giving less information, encouraging problem solving by supervisees, and asking more questions that require thinking by the supervisee.

Some supervisor objectives will be directly related to the objectives set for a specific supervisee. If an objective for the supervisee has been to engage in more problem solving, then the supervisor may set an objective that directs him or her toward the asking of more broad, thought-provoking questions and the elimination of the practice of giving solutions and strategies before the supervisee has an opportunity to problem-solve. Participation by supervisees in planning the supervisor's objectives adds to the collaborative nature of planning.

Planning for supervisors, which includes the setting of objectives and planning procedures for observation, data collection, and analysis, should provide direction for the supervisory process. If objectives are set appropriately, the domination and control of the supervisory process by the supervisor should be reduced. Activities should be planned so that supervisees know what to expect, so that their needs will be reflected through the supervisor's objectives as well as through their own. Their involvement in this planning adds to their understanding of the supervisory process. It also should reduce anxiety since there will be less of the unknown, erratic, or unpredictable type of supervisor activities discussed elsewhere as a threat to supervisees.

REALITIES OF PLANNING

The immediate reaction of many supervisors and clinicians to this discussion of planning may well be "How can we find the time to do one more thing?" In a world where supervisors are assigned too many supervisees, and clinicians too many clients, where there are more and more professional demands, such a question may be supportable. Rather than thinking of this procedure as additional work, however, it seems more accurate to think instead of a different *direction* for supervisor/supervisee interaction. It would require, for some, a shift of emphasis and a more structured approach to supervision. What are the realities of implementing such an approach?

Where supervision takes place, it is assumed that some time is spent in face-to-face interaction, usually a conference. If not, it cannot be considered supervision and nothing that has been said applies. In educational programs, time is usually assigned for regular conferences, although one does occasionally hear of a program where conferences are arranged only as need for assistance is perceived by clinicians. This is appropriate for the Consultative Stage but, filtered through this writer's "square box," it can scarcely be considered adequate supervision, particularly for students who may not know how to identify their own needs in training. But, even where that is the case, the principles presented here are still applicable for the times that they do meet.

Assuming then that time has been allotted for conferencing, how can the four-fold planning described here be implemented? The setting of clinician and supervisee objectives is basically a matter of broadening one's thinking about planning to include this concept, if it is not already a part of the supervisor's approach. Decisions about what the clinician will do to help the client attain the stated objectives are implied in any planning. Four-fold planning only suggests that objectives for the other participants be stated clearly and behaviorally at the same time and in the same way as client objectives. If this is done, clinician behaviors can be observed and recorded, and growth measured. Supervisee objectives come naturally from clinician objectives—What will be done with the data about clinician and client from the clinical session? How will the supervisee participate in the supervisory process?

Studying the supervisor's behavior and setting subsequent objectives may be an additional activity. It can involve varying amounts of time, ranging from listening to an audiotape of a conference and targeting certain areas for change, to extensive analysis of ongoing interactions. People find time for those things that they are really motivated to do. Supervisors who are seriously interested in examining their behavior will find a way to do it and, hopefully, the content of this book will not only encourage them but assist them in doing so. The chapter on studying the conference will deal with this in greater detail.

Additionally, it should be stated that such changes in the approach to supervision will be more easily accomplished if taken one step at a time. Clients are not expected to change all behaviors simultaneously; supervisees and supervisors should have the same option.

SUMMARY

Planning for the client in speech-language pathology and audiology has always been considered an essential part of the responsibilities of the clinician and the supervisor. This chapter has extended that responsibility to include four-fold planning for all participants in the supervisory process. All the principles that have been applied to planning for the client are equally relevant to the clinician, supervisee, and supervisor.

Observing the Supervisory Process

A supervisor can waste a professional lifetime trying to reconstruct a teacher's performance with him by talking about it from recollections.

—Cogan (1973, p. 136)

Webster (1984) provides several definitions of observation, two of which are, "The act of noting and recording something, as a phenomenon, with instruments" and "the result or record of such notation." Also included is the following definition: "A judgment or inference based on observing" (p. 811). It is exactly the difference between these definitions that will be the theme of this and the next chapter. At the risk of taking liberties with Webster, it will be argued that, for supervision, the first and second statements are appropriate definitions of *observation* and will form the foundation of the discussion in this chapter. The latter definition, however, which includes inference and judgment, will be considered to be the basis of the Analysis component of supervision and the later Evaluation aspect.

Observation to some *is* supervision. The literature about supervision and the language used by many in discussing supervision makes it clear that *observation* and *supervision* are often used interchangeably. "I am supervising at 9:30" may mean "I am observing at 9:30." Even the language of ASHA requirements for the Certificate of Clinical Competence until recently added to the lack of precision in the use of both words. 'Direct supervision" was frequently used without definition in early requirements for certification and accreditation and it was often interpreted to mean observation. Currently, these ASHA requirements (ASHA, 1985c) define direct supervision as "on-site observation or closed-circuit TV monitoring of the student clinician" (p. 44), still implying that observation is the sole component of supervision. Later the document does say, "In addition to the required direct supervision," that is, observation and TV monitoring, that supervision should also utilize "ways to obtain knowledge of the students' clinical work such as conferences, audio- and videotape recording, written reports, staffings, and discussions with other persons who have participated in the student's clinical training" (p. 44). This suggests some progress in viewing the many facets of supervision, yet there is still an equating of supervision with observation that distorts the definition of both. For example, Educational Standards Board requirements recognize only hours spent in observation by supervisors, not the many hours spent in other activities. In stating requirements for supervision of the Clinical Fellowship Year, on-site supervision, presumably meaning observation, is only one of the listed "monitoring" activities (ASHA, 1985c). Such recent indications that supervision is perceived as more than observation have begun to clarify the various roles of the supervisor in meeting ASHA standards, and for purposes of this discussion, support the concept of observation as only one entity of supervision.

Goldhammer and colleagues (1980) considered observation synonymous with data gathering and stated, "Observation is the activity through which a supervisor becomes aware of the events, interactions, physical elements, and other phenomena in a particular place. . .during a particular time" (p. 70). Cogan (1973) called it the "Operations by which individuals make careful, systematic scrutiny of the events and interactions occurring during classroom instruction. The term also applies to the records made of these events and interactions" (p. 134).

It is assumed for purposes of this book that data collection is inherent in observation, observation without data collection is a waste of time, data collection without observation is of course impossible, and that it is unnecessary to use both terms in describing this component of supervision. Therefore, the terms will be used interchangeably in the text that follows.

Additionally, as with each of the other components of supervision described here, observation is a four-fold activity—each participant becomes the object of some type of observation at various times during the process. Further, the assumption in the Collaborative and the Consultative Styles is that clinicians, supervisees, and supervisors will all be involved in self-observation followed by self-analysis. This chapter will concentrate on general principles of observation and observation of the clinician and the clinical process, leaving the discussion of observation of the supervisory process for another chapter.

PURPOSES OF OBSERVATION

Perhaps the first question that should be asked about observation is its purpose. True, a certain number of hours of observations of clinicians by supervisors is required in educational programs in speech-language pathology and audiology (ASHA, 1985c). Also, in some service delivery programs, supervisors are required to perform a certain number of observations before a formal evaluation of an employee is written. Real as these requirements are, they scarcely constitute a meaningful purpose.

There are a variety of possible purposes for observations at all levels. The observation may be conducted to collect data to be used in the analysis of behaviors for teaching purposes during the supervisory conference (Dussault, 1970). The purpose may be solely to collect information for a formal evaluation.

It may be for the purpose of monitoring to assure quality services, especially relevant to the observation of assessment services in programs where they are a one-time activity. Or it may be for the purpose of collecting baseline data to determine future plans. These are broad and general purposes. Supervisors should ask themselves very specific questions about their own personal agenda when they enter the observation activity. Do they have a clear concept of their purpose? Is it to identify strengths? Or weaknesses (Cogan, 1973)? Is it to measure progress toward objectives? Is it to identify behaviors of clinicians? Clients? Or the interaction between the two (Goldhammer, 1969)? Is it "an inspection trip involving only the crudest of procedures, a single 'rating scale' and the dreaded judgmental feedback" (Harris, 1975, p. 165)?

According to Goldhammer (1969), the principal purpose of observation is to collect objective and comprehensive data in such a way that each lesson can be reconstructed validly enough to analyze it. He emphasized that the observer should write down what he *sees*, not how he *feels* about it. The following simple and straightforward guideline should probably be posted in every room where observation takes place, and on the front of every supervisor's notebook or clipboard: *Perceptions—not inferences; description—not commentary!* Inferences and commentary should be saved for the analysis phase.

Observation is discussed frequently in the literature about applied teaching—education, counseling, psychology, social work—as well as in speech-language pathology and audiology. Two levels of observation become apparent. One level is the observation of the student, counselee, client, or in other words, the "less-knowing" or the "helpee" of the dyad. The other level is the observation of the teacher, counselor, or clinician—the "helper" or "more-knowing." Although the principles and techniques of observation may be similar for both, one needs to differentiate between the two, because the content and procedure will vary. "When our purpose is to gather evidence on learning, the focus is logically on the learner. When our purpose is to gather evidence about teacher behavior, the focus is on the teacher. When our purpose is to gather evidence on the teaching-learning process or instruction, the focus must be on interactions among teacher(s), pupil(s), and things" (Harris, 1975, p. 166). This is further support for knowing the purpose of the observation.

In reality, the purpose may be any or all of these and many more. Surely, the subsequent analysis of the clinical or diagnostic process will be more productive and the conference more meaningful if it is assumed that the fundamental purpose of the observation is to collect data. Further, the data should be collected in a manner that will enable the observer, or someone else, to relate the behavior of the clinician to the consequences of that behavior in the client. Later, in the case of the observation of the conference, the importance of relating the behavior of the supervisor to the consequences of that behavior on the supervisee will be considered. In other words, does the action of the clinician or supervisor appear to make a difference, positive or negative, in what the client or supervisee achieves? Can inferences or assumptions be made about the situation that has been observed? What data have been collected to support the inferences or assumptions made about those behaviors?

CHARACTERISTICS OF OBSERVATION

Two main characteristics of observation are of importance. One is its scientific nature; the other is the fact that, to be of value, observation must be an active process.

Observation Is Scientific

The observation component is the point at which supervision begins to move from the realm of a somewhat undefined art to the utilization of a scientific base. It is the objective collection of data in the observation that changes supervision from being solely an art to being closer to a science.

It is here that supervision assumes an objective approach, where quantifying procedures begin to be utilized, where data are collected which will be submitted to much the same type of analysis required for research projects. Researchers describe data as numerical and verbal descriptions of attributes and events (Silverman, 1977b), not a new concept to supervisors. Data from the observation provide the raw material for the conference. If they are not accurate, objective, and reliable, all subsequent stages of the process will be distorted or ineffectual. Without behavioral data as a foundation, the conference will become a potpourri of supervisee reports about what happened in the assessment or treatment session, supervisor attempts to recall the events, general discussion of treatment or assessment principles, guesses about the direction to take in further sessions, and subjective evaluations by supervisors.

The science-art continuum is an important concept. Cogan's (1973) general statements about supervision as a science are relevant here. Although not a science, he maintained that supervision is in part committed to science and that "whatever relevant science is available is needed to set proper constraints upon the claims of art, experience, and instruction." Certainly at the observation level principles can be borrowed from the behavioral sciences, as Cogan suggested. "Supervisors need to apply the intellectual rigor and discipline of science" and "to internalize the standards of evidence and proof that are characteristic of science" (pp. 18–19).

Emerich and Hatten's (1979) discussion of the science-art issue in relation to assessment activities is an appropriate backdrop to a similar view of supervision. They said that the scientific and artistic approaches each possess their own set of characteristics. The scientific approach leads to, among other factors, "more rigorous adherence to standardized procedures" and "objectivity, quantifiability and structure." The artistic approach, on the other hand, depends more upon "casual and non-structured scrutiny. . .the hunch, or clinical intuition." Emerich and Hatten presented the weaknesses of each approach and the need for a mixture of both and said, "Diagnosis is a unique blending of science and art" (pp. 12–13).

This continuum of art and science is certainly as real in relation of the supervisor's approach to observation as it is to assessment. The fact that the preferred style in traditional supervision seems to have been closer to the subjective end of the continuum makes it tempting to stress the scientific approach as an antidote to what appears to be the usual practice. Yet, it is easy to err too far in this scientific direction in observations and to miss certain important factors. The goal must be the blending of art and science similar to that suggested for assessment by Emerick and Hatten.

A clear distinction must be made between *data collection, analysis,* and *evaluation.* The purpose of the observation in the Collaborative and Consultative Styles is not "instant evaluation," but rather, to collect data. Inferences will be made from these data which will lead to interpretation, to further planning, and eventually, to evaluation. The inferences are determined jointly to provide an opportunity for learning by the supervisee.

Many supervisors may find it difficult to resist writing instant evaluations during the observation, but such comments should not be considered the primary product of the observation. The fallacy of such instant evaluations can be recognized by supervisors who recall how many times, in the darkness of the observation booth, in front of the videotape, or in the corner of the room in which they were observing, they have written an evaluative statement on the basis of one event or a few behaviors, only to erase the statement later, when subsequent events invalidated the previously written evaluation.

Although there may be occasional times when the instant evaluation is appropriate or expedient, the data collected during observation should not be mainly evaluative and judgmental, but should be a behavioral, descriptive record of what happened during the clinical session. The writer has had repeated experiences that reinforce the need to emphasize this point. In teaching courses or presenting workshops on supervision, it has become obvious that supervisors, or those studying supervision, tend to perceive evaluation as their primary role. When conducting practice experiences in behavior recording, for example, it has repeatedly been difficult to get even experienced clinicians or supervisors to refrain from stating evaluations while supposedly recording behaviors. This happens despite the emphasis that has been placed in clinical training on the importance of objectivity in description of behavior. It seems that, given the opportunity to watch a clinical session on videotape, supervisors or would-be supervisors cannot resist evaluating, often on the basis of very limited observation and information. This self-image of the role of the supervisor is consistent with the Direct-Active Style but not with the Collaborative Style. To change such perceptual sets about a role is not easy. It may be the point at which it is most difficult for supervisors to exercise what Cogan (1973) called "professional control."

Observation Is Active

Observation is more than just looking at what is occurring, and to be done well, it demands attention, practice, and precision. Let no one say of supervisors, in the words of Sherlock Holmes, that they see, but they do not observe. Observation is an *active, systematic process.* It may be done by supervisors during the actual clinical or diagnostic session within the room, through an observation window, or later, by way of listening to an audiotape or viewing a videotape of the session. Data may also be recorded by clinicians themselves during sessions or through later observation of audio- or videotapes of their own activities. Observation may include data gathering by colleagues in the case of team therapy, the teaching clinic (Dowling, 1979a; Dowling, 1983a,b; Dowling & Shank, 1981), or peer review and peer evaluation. Whatever the circumstances, the observer will be actively involved in the careful recording of events. As indicated in the planning section, the data to be collected will have been identified based on the objectives that have been set, and the method of data collection will have been determined. Such planning provides guidance for the activities of the supervisor during the observation, or for the supervisee during self-observation. The end product, then, is a set of carefully recorded data which can be utilized for a variety of purposes during the analysis and evaluation processes.

IMPORTANCE OF OBSERVATION

Observation, ranging from informal and nonstructured to structured, has long been considered of importance in any teaching or therapeutic process. Berne (1966) suggested that observation of the client is the most important tool of the counselor, a time when he or she is attuned to overt and subtle behaviors. In the classroom, observation techniques have been used for many years to answer questions about the critical dimensions of interaction between teacher and student with emphasis on student learning (Brandt, 1975; Harris, 1975).

Observation in Speech-Language Pathology and Audiology

Observation of the "Less-Knowing"

In speech-language pathology and audiology, the clinician's ability to observe the client has always been of concern, as evidenced by the inclusion of items related to observation on evaluation forms. Probably no existing evaluation forms are without items that assess observation and data collection skills in clinicians. Teaching these skills has been one of the responsibilities of supervisors, a fact that is supported in the ASHA list of competencies for supervisors (ASHA, 1985b): "Ability to assist the supervisee in using observation and assessment in preparation of client goals and objectives" (p. 58).

Skills related to the observation of the client have received greater emphasis than has observation of the clinician in the literature in speech-language pathology and audiology. Darley and Spriestersbach (1978) said that speech clinicians should become special kinds of observers who must be reminded of three principles: (1) observe and report enough, (2) observe and report objectively, and (3) observe and report precisely. Discussion of the techniques and skills of observation of clients are found in various texts on evaluation and assessment of communication disorders (Darley, 1964; Darley & Spriestersbach, 1978; Emerich & Hatten, 1979; Johnson, Darley, & Spriestersbach, 1963).

Mowrer (1977) devoted several chapters to an in-depth treatment of observation and behavioral assessment of speech behaviors and stated, "*How* we observe, *what* we observe, *where* we observe, and *when* we observe, and what we *do* with the observations is, as you will discover, a very complex process" (p. 46).

Skilled observation of communicative behavior is the basis of all effective efforts in evaluation and treatment of disorders, according to Kunze (1967), who stated that "techniques in the observation of communicative behavior should be systematically taught as the first step in our clinical training program and the student should have obtained observational skill before he faces his first practicum assignment." Kunze then outlined a program for helping students obtain these important observational skills that includes: (1) differentiation of behavioral events and behavioral impressions, (2) systematic data recording, (3) opportunity for recording practice, and (4) analysis of data.

The scientific approach to teaching/treatment/counseling, the need to validate techniques and strategies for learning, and the current emphasis on accountability actually mandate the systematic collection of data. The need for the supervisor to teach the supervisee the techniques of scientific observation and data collection is increased, and responsibility is placed on supervisors to model a similar approach to observation themselves in observation of the clinician.

There are many sources of information about collecting and utilizing data on client behavior that the supervisor can use in assisting supervisees and themselves to attain or improve observational skills. These sources also provide a basis for the evaluation of the observational competencies of students so necessary for competent evaluation and treatment (Diedrich, 1971b; Elbert & Geirut, 1986; Elbert, Shelton, & Arndt, 1967; Golper, McMahon, & Gordon, 1976; Hegde, 1985; Johnston & Harris, 1968; Mowrer, 1969, 1972, 1977; Shelton, Elbert, & Arndt, 1967).

Observation of the "More-Knowing"

Although not much has been written in speech-language pathology and audiology about the importance of observing the *clinician*, writers of textbooks on supervision in other areas have assumed that observation of teachers, counselors, social workers, and others of the "more-knowing" category is a primary responsibility of supervisors (Blumberg, 1980; Boyd, 1978; Harris, 1975; Hart, 1982; Kadushin, 1976; Kaslow, 1977; Kurpius et al., 1977; Munson, 1983). The work of Cogan (1973), Goldhammer (1969), and Goldhammer and colleagues (1980) particularly focused attention on observation of the behavior of the teacher, as well as the interaction in the classroom. Harris (1975) devoted an entire chapter of a book on supervision in education to observation and analysis of behavior in the classroom, in which he stated that classroom observation is "a complex activity but indispensable in the work of any supervisor" (p. 196). Systematic observation of supervisees, be they teachers, clinicians, counselors, social workers, or others, is crucial in the process of supervision. Observational techniques make the work of the supervisor more viable and meaningful, and lead to change in the supervisee through the use of data as feedback (Fleming, 1973). It is a most important activity, upon which the effectiveness and accuracy of the remainder of the supervisory process are dependent.

MYTHS ABOUT OBSERVATION

Certain myths seem to exist regarding observation as it relates to the interchange between supervisor and supervisee. Three common assumptions are (1) the supervisor has observed what happened in the classroom, treatment, assessment, counseling, or interview session prior to the interaction with the supervisee, (2) what the supervisor observed was accurately perceived and recorded, and therefore forms a valid basis for subsequent supervisor-supervisee interaction, and (3) observation is a simple act of looking and that the ability to observe "comes naturally"—at least as far as supervisors are concerned. These assumptions need examination.

Myth #1—Actuality of Observation

Conferences with supervisees are not always preceded by adequate observation. Excessive caseloads of supervisors or higher priorities for time for other activities may result in some supervisors meeting only the minimal ASHA requirements for observation in educational programs, which may not be sufficient for some supervisees. Sometimes only segments of the supervisee's activity are observed or the observation is intermittent. In the service delivery setting, such variables as the work load, the specific setting where treatment takes place, and other responsibilities of the supervisor may make it difficult or impossible for supervisors to observe consistently or adequately.

The supervisor who has not observed is at a disadvantage in most cases. All supervisors have heard glowing comments about what happened last week or in a previous session when they were not observing. Like the fish that got away, these reports may cover the gamut of accuracy. Whatever the particulars of the situation, if the supervisor has not observed the particular experience being discussed, then the data will come from the reporting of the supervisee. Its value will probably depend upon how well the supervisee has been trained in objective observation. If the clinician is not skilled in collecting and reporting such data, the discussion may take the form of a treatment of generalities. This does not necessarily imply that such interaction is useless, but it will be different from the interaction that utilizes carefully and systematically collected data.

Myth #2—Accuracy of Data

The second assumption, that the supervisor's data are accurate, is related to the larger topic of perception. It is well known that perceivers attend to different aspects of situations and of behavior. Their needs, values, purposes, and past experiences affect their categorization or coding of events or the way they describe them. Additionally, physical, cultural, and social contexts influence the perceiver's interpretation of behaviors and determine the kinds of inferences drawn from their observations (Schneider, Hastorf, & Ellsworth, 1979). Andersen (1981) found biases in supervisor ratings based on prior information about the supervisee. Familiarity with the supervisee was hypothesized to be a source of bias in Blodgett and colleagues' (1987) study of supervisor ratings. Hatten, Bell, and Strand (1983) and Runyan and Seal (1985) found lack of agreement among speech-language pathologists viewing the same clinical sessions.

Total objectivity is a myth (Goldhammer et al., 1980). The eternal struggle of supervisors is to minimize errors in perception and to exercise professional restraint to avoid making value judgments when their objective is the recording of observational data (Cogan, 1973). Nowhere is the admonition to "know thyself" more important to the supervisor than it is at the observational stage. The supervisor "needs firm knowledge about the effects of his perceptual sets, biases, and predispositions upon what he sees, how he responds to these events in the world around him, and how he forms inferences and hypotheses and judgments about them" (Cogan, 1973, p. 35).

Several realities come between the supervisor and objectivity in observation. Supervisors' own perceptual screens or inferential sets change the perceived events because supervisors see what they wish to see, make errors in perception, search for certain events, project into them, or are influenced by what makes them comfortable or anxious (Cogan, 1973). The human inclination to label, categorize, select events, and make judgments that support biases or strengthen beliefs is a constant threat to the ability to be objective in observation. Snap judgments may be made in which premature inferences are drawn. Such judgments are not a result of complex hypotheses, frequently are related to negative qualities, and are not usually conscious efforts (Schneider et al., 1979). These judgments may be difficult to control—it is what is done about them that matters. Someone has said that no one can keep people from making judgments. People can, however, control how they *act* as a result of the judgments they make.

A further problem in relation to objectivity and accuracy of data collection is the question of reactivity, usually referred to as the response of subjects to participation in research. The very presence of the supervisor may be a factor in changing the behaviors being observed. Research has consistently indicated that subjects change their behavior while being monitored, thereby affecting assessment and intervention (Hartman, 1982; Kazdin, 1982). Ventry and Schiavetti (1980) warned that the researcher should be alert to the reactive effects of tests, inventories, rating scales, videotapes, and tape recordings. "The act of observation may produce changes in the phenomenon under investigation" (Neale & Leibert, 1973, p. 165). Campbell and Stanley (1963) referred to the "play-acting, outguessing, up-for-inspection, I'm a guinea-pig, or whatever attitudes" (p. 20) that may be generated in such situations. Further, "The more novel and motivating the test device, the more reactive one can expect it to be" (Campbell & Stanley, 1963, p. 9). Ingrisano (1979) determined that audio- and videotape observations were reactive data-collection procedures in speech-language pathology research.

Brooks and Hannah (1966) suggested that "the presence of the supervisor in the classroom is visually distracting, inhibits the development of a close interpersonal relationship between the client and the student clinician, prohibits the atmosphere of personal privacy, and tends to subordinate the role of the student clinician in the eyes of the client" (pp. 383–384).

In attempting to become more scientific in their techniques, supervisors should assume that the basic facts on reactivity are as valid for supervision as they are for research. In an exhaustive chapter on the methods and tools of observational research, Borg and Gall (1983) presented information that would be extremely useful to supervisors who wish to explore this issue. Ingrisano (1979) applied the implications of his study of clinical reactivity to the supervisory process and suggested that supervisors may need to search for less reactive data collection procedures than audio- or videotaping. On the other hand, he said that it is possible "that a reactive response to observation may be desirable in the supervisory process. For example, a student clinician might monitor her or his own verbal behavior more carefully with the knowledge that she or he is being observed. For some student clinicians in practicum, a reactive response to observation could become a positive training device of the supervisor" (pp. 87–88). This is an important point in relation to the planning of the observation as advocated here.

Ingrisano further suggested the possibility of adaptation or desensitivity to observation over time. According to Kazdin (1982), however, there is no clear evidence that reactivity can be controlled by adaptation and, although a period of adaptation may be wise, it is not known how much time it requires. The researcher or decision-maker must collect enough data to ensure that the description is as accurate as possible (Evertson & Green, 1986). Thus, supervisors are left, as they are so often, with the alternative of saying that the truth may never be known. Reactivity is an important phenomenon for supervisors to consider in terms of the results of their observations, but there is little assistance offered for dealing with it.

Myth #3—Observation Skills Are Innate

The third assumption of the simplicity and the innate nature of observation is related to the lack of attention to supervisory methodologies in general. Specifically, it is related to the lack of education in observation and data-collection techniques for supervisors. Lack of such skills may make observation ineffective.

Speaking of the complexity of observing teacher behavior, Cogan (1973) said that there are no definitive inventories for supervisors to rely upon, rather, they must operate from "disciplined intuition" (p. 146). But is this enough? It has been shown that clinicians and supervisors can be trained to observe. Irwin and Nickles (1970) and Runyan and Seal (1985) suggested education of supervisors in observation techniques.

There is a clear analogy between the supervisory process and the research process at this point. The training of researchers has always emphasized the importance of precise data collection. If training and monitoring of observers are crucial in research (Borg & Gall, 1983; Frick & Semmel, 1978; Neale &

Liebert, 1973; Reid, 1982; Ventry & Schiavetti, 1980), is it any less important to attend to the observational skills of supervisors?

Even with such preparation, the large volume of behavior that surrounds the supervisor may be so great as to be unmanageable. The limitations on the supervisor's ability to see and record all important events becomes an issue. Kounin (1970) maintained that a good observation record should tell not only the truth but the whole truth. The difficulty of accomplishing this is obvious, but there is a further complication for supervisors. Even if all important events could be captured in notes or recordings of some kind, it is very probable that neither the supervisor nor the supervisee would be capable of utilizing or integrating all the data that might be obtained from a single observation. Supervisors need to learn how important it is, as a part of the planning component, *to limit the extent of the data collection* by deciding which behaviors will be the focus of the observation, how the observation will be conducted, and how and by whom the data will be recorded.

STRATEGIES FOR OBSERVATION

Variables in the selection of the method of observation include the setting; the philosophy, objectives, or personal preference of the participants; the availability of equipment; the time; and the training and experience of the supervisor and supervisee.

Observation Concurrent with the Treatment or Assessment Session

Probably the most frequently used form of observation is on-line recording, in which the supervisor is observing at the same time that the treatment or assessment session is being conducted. Observations may be done with the clinician and the client in the room or in an adjacent observation room.

Based on the previous discussion of reactivity, it is apparent that observers in the room with the clinician and the client will have some effect upon them. At the same time, clinicians and clients are usually conscious of the ever-present possibility of a live body on the other side of the window or at the video monitor. So, again, supervisors are left with the question of whether or not there is any way to observe the "real thing," and with the need to be sensitive to the possibilities of variations from the norm in behaviors during observations.

Videotape or Audiotape Recording

Speech-language pathologists and audiologists have used audio- and videotaping equipment to enhance the learning process with clients and clinicians since both types of equipment first became available (Mullendore, Koller, & Payne, 1976; O'Neil & Peterson, 1964; Schubert, 1978). Despite this long period of use, there is only a small amount of published research to demonstrate the usefulness of this equipment or to support any specific methodology or procedure.

The most extensive study of the use of videotape in the preparation of speech-language pathologists was conducted by Boone and Stech (1970). They reported that both audio- and videotape confrontation, viewing or listening, were useful in changing the behavior of clinicians. They also indicated that mere listening or viewing were not as powerful as when accompanied by the use of an analysis matrix on which clinicians recorded their behavior. Further, Boone and Stech found audiotape and behavioral scoring to be as effective in changing *verbal* behaviors as videotape confrontation, because, they said, 80 to 95 percent of the therapy process occurs at the verbal level. They added that this does not imply that videotape confrontation is not more effective in studying therapy. Rather, viewers of videotape should concentrate more on the nonverbal level—facial expressions and gestural cues, attending to the client, and behaviors used to punctuate therapy interaction.

Videotape recording as a teaching device in speech-language pathology was investigated by Hall (1971), Irwin (1972, 1975, 1981a,b), Irwin and Hall (1973), and Schubert and Gudmunson (1976). Most of their studies incorporated the microteaching techniques developed in education by Ivey (1971) and used in educating teachers and, later, counselors (microcounseling) (Kagan, 1970). This technique varies in its use but essentially follows this pattern: a short microlesson is conducted and videotaped, the tape is observed by clinician and supervisor, behaviors to be modified are identified, the lesson is redone and videotaped, another observation and analysis by supervisor and clinician is conducted to determine if behaviors have changed. Irwin (1981a) recommended this method for speech-language pathology and audiology education and made a case for further study of its use.

Schubert (1978) devoted several pages to the use of videotape recording for teaching, demonstration, and for self-analysis. He stated clearly that the videotape recording should not become a substitute for supervision (meaning, it is assumed, on-line observation), but should be used in conjunction with it. The quantification of behaviors from videotape provides an invaluable method of analyzing change in the clinical process.

Videotape equipment is no longer the exclusive tool of college and university programs. It is now found at many service delivery sites and can be used in the supervision of off-campus practicum, employees of the site, and Clinical Fellows. Butler (1974) reported on a model that used video- and audiotaping during his CFY in a school program and suggested that use of such a system enhances accountability in the work setting, as well as professional growth of the individual clinician. "The possibilities of field application are limited only by the imagination of the clinician and his willingness to use them" (p. 167).

As with any type of observation, audio- or videotaping is only as useful as the data that are collected and analyzed. Much listening to audiotapes or observing of videotapes by clinicians is probably a waste of time and tape because they have not been trained to observe or because the data collection has not been well planned. Farmer (1987) reviewed the literature on visual literacy and offered suggestions on more effective use of videotape recordings as well as suggestions for training in its use.

The video camera is a powerful teaching tool which has probably never been fully utilized in speech-language pathology or audiology—at least not as reflected in the literature or in the personal experience of the writer. Its use in observation, particularly self-observation, deserves much more in-depth study and experimentation by supervisors. Just looking at a videotape is not enough— observation must be directed, purposeful, and goal oriented.

Live Supervision

The term *live supervision* has come to have a special meaning in counseling and psychotherapy. As practiced in that discipline, or as it might be adapted to other disciplines, it becomes a combination of observation and feedback. In terms of observation, its relevance is that it implies not only the presence of the supervisor in the room but the actual participation of the supervisor in the therapy session. Personal experience with supervisors leads the writer to the conclusion that this type of supervision exists in speech-language pathology and especially in audiology. There are no definitive data to support this conclusion, however. A form of live supervision that has been given some attention in the literature is the "bug-in-the-ear" technique, an electronic device that allows the supervisor to communicate directly with the supervisee. (Boyiston & Tuma, 1980; Brooks and Hannah, 1966; Byng-Hall, 1982, Engnoth, 1974; Kadushin, 1976; Korner & Brown, 1952). Live supervision will be treated further in the discussion of feedback.

DEVELOPMENT OF OBSERVATIONAL TECHNIQUES

It is not the intent of the writer to detail the evolution of the use of observation in scientific efforts of the past, as interesting as it is. It is important, however, to recognize that the techniques of observation are a part of the scientific heritage, and have long been the tools of scientists who have studied behavior in anthropology, education, ethnology, sociology, psychology, and industry. Darwin, Freud, Piaget, Mead, and many others whose classic works are well known were all forerunners in the use of the now somewhat more sophisticated methods of observation used today in many disciplines. Given added impetus, particularly in education and in speech-language pathology and audiology, by the behavior modification movement, the approach to observation of behavior has become more complex and more structured than when the early scientists gathered their data. Over the past 25 years structured observation systems have proliferated and have had a powerful impact on the study of many types of interactions. (Simon & Boyer, 1970a,b, 1974) Currently, the emphasis on naturalistic or qualitative research is introducing still another approach to data collection that is important to supervisors. (Lincoln & Guba, 1985).

METHODS OF DATA COLLECTION

The understanding and appropriate use of systematic observation and data collection methods by supervisors is important to those who wish to see supervision raised to a more thoughtful, scientific, and validated process. Supervisors need to be skilled observers, but more than that, they must also develop efficient, practical procedures for recording their observations for later use.

The literature from many disciplines contains classifications of methods for recording data from observation. Some have application for speech-language pathology and audiology, many do not. The following discussion of data collection methods contains some already in use by supervisors and others that supervisors may wish to try for some variation in their current observational techniques.

Recording Evaluative Statements

The most traditional procedure, and perhaps the method of least effort or the most expediency for supervisors, is to simply write evaluative statements reflecting their perceptions of the appropriateness of the behaviors in the treatment or assessment session as they view it; for example, "Your directions were too difficult for the client" or "You did a good job of motivating him today." Such action is consistent with the Direct-Active Style of the Evaluation-Feedback Stage. This procedure may be expanded slightly as supervisors record behavioral data selected to support their judgments or to illustrate to the clinician what they perceived as good or poor clinical practice. This methodology is neither appropriate nor inappropriate *per se*. It may be decided during the planning component that there is a need for such direct evaluative procedures, if not in the entire session, at least in certain parts of it. As stated previously, however, it is these active, direct behaviors of the supervisor that do not *en*courage, in fact will probably *dis*courage, analysis of their own procedures and creative thinking on the part of supervisees.

It is not suggested that supervisors should never record evaluative or judgmental statements. If it has been determined that there is a need for such judgments at certain times, however, the aim of supervisors and supervisees should be to reduce their numbers as rapidly as possible and to involve the supervisee in more self-evaluation procedures. There are times when it may be decided that this is a more efficient procedure in a certain situation, that the behavior is too trivial for extensive data collection yet needs to be identified, that the clinician is trying to modify a specific clinical behavior but is unable to identify change as yet, or that it is appropriate for other reasons. The caution here should not be against occasional, but rather against habitual, use of the instant evaluation without rationale.

Tallies of Behaviors

Collection of baseline data or recording of data on clinician behaviors selected during the planning session by supervisors and supervisees may be done by a simple tallying by one or both—exactly the type of tallying and charting suggested earlier for clients. For example, if the clinician is working on a simple, straightforward goal such as decreasing the number of utterances of *O.K.* in his or her vocabulary, a simple tally by the supervisor over a period of time will measure the progress toward that goal. As clinicians gain more experience, they may be able to tally their own behavior within the session themselves, as well as using tapes. Certain reinforcement techniques, accurately or inaccurately evaluated target sounds, responses to clients, or other specific behaviors can be tallied in this manner. It may appear gratuitous to discuss this method since most supervisors and supervisees do this at some time. The important point for the Collaborative or Consultative Styles is that data collection on the behaviors of clinicians is planned jointly; that both participants are involved in some portion of the record keeping; and that it is done systematically, not occasionally at the whim of the supervisor.

Rating Scales

Rating scales may be used in observation when behaviors to be observed are known ahead of time and there is a need for qualitative data. In such instruments, behaviors or events are listed and value judgments are made as to the quality of the behaviors, that is, the degree to which the rater perceives that the behavior has been performed adequately or inadequately, appropriately or inappropriately. Rating scales direct the observation toward specific dimensions of behaviors and provide a way of recording judgments when this is desired (Cartwright & Cartwright, 1984). Rosenshine (1970) called them "high-inference systems" because they call for inference and judgment on the part of the observer, as opposed to analysis systems, which he called "low-inference" because of their relatively more objective nature. Many rating scales are of very poor quality, reflect the bias of those who constructed them, and have not been validated.

Rating scales of the type used for evaluations in speech-language pathology and audiology are usually not appropriate for tallying behaviors in the clinical sessions although they may sometimes be used in that way. If the descriptors are specific and are stated behaviorally they might be modified for data collection, which would then feed into the analysis and the evaluation. Generally, however, rating forms used for evaluation are not useful for data collection because of the global nature of the items and the inherent judgmental factor that is built in.

In addition to providing qualitative data on previously identified behaviors, rating scales are useful for making summary statements about performance over time. When used in this way, they should follow discussion of data collected during observations. The criteria for rating items should be clear to both supervisor and supervisee, and both should recognize the high-inference nature of the instrument. The use of rating scales should be discussed as a part of the total planning for the supervisory interaction. Used in this way, rating scales can be a profitable basis for discussion between supervisor and supervisee.

Verbatim Recording

Goldhammer (1969) dismissed audio- and videorecording, as well as rating scales or analysis systems, in favor of written recordings—not descriptive records, but *verbatim* transcripts that contain everything spoken or done during the lesson. These transcripts are then examined in the analysis stage. Goldhammer's reasoning is sound—observation schedules or rating scales force behavior into *a priori* categories, record supervisors' interpretations or perceptions, are often not reliable or valid, and may miss important behaviors. Audio- or videotapes are unmanageable unless submitted to extensive analysis. The practicality of Goldhammer's suggestion must be examined. The thought of recording everything that happens in an observation, making comments and questions in the margin, recording descriptions of nonverbal behaviors, identifying individual pupils and diagramming teacher and pupil positions, as recommended, is mind-boggling. One feels that Goldhammer's approach is more easily discussed than accomplished! Despite this, Goldhammer has made a contribution in his discussion of the need for *totality in recording* of the activities being observed and it is certainly not impossible, and in fact, is desirable for some purposes. Goldhammer and colleagues (1980), in their revision of Goldhammer's original book, modified Goldhammer's stance considerably, and stressed mainly the skill needed in note-taking and the suggestion that symbols, abbreviations, diagrams, schedules, and charts be used and that supervisors learn some type of shorthand or speedwriting—something that most supervisors have probably done already for self-preservation!

Selective Verbatim

Selective verbatim is an alternative to Goldhammer's method suggested by Acheson and Gall (1980), in which a verbatim transcript is made of only certain events or categories of events selected during the planning component by supervisor and teacher for study and analysis. Such recording can be done either concurrently with the lesson or from tapes. Supervisees may participate in such recording from tapes. Acheson and Gall listed the advantages of this system as (1) the teacher becomes sensitized to the verbal process in teaching, (2) the teacher does not have to respond to all aspects of the teaching-learning process, only those that have been selected, (3) an objective, noninterpretive record of behavior that can be analyzed is provided, and (4) it is a simple procedure. However, these advantages may also be problems, according to Acheson and Gall. The teacher, knowing what is to be recorded, may become self-conscious in using the behaviors or may use more of the target behaviors during the observation only. Other problems are the possibility of bias in the selection of behaviors and the way they are analyzed and interpreted, the possibility of selecting trivial behaviors, and the very real difficulties in keeping up with the verbal behaviors. Nevertheless, this is the type of data collection that can be planned jointly during the planning time based on the objectives. Logs, anecdotal reports, time samplings, or similar methods of capturing the events in the clinical session are also forms of selective verbatim recording.

Selective verbatim recording from tapes is a useful tool for self-analysis. Nothing reveals the inaccuracies, monotonies, ambiguities, and irregularities in a person's own verbosity as quickly as a written script. Although time-consuming, it is a potent tool for behavior change. For example, some clinicians have difficulty providing clear directions to their clients. This behavior may be treated as follows: The clinician makes verbatim transcriptions (from a tape) of a series of directions used in a session. Specific verbalizations that contribute to lack of clarity are identified and rewritten to obtain clarity. The modified behaviors are transferred to the next session and the process repeated until the objective of clear directions is reached.

In speech-language pathology, an innovative method of recording was devised by Block (1982) (Appendix E). Called the *Pre-Conference Observation System* (PCOS), it is a coding system that enables supervisors to record objective data which will become a basis for the feedback in the conference. Block stated, "Because of the objective nature of the supervisor's notes, the supervisory conference becomes an interchange of shared information rather than a monologue of rights versus wrongs from the supervisor's point of view" (p. 2). The PCOS utilizes to some extent the selective verbatim method of Acheson and Gall for recording certain client and clinician behaviors such as giving directions, models, responses and verbal reinforcements. Block also used other techniques such as a standard set of symbols, initials, abbreviations, and various placements on the page, all of which make up a kind of shorthand. Block found positive attitudes toward the system in a study of its use by 14 supervisors in clinic and school practicum settings. These supervisors listed the following advantages of the system: (1) improved recall of incidents in the clinical session, (2) a better basis for agreement with students when perceptions of events differed, and (3) improved concentration during the observation. A significant number indicated that they would use the PCOS again. One hour was deemed sufficient to train supervisors in the use of the system. The system could also be used for self-analysis by clinicians. Supervisors could also add their own symbols to this system to fit different situations.

Interaction Analysis Systems

The most structured form of recording observations is the interaction analysis system which has been used for many years in several disciplines, especially education, counseling, and psychotherapy (Amidon & Flanders, 1967; Bales, 1950; Simon & Boyer, 1970a, b, 1974).

Interaction analysis systems developed out of a need for discovering the relationship between events and the desire to correlate those interactional patterns with certain outcomes (Brandt, 1975). They are more highly structured examples of the checklists for tallying events, which were discussed earlier, but are different in that they are constructed in such a way that interactions *between* events can be analyzed and patterns identified. They have been developed by taking the behaviors that occur in teaching or in clinical sessions and categorizing them into sets that are distinguishable from each other, relevant to the purpose of the observation, and mutually exclusive, that is, all behaviors with common characteristics are placed in a category. Although most of the interaction analysis systems seem to have been developed originally for research purposes, they are also useful in supervision.

The use of such systems by supervisors or in self-study by the supervisee is based on the assumption that the supervisee will change behavior as a result of feedback. These systems are useful and, in some instances, indispensable; but they should not be seen as a panacea, as they have been by some.

A few systems have been developed in speech-language pathology and audiology, but they do not seem to be used as frequently as they were at one time. They are presented here because of their potential for use in supervision, research, and self-study in structuring observations and data collection. Before discussing the systems themselves, the advantages and disadvantages of their use will be presented. (Several interaction analysis systems for use with the supervisory conference are available and will be discussed later. The advantages and disadvantages of the systems listed here also apply to those used for the conference.)

Advantages of Interaction Analysis Systems

There are many advantages in the use of interaction analysis systems. The quantity of behaviors in most situations where observation takes place is usually so great that it must be structured in some way that enables the observer to analyze the total. Some people may be able to do this without observation systems, but certainly they make such analysis quicker, easier, and relatively more reliable. The systems also help establish a baseline and a record of progress for included behaviors. Analysis systems are helpful in training students or supervisors in the observation process—to sort individual behaviors out of the global mass of new behaviors they may be encountering as they take on clinical or supervisory tasks (Golper et al., 1976). They help observers focus their attention. They allow comparisons between sessions and simplify both the recording of data and the feedback. They also provide "grist" for the analysis component. When used by clinicians themselves, analysis systems help them become aware of components of clinical sessions as well as their own behaviors—perhaps one of the best uses, in fact, is for this self-recognition and self-analysis. They may contribute to clearer communication between supervisors and supervisees about the clinical session, especially if the behaviors are described specifically and unambiguously. They are more objective in their classification and identification of behaviors because the behaviors are operationalized and ground rules usually given for categorizing ambiguous behaviors. Certainly they reduce a large amount of the opinion, judgment, some of the inaccuracies, impressions, misinterpretations, and plain poor memory which may go into a less structured observation. One reads occasionally that observations where systems are used are less threatening to the observed, because the evaluation component is lacking. However, this seems questionable. One must ask what it is that presents the threat—the presence of the observer or the methodology?

Disadvantages of Interaction Analysis Systems

The disadvantages of interaction analysis systems may be found in their construction, their use, or their interpretation. The assumption that they are "objective" is a dangerous one. It is true that they do force a certain amount of objectivity onto the observer because the behaviors are preselected and defined. However, that very selection may be reflective of the bias of those who constructed it or it may reflect a specific theoretical approach. Additionally, the possibility of subjectivity in the process of using the system, that is, interpretation, selection of one category over another, or perceptual errors, is ever present.

Some analysis systems for the clinical process focus on the process but not on the content, giving incomplete information. Thus, a question may be checked as a question but nothing is known about the type of question or its appropriateness without further analysis. Further, they usually do not relate to the efficacy of the treatment. What happened is identified and quantified, but its effectiveness is still open to the judgment of the observer. Additionally, most systems do not account for nonverbal behavior.

The volume of behavior included in the system may be so great that it is not only difficult to record all of it, even with an analysis system, but it may then be impossible to manipulate it to make it meaningful. At the same time, the types of behaviors are limited; therefore, many important behaviors may be missed.

Supervisors or clinicians may become too dependent on such systems, limiting their ability or opportunity to look at the "large picture." Many analysis systems are poorly constructed and have not had their reliability and validity established. But perhaps the greatest sin against such systems is that they are often equated by their users with evaluation procedures, which they are not, nor were they ever intended to be. The writer has often heard the *Content and Sequence Analysis System* devised by Boone and Prescott (1972) referred to as the "Boone evaluation form" or has heard a supervisor say "I evaluated her on the Boone." This misconception was clear in a survey in which, when supervisors were asked to indicate the evaluation instruments they used, they listed the Boone and Prescott (1972) system and the ABC (Schubert et al., 1973), which are both interaction analysis systems, with such evaluation instruments as the Pennsylvania State Practicum Evaluation Form (Klevans & Volz, 1974) and the W-PACC (Shriberg et al., 1975), which are truly evaluation forms (Schubert & Aitchison, 1975). In a later discussion of these systems, the differences will be identified and more information provided about how analysis systems should be used.

Despite the seeming greater weight of the negatives listed previously, interaction analysis systems are invaluable tools in the supervisory process when chosen well and used properly. The next section will provide guidelines for choice and evaluation of the instruments.

Selection and Use

Certain guidelines must be followed in choosing and using interaction analysis systems. They are only as good as the reason for which they are used, the way they are constructed, and the way they are used. In other words, one must know what data one wishes to collect and select the analysis system accordingly. Users must be constantly alert to the strengths and weaknesses for the particular situation.

A valuable outline of criteria for the developers and users of interaction analysis systems has been provided by Herbert and Attridge (1975), which includes three categories of criteria: identifying, validity, and practicality.

Identifying criteria are those which enable users to select the instrument that is correct for their purpose and application. These include such items as appropriateness of the title to the system's purpose, the rationale or theoretical support, the specificity of its uses, and the behaviors included.

Validity criteria include characteristics such as clarity, lack of ambiguity and consistency with theory. Under this heading, Herbert and Attridge suggested questioning whether the items are exhaustive (that is, include all behaviors of the kind being studied, even if it is labeled "other"), are representative of the dimensions of the behavior being studied (related to sampling and generalizability), and are mutually exclusive (Can behaviors be classified into one category only?). They also stated that, in addition to procedures for use, ground rules should be provided to assist the coder in making individual decisions about borderline or unusual behaviors. Other characteristics related to validity are nature and degree of inference to be made from items, context, observer effect, reliability, and validity measures.

Practicality criteria include relevance of items, method of coding, qualifications and training for observers, and provisions made for collection and recording of data.

Unfortunately, no interaction analysis systems known to the writer meet the high standards of Herbert and Attridge. Nevertheless, users who are knowledgeable about the criteria will at least know the strengths and weaknesses of the systems they are using and will be able to make adjustments accordingly. Further, preparation and practice with the systems is crucial to their effective use. Anyone wishing to utilize interaction analysis systems, especially for research, should become familiar with the Herbert and Attridge criteria.

ANALYSIS SYSTEMS IN SPEECH-LANGUAGE PATHOLOGY AND AUDIOLOGY

Although interaction analysis systems have not proliferated in speech-language pathology and audiology as they have in some other disciplines, there was a surge of interest in this methodology during the late 1960s and early 1970s, coming out of the behavioral paradigm originally described by B. F. Skinner

(Johnson, 1971). Systems for use in studying the clinical process were developed by Boone and Prescott (1972), Diedrich (1969, 1971a), Johnson (1970, 1971), Schubert and colleagues (1973), Conover (1979), and Brookshire, Nicholas, Krueger, and Redmond (1978). Other systems for studying the nonverbal behavior in interviews have been developed (Farmer, 1980; Klevans & Semel, no date; Shipley, 1977).

Even though the use of these systems is not as common as it once was, they are presented here because of their potential as tools for supervisors. Later there will be a discussion of this potential as well as other methods of recording behavior.

Content and Sequence Analysis of Speech and Hearing Therapy

The Content and Sequence Analysis of Speech and Hearing Therapy (Boone, 1970; Boone & Prescott, 1972; Boone & Stech, 1970; Prescott, 1971), based on an operant model, provides a method of quantifying certain behaviors of clinicians and clients in the clinical session. For clinicians, the behaviors are (1) Explain, Describe; (2) Model, Instruction; (3) Good Evaluative; (4) Bad Evaluative; and (5) Neutral-Social. For clients, the behaviors are (6) Correct Response, (7) Incorrect Response, (8) Inappropriate Social, (9) Good Self-Evaluative, and (10) Bad Self-Evaluative. In their presentation of the instrument, Boone and Prescott (1972) listed the values to be obtained from its use: clinicians in educational programs can (1) analyze the content and sequence of events in their own therapy, (2) study the therapy of master clinicians, and (3) study various parameters of the clinical process. Experienced clinicians can study their own interaction with their clients in their own work setting. A new focus is placed on the therapy process, rather than the historically common practice of concentrating on pre- and posttherapy evaluation. All behaviors are recorded on a matrix and a summary form is available for analysis of the collected data.

The publication of *The Content and Sequence Analysis of Speech and Hearing Therapy* had a major impact on supervisors and clinicians in speech-language pathology and audiology. It was probably the first time that an instrument had so clearly "dissected" the clinical process. Supervisors in educational programs found it useful in preparing students to observe and identify components of the clinical process, to quantify the behaviors included in the system, to keep records of changes in those behaviors, to identify patterns of interactions and a multitude of other clinical activities. Its appeal also contributed in some instances to misuse, overuse, and overinterpretation. The writer recalls hearing one off-campus supervisor complain that some students assigned to her had been "Booned-to-death" in a university program—an interesting example of "verbing"! But it did point out a very real problem. The categories are limited in number and what this frustrated supervisor meant was that the students were unaware of the importance of behaviors other than those included in the system.

An additional misuse is the assumption that the system is the equivalent of an evaluation form. Inferences and assumptions can be made from the data collected by using the system but, in itself, it does not contain the rating aspect of an evaluation form. The feedback is quantitative, not qualitative.

The system meets many of the criteria stated by Herbert and Attridge (1975), but not all. Users of the system, particularly for research, might wish to evaluate it more thoroughly on the basis of these criteria. It is useful in the clinical session for collecting data on clinician/client interaction. It is also easily learned, practical, and quantifies behaviors particularly important to an operant approach to therapy (although not totally irrelevant for other types).

The Analysis of Behavior of Clinicians (ABC) System

Probably the next most familiar interaction analysis system for use in speech-language pathology is the *Analysis of Behavior of Clinicians (ABC) System* (Schubert, 1978; Schubert et al., 1973). The ABC is an example of a timed system. Behaviors are recorded at 3-second intervals or when a behavior changes within a 3-second interval. by writing down the numbers assigned to that behavior.

The ABC categories are directly derived from the categories of the original Flanders (1970) system, which was based on behavior of teachers and children in the classroom. They include the following clinician categories: (1) Observing and Modifying Lesson Appropriately, (2) Instruction and Demonstration, (3) Auditory and/or Visual Stimulation, (4) Auditory and/or Visual Positive Reinforcement of Client's Correct Response, (5) Punishment, (6) Auditory and/or Visual Positive Reinforcement of Client's Incorrect Response, (7) Clinician Relating Irrelevant Information and/or Asking Irrelevant Questions, (8) Using Authority or Demonstrating Disapproval. Client categories include: (9) Client Responds Correctly, (10) Client Responds Incorrectly, (11) Client Relating Irrelevant Information and/or Asking Irrelevant Questions, Category 12 is Silence.

The system has the same purpose as the Boone and Prescott system—to quantify behaviors in the clinical session so that supervisors and clinicians can more accurately recognize, recall, and analyze the behaviors and sequential patterns.

The ABC system provides information similar to that obtained by the system developed by Boone and Prescott. In a comparison of the two methods, Schubert and Glick (1974) found that the two systems obtain essentially the same information when the therapy consists mainly of stimuli, response, and reinforcement. However, in a long occurrence of one behavior, such as reading a story in a language lesson, the ABC naturally gave a much clearer indication of the length of time spent on this category. The final conclusion was that both systems provide useful, objective information about the clinical session.

The ABC should also be evaluated against the Herbert and Attridge (1975) criteria to determine its appropriateness for the particular situation in which it is used. The same statements can be made about the ABC that were made about the Boone-Prescott system—behaviors are limited and the same opportunities for misuse exist.

Multidimensional Scoring System

The *Multidimensional Clinical Process Scoring System* developed by Diedrich (1969, 1971a) and Johnson (1970, 1971a) was the result of a long and extraordinarily detailed probing of the dynamics of the clinical process. Relating the clinical process to the communication process, they drew from the literature on both verbal and nonverbal interaction in communication, information on interaction analysis systems from education and psychology, the behavioral paradigm of Lindsley (1964), and the work of Porch (1967) to develop a training and research tool in speech pathology. Forty categories of behavior were included in the system and a protocol for scoring was included. The complexity of the system made it impractical for use as a supervision tool and the authors have recently indicated (Diedrich, personal communication, 1986; Johnson, personal communication, 1986) that work on the system was terminated. This is unfortunate because the instrument, if it had been refined further, could have been invaluable both in clinical research and in supervision.

Quantification and Description of Clinical Interaction with Aurally Handicapped Children

Another system was developed by Prescott and Tesauro (1974) for quantifying interactions in a parent-child-clinician therapy session in a simulated home environment. Seventeen behaviors that accounted for both manual and oral communications and combinations of the two are included in the system. Scoring and analysis procedures are similar to the Boone-Prescott system. A high degree of intra- and interjudge reliability was reported. It is not known how widely this system has been used, but it appears that it would produce useful information for parents and clinicians.

Conover Verbal Analysis System

An alternative to the Boone-Prescott and the ABC systems was developed by Conover (1979). The system is presented as more easily used than the others. Each of the seven clinician categories and the four client categories are assigned symbols: *Clinician*—Authority (A), Information (I), Model (M), Stimulate (St), Reward (R), Punishment (P), Social (So), and *Client*—Question (Q), Correct Response (CR), Incorrect Response (IR), and Social (S). The behaviors can be charted, recording the symbols in either a linear or a horizontal manner, so that interactions or patterns of responses can be identified. Frequency and percentages of behaviors can then be summarized and interactions noted. Conover suggested that it be used as a tool for clinical training from the beginning of the students' training sequence—as a means of helping them learn to observe and later for their own use in self-supervision. Many of the categories are similar to those found in other systems, and as with many, reflect the interest of the developer. Reliability and validity data are not provided for the system and it is obviously also limited in the behavior it includes. A rationale is given for the choice of each behavior. The system has use in recording behaviors in supervision but unless validated, is not suitable for clinical research.

Clinical Interaction Analysis System (CIAS)

Brookshire and colleagues (1978) developed a system specifically to identify the interaction in aphasia therapy. They addressed what they believe is a major weakness of other interaction analysis systems, namely, that they provide means of recording client and clinician behaviors but not the parameters of the treatment program—the nature and complexity of the treatment tasks, and the adequacy of the client's responses to those tasks. They maintained that, in order to evaluate the efficacy of treatment, the coding system should include records about the task, the client's responses, and the behavioral interaction between clinician and client. Thirty-nine events categories are listed under eight major categories: (1) Type of Clinician Behavior, (2) Complexity of Request, (3) Manner, (4) Materials, (5) Expected Response, (6) Support, (7) Patient Response, (8) Clinician Feedback. A shortened version of 26 events for easier use in live supervision has been constructed and validated, and reliability data have been presented for each item. Brookshire (personal communication, 1986) recently revealed that, despite efforts to further reduce the length of the system and to include a more evaluative component, the system did not capture as much of the subjective nature of the clinical interaction as the developers had hoped. They, too, have discontinued work on the system.

Systems for Recording Behavior in Interviews

Skill in interviewing is certainly an important component of the clinical process and one in which most supervisors find their clinicians involved at some time. Three systems for scoring interview behaviors are known to the writer.

Shipley (1977) presented an observation method for the interview which included a mixture of verbal and nonverbal categories with their definitions as follows: Encouragement, Orientation, Information-Seeking—high (requires high level response), Information-Seeking—low (requires low level response), Interpretation/Evaluation, Neutral/Social, Positive Head Nod, Negative Head Nod, Forward Body Lean, Backward Body Lean, Smile, Touch, Guggle/Interruption (*guggle* is a term that describes less overt behaviors than interruptions and which decrease or redirect the interviewer's utterances), and Silence. Descriptions of each behavior are included.

Shipley reported high intraobserver reliability but generally lower interobserver agreement, suggested that the results were encouraging for clinical use, and that clinicians using the instrument have increased their awareness of the behaviors that facilitate or inhibit communication. There are limitations in this system, but it is included here because it is another example of a set of behaviors assumed to be important in the clinical activities of speech-language pathologists and audiologists and because it introduces certain nonverbal behaviors.

Farmer's *Interview Analysis System* (1980) was modified from the Conover system and is a combined objective recording system and subjective rating form. The interviewer records an entire interview, transcribes a 15-minute segment, and then codes each response in the dialogue between the interviewer and the informant. For the interviewer, categories include Authority, Information, Open Question, Specific Question, Reward, Punish, Social, and Miscellaneous. For the informant, categories include Question, Desired Response, Undesired Response, Social, and Miscellaneous. A coding system is provided as well as a lengthy critique section. No reliability or validity data are given, but Farmer recommends it as a useful procedure for looking at interaction behaviors, understanding why the interview did or did not work, and becoming more proficient in interviewing.

A more extensive system for observing verbal interaction in the interview is the Molyneaux/Lane Interview Analysis (Molyneaux & Lane, 1982). The authors have developed a system for identifying 64 types of utterances made by interviewers and respondents, which also includes a method of identifying *expressed* feelings about the utterances—positive, negative, or ambivalent. The numerical coding system makes computer analysis possible. Included are training exercises for students as well as procedures and forms for analysis of the collected data. High student inter- and intrarater reliability are reported. The book contains a thorough discussion of interviewing skills in addition to the analysis system.

Observing Nonverbal Behavior

The tendency to concentrate on verbal behavior makes it easy to forget the importance of nonverbal behavior, especially as it relates to affective components of interaction. Certainly interaction between persons cannot be discussed without acknowledging the importance of nonverbal behavior in communicating meaning, either through facial expressions, body position, or gestures (Darley, Glucksberg, & Kinchla, 1986). Many of the current studies on nonverbal communication consider it as the analogue of the state of the mind. Nonverbal behavior is assumed to be less consciously controlled than verbal behavior. Nonverbal behavior may either support, contradict, substitute for, complement, accent, or relate and regulate verbal behavior. Where there are inconsistencies between the two, the listener is more likely to believe the nonverbal (Condon, 1977). Many scholars have researched the intricacies of nonverbal communication and all clinicians and supervisors should be aware of the importance of this phenomenon (Birdwhistell, 1952, 1970; Hall, 1959, 1966, Knapp, 1972, Mehrabian, 1969; 1971).

Unfortunately, popular literature in the past few years has encouraged an overemphasis on and overinterpretation of nonverbal behavior. Many of the "how-to" books related to interpersonal interaction, communication, or success in life, careers, and social life have oversimplified the meaning of nonverbal communication. It is tempting to move ahead of complex scientific analysis and speculate about such behavior. "If we are at all serious about understanding our nonverbal expressiveness in interpersonal communication, we must be somewhat cautious. There is a great difference between reading and reading *into* the expressions of others" (Condon, 1977, p. 106).

This is a particularly important warning for the supervisor. It is difficult, if not impossible, for individuals to interpret most of the nonverbal cues directed at themselves. How much more difficult it is to interpret as an observer! Not everyone reacts in the same way to nonverbal cues. Much interpretation is dependent upon the context as well as the observer's own perceptual processes, attitudes, beliefs, and expectations (Stewart & D'Angelo, 1975). Cultural factors may also account for differences in nonverbal behaviors, which lead to misunderstanding. Therefore, for the supervisor to interpret the meaning of the clinician's behavior to a client or its effect on the client, or vice versa, is folly.

Nevertheless, such behaviors are an important part of clinical interaction and, no doubt, are frequently recorded by supervisors, whether or not they can be interpreted accurately. Often they are obviously distracting; at other times the effect on the client can be observed in backing away from a clinician, facial expression, or other movement.

Johnson (1970, 1971) and Diedrich (1969, 1971a) incorporated several nonverbal aspects of behavior into their *Multidimensional Clinical Process Scoring System*—postural-gestural, facial affect, tactual contact, vocal quality, and intonation. Shipley (1977) considered the nonverbal component important enough to include six nonverbal behaviors and one that might be either verbal or nonverbal in his interviewer behavior categories.

The writer is aware of only one system specifically developed to identify nonverbal and implicit verbal behavior in the clinical interaction in speech-language pathology—*Nonverbal Behavior Systems* (Klevans & Semel, no date). Based on the work of Mehrabian (1969, 1971), the system has not been published. It includes both a scoring component and a five-point rating scale which includes a list of desirable and undesirable nonverbal actions. Categories in Part I of the system, which is scored live or with the use of videotape, include Immediacy Dimension (distance, body lean, facial observation, touching), Relaxation Dimension (arm symmetry, hand relaxation, leg symmetry), and Responsiveness Dimension (facial activity, head movement, gesticulation, self or object manipulation, leg or foot movement). Part II includes implicit verbal behaviors which are coded from audiotape recordings. These include syllables spoken, total talking time, speaking rate, pronounced silence, speech volume, and thought units. Reliability and validity data and scoring sheets are included, as well as rationale and instructions. No further information is available on the use of the system. It is included here as an example of the type of analysis that might be utilized for nonverbal behavior.

WHERE HAVE ALL THE SYSTEMS GONE?

Methodology for collecting data is a crucial variable in the supervisory chain of events, particularly in moving it toward the realm of the scientific. In actuality, the efforts to approach observation of the clinical process, and therefore, its assessment, more scientifically through the development of interaction analysis systems, seem to have had a brief history and limited attention in speech-language pathology and audiology. Most of the systems were never published; others have apparently been abandoned by the developers for such reasons as loss of interest, complexity of the task, cessation of funding, or higher priority of other interests. Some enjoyed a brief era of popularity and now seem to have been forgotten. At the same time, other disciplines, particularly education, have continued to examine the specifics of the teaching/learning process through the development and use of interaction analysis systems (Evertson & Green, 1986). Speech-language pathology and audiology, however, has been left with relatively the same type of systems available since the 1970s and even these seem to be used infrequently.

This raises several questions. Is this a reflection of the lack of concern in the profession about the clinical and supervisory *processes* resulting in a modicum of research on or with analysis systems? Does the decrease in the use of these systems reflect a lack of interest by supervisors in a more structured form of data recording? Do such systems seem to involve too much work? Is it a rejection of the place of analysis in the supervisory process in favor of direct evaluation? Did the systems not tap important dimensions of the clinical process? Or are they perceived not to be useful? Are researchers or supervisors any worse off for not having more structured or more validated ways of observing and recording those observations? Are such methods any more reliable than the "old-fashioned" way of observing? Are they considered only another form of tallying, albeit more structured, providing more information, and slightly more objective?

Has anything been lost then, in not continuing to develop or validate analysis systems? Is this a direction for clinical research? There are no data at this time to indicate the important components of the clinical process. Are such systems the way to obtain this information? Are they of enough value to supervisors and researchers to continue their development? Even when observation systems are used, the user is left with the need to make subjective analyses of the data. And, although several of the systems include a matrix of some type for analysis, they are still subject to the biases of their developers and their users. This issue of subjectivity in the development and use of the systems and the high inference necessary in recording the behaviors and in making meaningful interpretations and assumptions from those recordings is monumental. But is that not comparable to the assessment process, where, no matter how many tests are given, there is still the necessity for subjective integration and interpretation of information?

The use of interaction analysis systems, as with each of the methods of recording behavior described here, must be seen as appropriate or inappropriate according to the variables in the situation. And supervisors, as well as supervisees, must constantly be alert to the limitations of each method.

The reader might ask at this point why such an extensive discussion of analysis systems is included if they are used so infrequently and have so many disadvantages. It is the writer's belief that the possibilities of interaction analysis systems were never fully explored and that because so few of these systems have been published, they probably are not well known to many supervisors. Despite the weaknesses inherent in each system, they have great utility for supervisors, particularly if used carefully with full knowledge of their limitations. Perhaps, as a result of reading this discussion, someone will become interested enough to pursue the intricacies of the clinical process further, will find such procedures a helpful beginning, and will improve upon the systems.

Other Methods of Recording Observations

Traditional approaches to clinical intervention and assessment techniques are being modified rapidly with the advent of new knowledge and technologies. These new developments in the clinical process have required changes of focus and methodologies for observation and data collection and for transcribing and analyzing client behavior (Fey, 1986; Gallagher & Prutting, 1983; Lund & Duchan, 1983; Miller, 1981; Prutting, Bagshaw, Goldstein, Juskowitz, & Umen, 1978; Snow, Midkiff-Borunda, Small, & Proctor, 1984). Current developments in the treatment of phonological disorders differ from the traditional approaches to articulation therapy (Bernthal & Bankson, 1981; Elbert & Gierut, 1986), with accompanying changes in emphasis on the recording of data. The focus on pragmatics and the ensuing methods of recording language samples, analyzing discourse, and describing conversational interactions has created new tools for the clinician (Prutting & Kirchner, 1983, 1987). The further development of naturalistic or ethnographic methodologies in research will surely provide insights that will be of value to the supervisor and supervisee in the collection of clinical data (Leech, 1976; Lincoln & Guba, 1985; Schieffelin, 1979). The use of computer technology in the clinical process (Palin & Cohen, 1986) has already brought major changes to the profession. Oratio (1979) described the use of a computer program for analyzing the clinical process in educational programs, research, and treatment. Multimedia such as movies, slides, videotapes, and filmstrips (Shanks, 1984), and the availability of a plethora of commercial materials and programs may in time change the focus and the methods of observation. It seems predictable that the future holds much that will require adjustment, flexibility, and innovation on the part of supervisors. Supervisors will surely adapt the new techniques for studying client behavior to analogous systems for studying clinician behavior, as well as the supervisory process.

PLANNING THE OBSERVATION

Observation should not "just happen." Given the vast amount of behavior available to supervisor and supervisee in the clinical session, and the variability in recording methods, some selection must be made to make the observation manageable and the later analysis meaningful. Like all other activities, the planning should be done jointly by the participants. At the Evaluation-Feedback Stage, the bulk of the decision making about observation will probably be done by the supervisor. As the participants move away from this stage, there will be more participation by the supervisee in deciding what behaviors are important enough for data collection. This moves the interaction away from the traditional style, where behaviors to be observed are selected by the supervisor, possibly after entering the observation situation. With planning, data collection can be more organized. Probably more happily, however, the observer will not try to cover the entire session, but rather its important components or those about which the supervisee has concerns.

Planning for observation should take place at different times during the supervision sequence. It certainly will occur at the beginning when long-range plans are being worked out and also throughout the supervision sequence as plans are being made for subsequent therapy sessions or conferences.

Early Planning for Observation

The teaching of observational skills for assessment experiences appears to be a given for student clinicians, but observation of clinical sessions has a slightly different focus. When supervisees begin their clinical experiences they may need specific assistance from the supervisor in data collection methods. Although they have encountered the academic treatment of data collection, the real clinical world application is another kettle of fish. This may be one of the first tasks of the supervisor—to teach data collection methods or assist in their application. Clinicians need to learn that certain observation tools exist for their use, but should not perceive such tools as the exclusive approach to data collection. This responsibility of supervisors is documented in Task 6—Assisting the supervisee in observing and analyzing assessment and treatment sessions—of the ASHA list of tasks and competencies (ASHA, 1985b).

At the beginning stages of planning for the supervisory experience, certain general principles about observation should be discussed as required by each supervisee. This discussion will cover such topics as the purpose and importance of data collection, the supervisee's past experiences and skills in recording data, potential methodologies for recording both client and clinician data and the possible reasons for selecting one or another of those methodologies, the responsibilities of the supervisor for observation, the responsibility of clinicians for data collection on the client and on themselves, and the preferences, biases, or feelings of each participant about observation. A thorough, rational, objective discussion of the purposes of observation at this point will encourage efficient and effective data collection; it may also relieve some of the anxieties of the supervisees if they know what is to be recorded.

Clinicians must be helped to see at a very early point in their education that, without complete, accurate, ongoing data collection on their clients, as well as on their own behaviors, there is no measurement, no accountability. They must learn that they, as well as the supervisor, have responsibilities for data collection that will benefit them as well as the client.

Mawdsley (1985b) developed a useful instrument that could be used at this point—the *Kansas Inventory of Self-Supervision* (KISS) (Appendix F). Mawdsley assumed that supervisors will be attempting to assist students in modifying one clinician behavior at a time. Thus, the instrument includes one page for use of O.K., clinician versus client talk time, positive reinforcement, corrective feedback, group management rotation rate, response rate, and clinician response to client social comments. Each page includes a different method for recording data on the specific behavior and a method for analysis. This creative approach to data collection and analysis could be expanded to other clinical behaviors, and to the supervisory process.

Data collection may seem to be a given, but even in educational programs where data collection is part of the clinical methodology taught to clinicians, supervisors often have to be vigilant in determining that it is actually done. Many clinicians, and indeed, supervisors, resist data collection. It is sometimes hard work, and is often tedious. It requires concentration and purpose. Clinicians often take great pains to collect objective data on the client during the diagnostic period but then do not continue the collection of the same kind of objective data to measure progress during therapy. Rather, comments about therapy may be subjective and evaluative (Turton, 1973). Long-range planning for observation of the clinical session makes it more meaningful to clinicians and results in a greater commitment to the task. A clear, specific intent to collect certain data will make the clinical process not only more purposeful, but more interesting. Tangible evidence of change is much more reinforcing than subjective guesses about results of therapy. Clinicians also need to understand that responsibility for data collection does not end with the receipt of their degree—it continues into the job setting, wherever it may be.

There are advantages for the supervisor, too, in planning the data collection. Tangible evidence of progress in the supervisees for whom they are responsible is also rewarding to them. Definite goals for data collection keep the observation more interesting. Any supervisor who has ever nodded off momentarily in the dark shadows of the observation room will probably welcome structure and direction in the data collection task.

Who Does the Data Collection?

Supervisors and supervisees will have different responsibilities for data collection, depending upon the situation. Basically, there is a natural division of labor between supervisor and supervisee in terms of data collection. The supervisee collects client data as a part of the treatment or assessment session or later via audio- or videotape; the supervisor usually collects data on the clinician or the interaction between clinician and client. There will be times when supervisors, to be truly collaborative, also will collect data on clients for certain purposes, for example, to check the reliability of the clinician's observations, to gather data about behaviors that cannot be collected during the session by the clinician, to identify behaviors not perceived by clinicians, or to record the unexpected. Particularly at the beginning of the interaction, both participants will want to collect baseline data on the clinician for purposes of establishing objectives, parallel to the process used for clients.

At some point, clinicians will need to be responsible for collecting data on their own behavior, as well as that of the client. Clinicians can develop an awareness of their own abilities through the analysis of their own audio- or videotape recordings (Boone & Stech, 1970). Some clinicians may reach the stage where they can collect data on certain of their own behaviors during the clinical session. This is one of the areas where supervisees must be involved if a true collaborative relationship is to develop and if they are going to learn the process of self-analysis and self-evaluation.

Ongoing Planning of Observation

A portion of every conference should be used for dual planning of the details of the observation of the next clinical session. Just as selection of client data to be collected depends upon the stated objectives, so does the collection of clinician data. Progress of *clinicians* toward their objectives must be measured just as client behavior is measured. Once again there is the blending of one component of the supervisory process into another. Establishing the relationship and determining needs leads to planning and setting of objectives. Data collection planning comes directly out of those objectives—with space left for serendipity! (Goldhammer et al., 1980)

Leaving space for serendipity is an important point. Despite the stress placed here on planning the observation, supervisors and supervisees must allow for the unexpected. Too much planning may be restrictive (Evertson & Green, 1986).

Observation that is not planned but left to the supervisor's choice, however, is then subject to supervisor bias. What supervisors will see and choose to record as they observe without planning will depend to a great extent upon their theoretical base, their own mood or feelings at the particular time, and the importance their own professional experience or expertise places on certain aspects of the clinical session such as direction giving, stimulation, reinforcement, modeling, client participation, expansion, and feedback (Roberts & Naremore, 1983). These parameters provide the framework through which every clinical interaction is visualized and can be just as limiting as some interaction analysis systems.

Unplanned, subjective observations also make it difficult to document change or to provide feedback other than evaluative judgments based on impressions. Supervisees, too, may have their own framework for the components of the clinical process which may differ from that of the supervisor. If this is true, care must be taken that both viewpoints are given consideration in the planning. If the supervisor's choice dominates and the supervisee's sense of what should be observed begins to conform as the interaction proceeds, some questions must be asked. Is the supervisor too active or direct? Is the supervisee too inexperienced, unknowledgeable, or passive? What other factors may be interfering with joint participation in this planning?

This ongoing planning of the observation activity includes planning what behaviors will be observed, how they will be operationalized, what kind of data will be collected, how it will be recorded (tallies, observation systems, verbatim recording, informal recording), the physical aspects of the observation (in-room, observation room, videotape, etc.), who will collect what behaviors, and when the data will be collected. The observation of the supervisory process will be discussed later.

Guidelines for Assessing the Planning of the Observation

The following questions need to be asked about the planning of the observation:

- Have the observation/data collection been jointly planned?
- Is there a rationale for the data collection?
- Are the data to be collected consistent with the long- and short-range goals of the client and the clinician?
- Do the data come out of the needs, concerns, or self-identified strengths or weaknesses of the supervisee as well as from the experience and impressions of the supervisor?
- Are options allowed for supervisor selection of behaviors for data collection which were not included in the plan?
- Are the plans detailed and specific and understood by both participants so the data can be collected as planned?
- Will the data be collected in such a way that they can be used effectively in the analysis stage?
- Does the plan allow for variance in the situation such as presence of the supervisor, interruptions, time of day, mood of client, unexpected learning by the client, etc.?
- Does the plan include the recording of behaviors of clinician or client or both, depending upon the situation?
- Is the amount of collected data sufficient to assist supervisors and supervisees in drawing inferences?
- Does the plan provide for data collection by the clinician on her or his own behavior?
- Have previously collected data followed the plan? Have they been appropriate? If not, can changes be built into the new plan?

All supervisors have experienced the frustration of losing some important observation while madly attempting to record previous ones or being unable to support a point because of insufficient data. Data collection on clinician behavior is so important that each supervisor must make a great effort to perfect systems for recording that they can use easily and efficiently. The same principles will be applied to the observation of supervisor and supervisee behaviors in studying the supervisory process.

SUMMARY

Observation and data collection are scientifically based procedures through which data are obtained for subsequent analysis and evaluation. All participants in the supervisory process have responsibility for participation in this component. This responsibility must be carried out carefully, purposefully, and consistently if the data are to form a solid basis for the remainder of the supervisory interaction.

Any supervisor, particularly those who are teaching course work on the supervisory process, will want to become familiar with some of the extensive literature on general principles of observation, training in observation techniques, and use of various tools for observation and analysis of behavior (Baer, Wolf & Risley, 1968; Beegle & Brandt, 1973; Campbell, 1975; Campbell & Barnes, 1969; Cartwright & Cartwright, 1984; Cronbach & Snow, 1981; Fleming, 1973; Hartman, 1982; Heward, Heron, Hill, & Trap-Porter, 1984; McAvoy, 1970; Medley, 1975; Medley & Mitzell, 1963; Murray, 1970; and Weinberg & Wood, 1975).

*A*nalyzing the Supervisory Process

Once the data have been gathered—whether qualitative or quantitative— they have to be organized, or structured, in a manner that will permit the question or questions posed by the investigator to be answered. Without such organization, the answers derived from the data may not be accurate.

Silverman (1977b, p. 165)

Although Silverman was writing about research, his statement is equally relevant to the supervisory process. The analysis component, like the observation component, demands a scientific approach.

Analysis is probably the most difficult of the components of the supervisory process to understand, to operationalize, and to write or talk about. It is the activity that makes more demands on the intellectual resources of supervisors than anything else they are required to do (Goldhammer et al., 1980). It is not to be equated with evaluation, although it often is. Evaluation, rather, should be seen as the result of analysis.

Simply put, analysis is the process of making sense of the data that have been collected. It is the time when the behaviors of the clinician are related to the behaviors of the client in some method more rational and defensible than acting upon clinical intuition or hunches. It is the time when the supervisor's "square box" is put on the shelf. It is also the time when the clinician/supervisee begins looking at her or his clinical activities with an objective eye.

The analysis process receives direct support in the ASHA list of competencies: Task 6—Assisting the supervisee in observing *and analyzing* assessment and treatment sessions and Task 8—Assisting the supervisee in observing *and analyzing* supervisory conferences (italics the author's). The latter task will be addressed later, but the basic principles of analysis are applicable to both clinical and supervisory sessions.

SCIENTIFIC ASPECTS OF ANALYSIS

In the supervisory process, as in the clinical and diagnostic processes or in research, scientific procedures must be used for answering questions—not only the large, global questions, of which there are many, but the day-by-day,

155

session-by-session, conference-by-conference needs for information. They must all be studied objectively, not only through systematic data collection, but also by applying similar scientific principles to the *analysis* of the data, followed by the drawing of conclusions and the making of inferences. This scientific approach to supervision underscores the importance of analysis to the total process. It also counteracts the superior role of supervisors solely as *evaluators* or *raters* or *overseers* or many of the other available roles, and highlights their role as that of scientific co-investigator—co-investigator because the supervisee will be involved in this endeavor as soon as possible.

Ventry and Schiavetti (1980) stated, "We see the practitioner as an applied scientist or a clinical scientist who uses the clinic or school as a laboratory for the application of the scientific method toward the end of providing the best clinical services possible. The scientific method, we think, is at the heart of the clinical enterprise" (p. 14). This "applied scientist" concept is as applicable to the supervisory process as it is to the clinical or research processes.

In a discussion of the clinician-investigator, Silverman (1977a) noted several benefits to the clinician who functions as an investigator which can also be applied to the supervisor. First, he said that it probably will make one's job "more stimulating, less routine, and would possibly increase the possibilities for positive reinforcement" (p. 14). Second, clinicians probably become more effective when they determine scientifically the answers to questions about their therapy or diagnostics—"asking questions that are 'answerable' and stating hypotheses that are 'testable'" (p. 14). There should be no difference, therefore, between methods for answering clinically relevant questions and methods for testing hypotheses for research purposes. Silverman stressed another feature of a scientific approach to clinical work which is equally relevant to supervision—"being aware of the *tentative* nature of answers and hypotheses is one of the most important, because it indicates that no answer to a question or test of a hypothesis is final" (p. 15). This is extremely relevant to the analysis component—no *one* answer will be found.

If research is a process of asking and answering questions, so are the clinical and supervisory processes. If data are collected to answer those questions, they must be organized in some useful manner. In research, data are analyzed through "statistical analysis, graphical display, tabular presentation and narrative description" (Silverman, 1977b, p. 166). Perhaps the need for data analysis in therapy and supervision is somewhat less ambitious than those words imply, but certainly supervisors and supervisees must *abstract* data relevant to their questions, and then *summarize, organize,* and *categorize* those data so that they are meaningful. And, if they have the skill and the motivation, there is nothing to stop supervisors or clinicians from submitting the data to more sophisticated statistical analysis. Organizing data for a research project may be more extensive or more formal than organizing the data from a clinical session or a supervisory conference, but the process is the same.

Careful adherence to the scientific method in analysis will ensure that supervisors come closer to objectivity and will provide organization and quantification that can lead to accountability. If data have been systematically collected and analyzed before inferences are drawn from them, supervisors will be in a better position to make judgments than if they do what Goldhammer and colleagues (1980) called "hunching our way through supervision" (p. 88).

Supervisors may come closer to leaving their biases at the door of the conference or observation room if they approach supervision within this analytical framework. It would be a mistake, however, to assume that objectivity is easy in the analysis component—it is not. Supervisors must constantly be conscious of their own "square boxes"—their "conceptual repertoire" as Goldhammer and colleagues (1980, p. 86) called it. It becomes very easy to look for patterns or categories of behaviors and draw conclusions that support a hypothesis or a bias, just as data collected during observations may support the observers' biases and represent their perceptual sets.

IMPORTANCE OF ANALYSIS

It is at the point where supervisors and supervisees begin to utilize analysis techniques, that their supervision style probably differs most from what has previously been called "traditional" supervision. It may even be the most important step of all in producing thoughtful, self-analytical professionals.

If supervisors are serious about what often seems to be platitudinous voicing of the goal of producing "self-supervising" clinicians, this is a crucial point in the development of that ability. An off-campus supervisor recently endeared herself to the writer by saying about her supervisee, "She'll never be able to self-supervise! She can't *analyze* her clinical sessions." This insight is an important one for supervisors. It *is* important for clinicians to be aware of their behaviors and the effect of those behaviors on their clients if they are to be modified or strengthened. The analysis process enables clinicians to extract from a mass of behaviors a design—a configuration—from which they can begin to see what is happening, to draw some inferences, to construct some hypotheses about what was effective and what was not, to test out these hypotheses, and then to plan for the future on the basis on their findings.

Organizing raw data on both clinician and client so that it becomes coherent and usable sets up the supervisor and supervisee for a more meaningful and efficient conference or other form of feedback. Also, when supervisors analyze clinician behavior they are modeling an approach that is transferable to the clinician's analysis of the client's behavior. Later, as they study behaviors in the supervisory interaction they will find the same techniques applicable. Such analysis shows supervisees a method for functioning within the supervisory process. They are learning how to utilize the scientific approach applicable to both processes and acquiring a tool for self-analysis.

Properly utilized, analysis—particularly joint analysis—should contribute in a major way to meeting the expectations of supervisees for fair and rational feedback and evaluation, since evaluation will come from objectively treated data and supervisees will be involved in analyzing and evaluating their own behavior.

If the analysis is done jointly, it offers supervisees some protection from the subjective judgments made by supervisors. It takes away some of the pejorative nature (real or perceived) of supervisors' input and focuses on behavior, not the individual. As a result, there may be less defensiveness, which, in turn, makes for better communication. It also places the emphasis on supervisees' participation in measuring progress toward their objectives over time, not spontaneous or intermittent input about their behavior from someone else. This is what Cogan (1973) called "organized evidence." Analysis that places responsibilities on supervisees prepares them for participation in the conference. If well-planned and executed, the analysis will enable supervisees to function as colleagues in the conference (Andersen, 1980b).

There is strong indication, however, that this stage is neglected or avoided by many supervisors, who go directly from observation to feedback. This feedback may be in the form of direct evaluation or it may be the provision of strategies. Studies have been cited previously that indicate that supervisees bring to the conference most of the information (i.e., raw data, reconstruction of the session, etc.) about the clinical interaction while supervisors provide suggestions for strategies to be utilized in the subsequent clinical session. Culatta and Seltzer (1976, 1977) found that 61 percent of all strategy statements were made by supervisors following provision of observation and information by the supervisee. In fact, providing observation and information was the only behavior in which supervisees were dominant. This finding was supported by Tufts (1984), Roberts and Smith (1982), and Schubert and Nelson (1976).

The reporting in conferences of a great deal of client behavior, often a reconstruction or "rehash" of the clinical session, is the antithesis of analysis, as in this statement from a tape of an actual conference:

> Well, one thing—he got out of his chair and then I couldn't get him to do anything. He was OK while he was sitting. So I was waiting for him to sit down. I said, "OK, I'll wait." He asked me something about my glasses and I answered him. I shouldn't have done that. Then he started talking about his mother's glasses. Finally, I asked him again to sit down. So he sat down but when I asked him to make his sound he just sat.

If this behavior had been what Cogan called a critical incident, that is, a onetime occurrence that affected the child's learning, it might have been appropriate to report it in this way. In this particular conference, however, a similar monologue continued in excruciating detail for over half of the conference, occupying nearly as much time as the actual events. It was then followed by "Well, why don't you . . . next time?" from the supervisor, a clear example of Culatta and Seltzer's (1976, 1977) findings. The pointlessness of this discussion is underscored by the fact that the supervisor had observed the entire session and was aware of what had happened. Had the session been submitted to some type of organized data collection and analysis, the supervisee or supervisor could have quantified the data on the basis of certain patterns and the interactions or sequences of behaviors rather than on a string of anecdotal reports. The provision of a solution to the problem by the supervisor deprived the supervisee of the opportunity to problem-solve and make inferences from the data.

If the analysis component is not taken seriously or, worse yet, not understood by supervisors who go directly to the feedback component, conferences will probably continue to consist of a mass of raw data or anecdotal reports used essentially to reconstruct the clinical session, evaluations communicated directly to the supervisee, or a collection of trivial items lacking in real significance to the learning process.

PURPOSES OF ANALYSIS IN SUPERVISION

The major purposes of analysis emerge from the works of Cogan (1973), Goldhammer (1969), Goldhammer and colleagues (1980), and Acheson and Gall (1980), who were the first to verbalize the concept of analysis as an essential part of the supervisory process. One purpose of analyzing is to distill the raw data to a point where it becomes coherent, manageable, and usable for the feedback component. Another is to organize the observational data in such a way that it can be used to draw conclusions and make rational judgments about what happened in the teaching/learning process. It then becomes the basis for further planning.

In discussing analysis of data collected on the behaviors of teachers and students in the classroom, Cogan (1973) lists the objectives of analysis:

1. Determining if objectives have been met
2. Identifying salient patterns in the teacher's behavior
3. Identifying unanticipated learnings by the student
4. Identifying critical incidents in the interaction (teacher behaviors that occur once but that appear to significantly affect the learning that takes place or the relationship between teacher and student)
5. Organizing the data to determine what was learned
6. Determining if what was planned really was carried out
7. Developing a data base for the rest of the supervision program

Cogan urged supervisors to look carefully at the interactions between the behaviors of students and teachers while being careful not to oversimplify the analysis or the cause-effect hypotheses. In addition, he discussed the identification of process learning, which he identified as "learning how to learn"—being responsible for personal learning, making better choices, self-initiating and accepting new ideas.

Goldhammer (1969) and Goldhammer and colleagues (1980) concentrated on the notion that all human behavior is patterned and stressed the point that it is the cumulative effects of those patterns that are important to the learning that occurs in the classroom. Therefore, supervision should concentrate on identifying *salient* patterns, not unusual or incidental variables. The aim of supervision, they said, is to strengthen, extinguish, or modify the salient behaviors. They defended this emphasis on such patterns not only because of their importance, but because they are more resistant to change than superficial or incidental behaviors. All of these points about the classroom are equally relevant in the analysis of treatment and assessment in speech-language pathology and audiology.

METHODS OF ANALYSIS

Analysis may be performed by the supervisor, the supervisee, or cooperatively by the two (Cogan, 1973). Each method fulfills a need at various times along the continuum of supervision.

Analysis by Supervisors

At the beginning of the supervisor/supervisee interaction, the supervisee's clinical repertoire may be a blank slate to the supervisor. If the supervisor is to determine the salient features of this repertoire, it will require a broad look at the data and a dedicated effort to determine a baseline of existing patterns. The hazards of structuring observations to support biases were an earlier topic of discussion. The same opportunities are available in analysis. Supervisors may see patterns that fit their personal prejudices or pet assumptions. They must constantly strive to keep in mind that they are concerned about the *documented effect* of the behaviors—not their assumptions based on their "square boxes." At this point, then, the task of the supervisor is to examine the data carefully, looking for patterns, critical incidents, behaviors related to the objectives or to the plan, the interactions between clinician and client, and the visible learning effects. This is *not a time for judgments.* It is a time for looking at the data to see what is happening. Evaluation will come later after conclusions are drawn, inferences made, hypotheses developed. For supervisors who have been accustomed to providing direct evaluations this will require a great amount of restraint until they begin to be aware of their own behaviors.

At the Evaluation-Feedback Stage, probably little or no analysis will be done, and supervisors will provide an evaluation based on their own perceptions and judgments. This is, in fact, the outstanding characteristic of the style used at that stage—judgmental statements from the supervisor's "square box."

Introducing Analysis to Supervisees

It is nearly certain that the inexperienced clinician at the beginning of the continuum will be unable to analyze alone, although the supervisor should not make a general assumption about that. Some clinicians may have more ability in this activity than others, but it is probable that analysis skills will have to be taught by the supervisor to most clinicians. Teaching procedures will depend upon the supervisee's level, but they should be involved in self-analysis procedures as soon as possible. Supervisees may be asked to read certain material about data collection and its analysis (Brookshire, 1967; Goldhammer et al., 1980; Mowrer, 1977). Supervisors may choose to demonstrate the analysis procedure after the observation by doing it alone at first and presenting the analyzed data as feedback during the conference. They may choose to perform the analysis *with* the supervisee, again modeling the behaviors that contribute to the analysis. They may use, or suggest that the supervisee use, interaction analysis systems and their summary forms to learn how to identify categories and patterns of clinical behavior. Supervisors and supervisees may also use these together or separately. Later, the supervisor may choose to present the data recorded during the observation to the clinician prior to the conference so that the clinician can do the analysis and bring the information to the conference.

Beginning supervisees should learn that there is a certain core of categories of clinical behaviors that are important to most clinical interaction—recording and charting of client behavior, reinforcement behaviors, direction giving, responses to clients, staying on-task, and others appropriate to the specific client. The supervisor and supervisee will first analyze these categories to determine the skill of the clinician. Mawdsley's (1985b) self-assessment instrument discussed in the chapter on observation would be useful here (Appendix F). This process is helpful to the clinician in learning to place behaviors in certain categories. From here, the analysis proceeds to a less-structured search for other patterns that affect the clinical interaction.

If interaction analysis systems have been used, the summary forms that accompany many of them will be useful. If no summary forms are included, they can easily be constructed. As with their use in observation, however, these systems do not cover all possible categories, interactions, or other behaviors, and supervisors must identify categories from the other data they have collected.

Whatever method is chosen to begin the analysis, the objective of the supervisor should always be increased responsibility on the part of the supervisee for self-analysis. If supervisees are involved initially with their supervisors and then gradually assume responsibility for themselves, they will develop skills with which they can continue to be self-analytical even when they are working alone or with no supervision. Supervisors who do all the analysis for supervisees inhibit and prevent their learning. Similarly, the supervisor who uses the analyzed data to develop all the conclusions and inferences and—even worse—to evaluate and provide the strategies, is abrogating the responsibilities of supervision. As they move along the continuum, then, the balance of supervisor/supervisee responsibility for analysis should be in a continuing state of progression toward increased supervisee participation.

Organizing the Data on Behaviors for Feedback

Once the data have been collected by either supervisor or supervisee, they are then maneuvered into categories or series of interactions that relate to learning. Behaviors to be strengthened, extinguished, or modified are identified. Decisions are made about achievement of objectives.

Goldhammer and colleagues (1980) discussed at length the principles of organizing the data to determine patterns related to learning. Although they stressed the importance of being able to demonstrate consequences of behavior in the data and the ability to support the patterns on the basis of theory, they also said that patterns may be selected simply because one has hunches about them. The latter principle is discouraged because it is less persuasive, most likely to be wrong, and implies that "hunching one's way through supervisory practice" (p. 88) is acceptable. Cogan (1973), too, warned against premature decisions when he said, "It is a temptation to jump to a conclusion: doing so saves so much time and labor" (p. 183). On the other hand, as with observation, some of the "art" may be lost if this aspect is excluded entirely.

Cogan (1973) suggested first analyzing the data on the behavior and the learning of the student (client, in this case) and relating both to the objectives to determine if they have been met; then analyzing the teacher's (clinician's) behaviors and forming hypotheses about the relationships between the behaviors and the learning. He also stressed the importance of dealing with interaction, not parts in isolation.

Some patterns identified in clinicians' behavior will be more obvious than others, some will be more important than others, and some will reflect biases and inaccurate perceptions. Professional control by supervisors will help them make inferences and form hypotheses rather than make assumptions and judgments.

Cogan (1973) suggested that critical incidents should receive a high priority in the analysis because, by virtue of its earlier definition, they do affect learning. His examples in regard to teaching are related to aggressive behaviors by the teacher, behaviors related to discipline, and incidents that have positive consequences—where students gain sudden insights that have lasting effects. Certain skills for managing clients affect the clinical interaction and may be analogous to such critical incidents for teachers. On the positive side, the clinician's ability to capitalize on spontaneous learning, for example, the sudden insight of the client, the unexpected accomplishment of a task, might be a favorable critical incident—indeed, one that the supervisor and supervisee might wish to turn into a pattern, once it is identified.

The supervisor may very well have seen important patterns of behavior emerge during the observation and recorded them. If not, analysis is where the search begins. Data are perused, categories of behaviors are quantified, and consequences of certain behaviors are identified, that is, when the clinician did X, the client did Y. Some questions to be asked in analyzing the data include:

1. How many times did this behavior or sequence of behaviors occur?
2. How many times did the clinician model, expand, repeat, or describe?
3. What was the response of the client?
4. How many accurate and inaccurate responses were recorded?
5. What was the percentage of correct to incorrect?
6. What behaviors of the clinician preceded the correct or incorrect? Did they form a pattern?

7. What behaviors occurred that "fell out" of the patterns?

8. What questions were asked? How were they stated and how were they answered?

9. What objectives were met?

10. If objectives were not met, are the reasons to be found in the data?

Gradually, the detective work will yield results and the data will fall into place. Out of this quantification and categorization both supervisor and supervisee begin to draw some conclusions, make some inferences, and state some hypotheses to be tested.

A common scene for any supervisor will serve to illustrate. The data reveal that 60 percent of the client's responses to the task presented by the clinician were incorrect. Incorrect responses increased in frequency as the sessions progressed. Two patterns are immediately obvious in the clinician's behavior: (1) He positively reinforced 35 percent of the incorrect responses. (2) Direction giving and modeling for all productions (accurate and inaccurate) followed the same pattern throughout the session. Incorrect responses by the client were followed 20 percent of the time by nonverbal reactions to his own productions—facial grimaces, head shaking, or sighing. The clinician did not respond to these reactions but presented the task again in the same way.

What follows such a session will depend upon the supervisory dyad's place on the continuum. In the Direct-Active Style at the Evaluation-Feedback Stage, the supervisor may or may not have recorded such data. In the purest form of the Direct-Active Style the recording will be in the form of evaluative statements. The analysis or, more accurately, evaluation will be done by the supervisor. The feedback may be delivered by the supervisor in writing or in the conference and will consist of value judgments and/or strategies which the supervisee can utilize during the next session.

In the Collaborative Style, there are a variety of ways to utilize the collected data. During the early part of the Transitional Stage, the supervisor will complete the analysis by categorizing and quantifying the behaviors, quantifying types of interactions, comparing clinician behaviors with client responses, summarizing client nonverbal reactions, and other methods. This analysis is then presented to the clinician in the conference. The method of analysis is described, and relationships between clinician and client behavior that can lead to further planning are suggested. As an alternative, the analysis might be done jointly to demonstrate the process. A bit further along the continuum, the supervisor will give the analyzed data, and later the raw data, to the clinician for study prior to the conference, and to bring significant issues to the conference. At whatever point it seems appropriate, the clinician will begin recording data from tapes in preparation for the later stage of self-analysis.

The clinician may be assisted in the beginning stages of the analysis by certain questions or suggestions that will provide structure for the task. 'What evidence is there that your objectives were met or not met?" "Please look at the client's responses and see what you can find in your own behavior that relates to his responses." Or more directly, "Can you see anything in your directions and modeling that related to the client's responses?" Perhaps the supervisor will want to have supervisees look at the data with a wide-lens approach, identifying patterns and their consequences themselves. Or perhaps the data will be looked at in terms of the clinician's long-range objectives.

Finally, as clinicians progress along the continuum, they will assume more responsibility for data collection and self-analysis. Supervisors and supervisees will then analyze data separately. The analyses are brought to the conference where they become the basis for the conference agenda.

One may ask "Why take the time to do all this when it is so much easier to tell them and get on to other matters?" First, the answer is obvious, if the importance of learners being involved in their own learning, the merits of the supervisee "owning" a bit of the action, and the negative impact on the learner of the superior-subordinate relationship in supervision, all of which have been discussed earlier, are recognized.

Second, although this first experience may take a bit more time than direct feedback, what about subsequent sessions? There should be a "pay-off" in terms of time when supervisees become increasingly independent and are able to do their own analysis and problem solving.

Third, time should not be the prime consideration. It is assumed that if supervisors and supervisees are assigned to each other for a learning experience that *some* time is spent together. The question then becomes one of the *quality* of that time. For the Collaborative Style, as described here, that time must be spent in some way other than direct, evaluative feedback.

Fourth, teaching these skills contributes to accountability in supervision. Analyzed data of the type discussed here can be compared with similar data from subsequent sessions. Clinician growth and learning are truly documented, not guessed at. More accurate hypotheses can be made about methodologies and their results.

Fifth, a skill is being taught in the analysis stage which clinicians must have if they are to continue to be growing, self-sufficient professionals. Previous discussions of generalization of clinician behaviors are appropriate here also. Further, this skill is absolutely essential if and when clinicians become supervisors themselves. A colleague recently said to the writer, "I think lots of supervisors don't know how to analyze." Unfortunately, this is probably too true. Even if they perceive it as important, the skills of analysis may not have been a part of their clinical training. The lack of training in the supervisory process for most supervisors increases the probability that they may not understand how to teach analysis skills to clinicians.

DETERMINING THE CONTENT OF THE CONFERENCE

One of the stated purposes of the analysis is to determine the content of the conference. Analysis that really reduces the data and places a priority on items to be discussed in the conference leads to an efficient, organized, and directed conference. It is the prelude to the conference. Here is another place where components overlap—analysis and planning flowing together.

The content of the conference will be discussed in a subsequent chapter but the possibilities for topics are almost limitless. Besides general topics, which may vary by situation, the infinite amount of behavior observed in most clinical sessions makes it reasonable to think that not everything observed or identified through analysis can be dealt with in the conference, although it often seems that participants in conferences try to do just that. The premise, here, is that conferences or other forms of feedback, must be *planned*. Observation of many hours of tapes of conferences has made it obvious to the writer that they frequently are not; rather, they often appear to be unplanned, unfocused, and disorganized. They contain an unbelievable amount of trivia. The analysis stage does not assure the elimination of trivia—trivia are trivia, even when quantified. But analysis does make it easier, if one wishes, to establish higher priorities for the discussion of some events or issues than others.

Three criteria for selecting items for the conference from all the patterns observed were provided by Goldhammer and colleagues (1980): (1) *saliency*— the frequency with which the behaviors are found in the data, their significance, their relationship to theory, their relationships to other patterns or to commonalities among teachers and, last but certainly not least in terms of joint participation, the relationship to what the supervisee sees as important or has requested to discuss; (2) *accessibility of patterns for treatment*—the patterns related to emotionally charged issues that may be too threatening for the supervisee; and (3) *fewness*—because time in conferences is limited, and supervisees may only be able to assimilate a certain amount of input, patterns of behavior can be selected or rejected on the basis of certain criteria. These criteria include easy and clear identity of patterns in the data, the subsuming of some patterns under others, the similarity or difference to other patterns, the emotional content of the patterns, the amount of time needed to cover the patterns adequately, and the orderly transition from one issue to another. In other words, each pattern of behavior does not stand alone. It is related to others.

There are other important decisions to be made during the analysis that directly influence the content and organization of the conference. The foundation for an organized, problem-solving, meaningful conference is built during the analysis. Questions that must be asked are:

Are there data on clinician strengths as well as weaknesses?

Are there appropriate data to measure the accomplishment of objectives?

Have clinicians participated in the analysis to an extent that will enable them to have meaningful input into structuring the conference? How much should they be expected to participate in the analysis?

Are there enough data for an analysis? How much data are enough? Although there is some indication that three to five minutes of observation and data collection are sufficient to represent the entire session (Boone & Prescott, 1972; Schubert & Laird, 1975), these findings came from the use of specific interaction analysis systems with limited numbers of behaviors. The same kind of information does not exist for other kinds of clinical analysis. The answer to this question may depend upon what clinical skills are being addressed.

Is the information from the analysis to be considered as infallible? Will there be times when it is nonconclusive? Will there be crisis times—or even noncrisis times—when the analyzed data will need to be discarded in favor of some more urgent issues?

It is possible to miss some important issues through the effort to be analytical. Supervisors need to be sensitive to the fact that over-utilization of analyzed data can lead to a conference that is too structured.

There are many factors that need to be considered in planning the agenda for the conference. The use of the analyzed data is only one facet, but it is an important one in promoting a scientific approach to supervision and in helping supervisees' to become aware of their own behavior and their own needs.

EVALUATION

What about evaluation? the reader is probably asking at this point. Is it eliminated entirely? Is it legitimate for supervisors to provide a direct evaluation? Certainly, in fact, it is the responsibility of supervisors to evaluate at appropriate times. This need for direct behaviors at appropriate times has been identified in several chapters throughout the book. It is unrealistic, and probably unprofessional, to assume that evaluation should never happen; it is not the intent of the writer to imply that. Additionally, studies about what supervisees want and expect indicate a desire for a critique, and identification of weaknesses, and guidance about specific techniques. Thus, expectations may not be met unless supervisees (1) receive some evaluation, or (2) understand the reasons why the supervisor is encouraging self-evaluation and not providing it all themselves.

When the supervisor goes directly from the observation to evaluation it should be done rationally, however. Clinicians who are at the Evaluation-Feedback Stage and are unable to participate in joint- or self-analysis, can be assumed to need some direction which must come through evaluation and direct feedback. If certain behaviors have been identified as needing specific attention and it has been agreed that the supervisor will provide a rating of these occurrences of the behavior, this type of feedback is essential. Sometimes the use of direct evaluation is a more efficient procedure and certain features of the situation make it reasonable to utilize direct evaluation: the seriousness of the impact of the behavior on the client may demand immediate evaluative feedback, the behavior may be too trivial or too obvious to justify any lengthy analysis procedure, the behavior may be one that is being dealt with on an ongoing basis and the clinician may need only a reminder, the significance of the issue may be too complex for the clinician at the moment either intellectually or emotionally. Supervisors must use their best judgment here as to when to provide direct evaluation as related to teaching or when to involve the supervisee in self-analyses or self-evaluation. The important point of decision should be, What will the supervisee learn and how will she or he learn it best?

The topic of feedback will be dealt with in greater depth in the chapter on Integrating. The broader topic of the formal, organizationally based evaluation is another issue. It will be included in the section on Accountability.

SUMMARY

The Analysis component of the supervisory process, like the Observation component, is a point where a scientific approach is essential. It is the time when the supervisor and supervisee utilize the recorded data to hypothesize about what has happened and to plan subsequent events. Analysis is not synonymous with evaluation, but it is a necessary step that leads to objective, disciplined judgments by the supervisor and to independence through self-analysis and self-evaluation by the supervisee.

*I*ntegrating the Components

> *It is a matter of some curiosity that, with a few exceptions (Mosher
> and Purpel, 1972; Goldhammer, 1969), a reader of supervisory texts is
> rarely confronted by what really seems to happen in the course of the
> inevitable meetings that take place between the parties to the
> supervisory process.*
>
> Blumberg, (1980, p. 1)

At some point, everything that happens in the supervisory process—the
preparation, the observation, the analysis—must be integrated through some form
of communication between supervisor and supervisee. This usually occurs during
a conference in which all the "energy and thought" of the previous components
come together to "result in the intended benefits" of the process (Goldhammer
et al., 1980, p. 142).

Traditionally, the conference has been seen as a time when the supervisor
provides feedback to the supervisee about the observation. This feedback has
been perceived to be something of a one-way street—from supervisor to
supervisee. The supervisor talks; the supervisee listens. Certainly, this is the
pattern that characterizes the Direct-Active Style of the supervisor and the Passive
Style of the supervisee at the Evaluation-Feedback Stage.

For the Collaborative or Consultative Styles, the broader term of *integrating*
seems more appropriate than *feedback* in describing the interaction that takes
place when supervisor and supervisee meet. Although feedback will be one aspect
of the integration component, it is here where the components of Understanding,
Planning, Observing, and Analyzing will merge. Since those components have
been discussed previously, the content of this chapter will be related to the
communication that takes place about them and their results and will suggest
a richer synthesis of ideas than the traditional concept of supervisor-to-supervisee
feedback. In addition to feedback about the clinical session, the conference will
also include discussion of procedural topics such as administrative issues or report
writing, the supervisory process, professional issues, personal concerns, and
general information relevant to the development of all the participants.

Feedback is seen as not just evaluative, not as just the end product of the supervisory process, or as coming solely from the supervisor. It is, instead, an exchange of ideas that occurs throughout the entire interaction, emanating in a variety of ways from all the participants in all directions. It may come during or immediately after the observation, or it may be delayed. It may be verbal or written. It may be in the form of data collected during the observation or it may consist of judgmental or evaluative statements. Whatever its form, it serves both as closure to preceding events and transition to further planning. Cogan (1973) believed that the conference, the vehicle for this interchange, is neither the culmination of the supervisory process nor even its most important event, but "a development of everything that goes on before and after it" (p. 196). Figure 10–1 depicts the totality of the feedback that forms a part of the conference. Supervisors and supervisees will be both recipients and providers of feedback for each other, their peers, and themselves. In some situations where peer supervision takes place, supervisees provide feedback to each other. Supervisee and supervisor also engage in self-feedback. Further, in the best of supervisory situations, a line would be added to indicate supervisor-to-supervisor input or peer interaction.

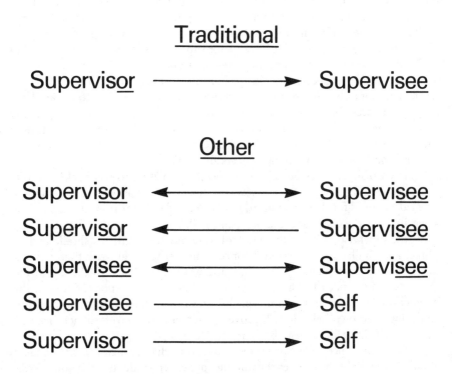

FIGURE 10–1. *TYPES OF FEEDBACK IN THE SUPERVISORY PROCESS*

Feedback is too limited a term for the total interaction implied here, but because the other components that lead to it have been discussed, this chapter will focus on feedback. The reader should keep in mind a broader interpretation of the integration component that includes such other activities as planning, problem solving, discussion of the supervisory process, analyzing, and the many other topics necessary to maintaining a profitable relationship.

EXPECTATIONS ABOUT FEEDBACK

Many of the expectations of supervisees about supervision are related to feedback behaviors of both supervisors and supervisees. In fact, it may be that feedback behaviors constitute a large portion of what many supervisees think of as "supervision."

The "Bill of Rights" (Gerstman, 1977) for supervisors and supervisees, prepared by a group of supervisors, reflects not only the twofold nature of feedback—teaching/guidance and rating—but also the concept of the totality of feedback as seen in Figure 10–1. The category in the Bill of Rights for supervisees is entitled *Right to Expect Supervisor to Provide Means and Method of Feedback*, and contains such feedback-related sub-items as systematic monitoring, ongoing mutual feedback, opportunity to express self, formal and informal conference time, honest appraisal of job performance, oral and written evaluations, the possibility of appealing decisions, and the opportunity to say "No." The category in the Bill of Rights for supervisors is entitled *Right to Offer and Get Mutual Feedback*, and includes the right to make justified criticisms, to expect staff to expect and accept criticisms, to judge and criticize effects of services, to honestly criticize and suggest other ways of operating, to get feedback from supervisees about supervision received, to expect supervisees to say, "You're a lousy supervisor," or even a good one, and to determine some of the ground rules of how often they will be observed. Obviously, this group of supervisors took a broad look at the many aspects of feedback.

How do supervisees perceive their needs in relation to feedback? A group of supervisees, in presenting their views on supervision in an ASHA presentation, stressed the need for demonstration, guidance, and support from the supervisor. They also saw the need for the supervisor to allow them to assume responsibility, while the supervisor still assumed the role of evaluator. Feedback should include "direct and challenging questions" concerning their clinical work that will lead to self-analysis, as well as constant oral and written feedback. At the same time, they stressed the need for supervisees to assume certain responsibilities in this interaction by formulating appropriate questions, defending their position, analyzing their own behavior objectively, and being open to feedback from the supervisor (Hatfield, Caven, Bartlett, & Ueberle, 1973).

Studies on expectations reviewed in an earlier chapter included several views about feedback. Both experienced and inexperienced students in Larson's (1982) study not only expected feedback from the supervisors, but they expected their supervisors to listen to them and accept what they had to say. They expected to take an active role in the conference and expressed a need to have supervisors provide them with information about their weaknesses, with the inexperienced expressing a greater desire for this type of information than the more experienced. However, they all expected some kind of critique.

Other studies have identified similar attitudes toward feedback. Three of the ten competencies valued most highly in a study by Russell (1976) were related specifically to the delivery of feedback to the supervisee by the supervisor (being fair and impartial in the evaluation of the clinician, providing the clinician with constructive evaluative information, and providing the clinician with direct feedback and evaluation), and two were related to the supervisor's treatment of the clinician's feedback: perceiving the clinician's feedback and evaluation and being responsive to it.

Dowling and Wittkopp (1982) cited feedback practices that supervisees like, including constructive evaluation of reports, evaluative feedback following an observation in either written or checklist form, positive and negative feedback about their clinical behavior, regular individual conferences, active involvement in problem solving, encouragement to use self-evaluation techniques and formal evaluation, and discussion of their clinical behavior. Feedback procedures they do not like include no comments on lesson plans, unannounced observation, and clinical experiences where there is no feedback.

This frequently expressed desire for direct feedback about their work—a critique, as it is sometimes stated, is the very issue that must be clarified in operationalizing the continuum. Supervisees must learn the appropriate balance between direct feedback from the supervisor and self-analysis. Unless this is clarified, it may be a source of frustration and dissatisfaction for the supervisee in the conference. Perhaps this is best exemplified by personal anecdote. In the very early days of the preparation program in the supervisory process at Indiana University, a doctoral-level trainee and an advanced, insightful clinician were paired in a supervision practicum and had established what the trainee and the program director both perceived as an excellent collaborative relationship—the supervision trainee was supportive, encouraged problem solving, and stimulated creative thinking; the clinician was self-analytical, creative in planning, self-evaluative, and participated productively in the conference. A supervisory dyad created in Heaven! Yet, about two-thirds of the way into the semester, as the two walked down the hall after a conference, the student said, "Well, when are you going to start criticizing me?" The implications in terms of expectations, unexplored and unmet, need not be belabored here, but the experience provided a valuable lesson for both the trainee and his supervisor, this writer.

If the sequence of events suggested in the chapters on understanding the supervisory process and planning is followed, each supervisor will be aware of what the supervisee is expecting by way of feedback. These expectancies will have been discussed in terms of their appropriateness for the supervisee and ways of meeting them will be incorporated into the planning.

PLANNING THE FEEDBACK

One of the basic principles of the clinical supervision model is the planning of the interaction between supervisor and supervisee to ensure its value as a teaching and learning experience. Cogan (1973) and Goldhammer and colleagues (1980) spent considerable time discussing strategies for the planning of the conference. This planning comes out of the analysis of the teaching, when decisions are made about what to do with the collected data or other information and priorities are set for the conference discussion. Goldhammer and colleagues discussed such issues as doing a full or partial analysis of the data; the order in which issues will be presented; dealing with strengths or weaknesses; the balance between the past (analysis of previous data), the future (planning), and the present (discussion of the supervisory process); how to record what is happening in the conference; reviewing the contract, if there is one, for possible modification; and how and when to end the conference. They suggested that, although there may be appropriate times for an open conference, it is easy to "squander an open conference on superficialities or on peripheral or irrelevant issues" (p. 136). The relationship between the analyzed data and planning the conference has also been discussed previously in the chapter on analysis.

Although most studies of the conference have centered on what has already happened, Peaper (1984) focused on planning for the supervisory conference. After completion of an opinion questionnaire about the conference, graduate students were divided into two groups. Students in one group were asked to plan agendas for their conferences after listing potential topics for discussion under three categories—client-centered, clinician-centered, and supervisor-centered issues. Students in the other group did not participate in such a listing. The opinion questionnaire was given again at the end of the semester.

Students in this study valued the conference, as opposed to the subjects of Culatta and colleagues (1975), who did not feel a need for regularly scheduled conferences. The group that preplanned agendas for their conferences felt more strongly after the experiment that they set the tone of the conference— not a surprising fact, but an important consideration for the supervisor who wishes to have the supervisee feel more "ownership" of the experience.

The type of feedback and the content of the conference should be planned as rationally as any other part of the supervisory process. Goals should be directed toward the supervisee's movement along the continuum. Whatever form it is to take, the feedback should be determined jointly by supervisor and supervisee during the planning component and should include feedback on both client and clinician. Such planning should include decision making about purpose, type, content, amount, timing, and rationale, as well as evaluation of the appropriateness of the feedback. This is when the supervisor can deal with the question of the supervisee's need for direct evaluation or for opportunity for self-analysis with self-evaluation. The feedback should usually result from the analysis of the data collected during the observation, although other content may be necessary. Feedback without analysis will probably become either presentation of raw data, or direct evaluation or suggestions by the supervisor. Although either may be appropriate, there should be a rationale for the selection of any procedure. It should be planned for maximum participation by the supervisee, which can be determined once the place on the continuum has been identified.

PROVIDING FEEDBACK

Feedback may be provided in a variety of situations using many different methods. Although the scheduled conference seems to be the most frequently used setting for the exchange of feedback, there are other procedures. They will be discussed briefly before the major topic of the chapter—the conference—is addressed. These procedures are mainly one-way delivery of feedback—supervisor to supervisee.

Written Feedback

Many supervisors use checklists, rating scales, evaluation forms, or messages written during the observation period which are given to the supervisee after the clinical session (Geoffrey, 1973); but type of feedback has received little attention in the supervision literature. Rees and Smith (1967) suggested that clinicians in the school practicum should receive written feedback in the form of a checklist and a narrative to be followed by oral communication between supervisor and supervisee.

Kennedy (1981) studied the effects of two types of preconference written feedback, subjective statements and verbatim transcripts of events, on verbal behaviors of supervisors in the subsequent conference. Both supervisor and supervisees showed differences in conference behaviors, depending upon which form of feedback had been used. The supervisor under the verbatim condition made more verbalizations in the categories of Supervision, Explanation, and Opinions, as measured by the *Multidimensional Observational System for the Analysis of Interactions in Clinical Supervision* (Weller, 1971), than the supervisor under the subjective condition. Supervisees also differed, with those who received the subjective treatment using more Justification of Opinions than the others. Other relationships were found between the type of feedback and verbal behavior in the conferences. Certain limitations to this study were noted by its author, but it addresses an important issue—Does type of feedback make a difference? More study is necessary, as answers to this question could make supervision more efficient and effective.

In a study of the nature of written feedback, Peaper and Mercaitis (1987) reported that it is more evaluative than that provided in conferences and suggested that either method is appropriate, depending upon the situation.

One place where written feedback is utilized is in relation to reports written by supervisees. In an investigation of such feedback, Gunter (1985) addressed the degree of consistency between supervisors' judgments of the most important constituents of a report and their evaluations of an actual clinical report. The components considered of highest value were related to content, as opposed to style. Analysis of comments on an actual clinical report, however, were inconsistent with this because they revealed more comments related to style than content. It is obviously easier to provide written feedback on style than content and Gunter pointed out the great need for a method to ensure that feedback on both style and content are provided. She also reported that supervisors' comments on the report were not consistent, indicating that important components of feedback may be left out. She urged some means of consistency, such as a checklist for supervisors to use in reacting to reports.

Although the written message may be justified on the basis of time or other reasons, it does seem that the content of the written message is of great importance in encouraging the collaborative approach to supervision. If the written message handed to the supervisee after the observation is observational data collected by the supervisor, it should be useful to the supervisee in the analysis that precedes the conference. Certain types of questions from the supervisor may also enhance self-analysis by the supervisee. If the written feedback is a direct evaluation, however, the opportunity or motivation for supervisee self-analysis and self-evaluation may be lost and the tone of the conference preset. If the written message is used without further verbal interaction, it may be misunderstood. The intent of the message may be clearer and the opportunity for misunderstanding not so great if the purpose and content have been discussed during joint planning.

Spontaneous or Unscheduled Verbal Interaction

Supervisors and supervisees have many opportunities for verbal interaction between the time of the observation and the conference. Regardless of setting, they meet in the halls, the lunchroom, or the classroom; they may be working together on other tasks; or they may interact in a variety of other ways. The opportunities and temptations to discuss fragments of the observed clinical session in such interactions may be great.

One must ask what purpose is to be served by such spontaneous interactions. If a very specific goal has been set for the supervisor to rate certain interactions during the session, feedback may be given to the supervisee immediately. If immediate reinforcement is the goal, then this type of feedback is appropriate. A brief interchange, however, may not do justice to the complexities of a clinical session. There may have been no time for analysis by either supervisor or supervisee. A quickly delivered message may be misunderstood. As with the written message, the probability is high that this type of interchange will take the form of an "instant evaluation" by the supervisor or a suggestion for future action, which removes the need for self-analysis or self-evaluation by the supervisee. On the other hand, if a session has been a devastating failure, the supervisee may be greatly in need of an understanding word that will sustain her or him until the time of the more formal, scheduled conference. Social rules usually encourage some kind of verbal interaction when two people meet—no one would wish to be met with a stony stare after a clinical session. A very specific goal may have been set for the supervisor to rate certain interactions during the session. As with all supervisory behaviors, such activities must be rationally decided and based upon planned objectives and specific needs of the supervisee. Supervisors should probably resist the temptation to respond automatically with a stereotypic positive or negative statement without giving some thought to its purpose or effect. As with the written message, if the supervisor has given approval or disapproval of activities in the session, it will appear that there is little need for further analysis or discussion. Whatever is said, the tone of the subsequent discussion may be influenced by the supervisor's words.

Cogan (1973) discussed this issue in the case of supervisors of classroom teachers when he said that the first sentence of the conference may actually be spoken before the conference ever begins, as the supervisor leaves the room after the observation. "What does the supervisor say as he passes the teacher? Most supervisors feel that they must make some favorable comment, whether the lesson merits it or not. If the lesson has been bad, they may mumble, 'very interesting.' Some will say, 'See you later,' and then pale at the inferences the teacher might draw. Others maintain that there has to be something deserving praise in every lesson, so they smile and say, 'Finished right on time!' and sidle out. Still others volunteer something like 'A good lesson,' planning to recapture the truth later, in the conference" (p. 205).

Although stated somewhat humorously by Cogan, the offhand remarks made by supervisors between observation and conference may be more important than they realize, especially in terms of the Collaborative Style. Such spontaneous remarks may take any of several forms, but certainly they deserve some thought by the supervisor and the supervisee and their goals and purpose should be an important part of the discussion in planning the supervisory interaction. If the activities that make up the observation and analysis components as well as the type of feedback have been planned previously, there will be less uncertainty about what to expect in the conference and probably less need for spontaneous verbal interaction.

Direct Feedback During Clinical Sessions

This form of feedback includes such behaviors as communication through the "bug-in-the-ear" referred to briefly in the chapter on observation, slipping notes to the clinician that suggest changes in activities, interruption of the session to make suggestions or to demonstrate, and other forms of attracting the attention of the clinician in an attempt to alter the direction of the clinical session.

Interruption of the Session

No data are available on the topic of interruption by the supervisor of the clinical session. Countless discussions with supervisees indicate, however, that there are mixed reactions to this technique, depending upon the supervisee's maturity, the supervisor's manner, the relationship between the two, the purpose and nature of the intervention, and the amount of planning that has preceded it.

Some clinicians report that they consider "swooping into the clinical session" without warning and taking over the work with the client to be the most reprehensible behavior supervisors can exhibit. There is a general feeling that, when supervisors enter the clinic space unexpectedly and begin to interact directly with clients or to make suggestions to the clinicians in the presence of clients, it threatens the professional status of the clinician, damages their credibility in the eyes of the client, and is demeaning. Other clinicians indicate that they welcome suggestions or demonstration. In fact, when present or former students are asked what was missing from their preparation, they often express a wish to have had more demonstrations from their supervisors. They do, however, rather consistently prefer to have some warning that it is going to happen.

In keeping with the theme of collaborative supervision presented here, such unannounced or unplanned intervention would be especially inappropriate. Sensitivity to the personal feelings of the supervisee and advanced planning would avoid the feelings of resentment and threat that may result from intervention in the session. The optimal way to deal with the question of intervention and demonstration is to include it in the planning activities, both long-range and specific instances, so that the supervisor's presence can be explained to the client. For example, the supervisee may indicate in the conference that she or he wishes a demonstration of how to execute a particular procedure and may request the supervisor to attend the next session. Or the supervisor may be concerned about the supervisee's evaluation and reinforcement of phoneme production and may wish to join the session to assist the supervisee in sharpening his or her listening skills. If this is a part of planning, the supervisee can then explain the supervisor's forthcoming visit to the client, or at least, be prepared to deal with the interruption. Without further study of this methodology, it seems safe to say that it may reinforce the supervisor/subordinate role in supervision and increase the dependency of the supervisee.

In the opinion of the writer, and to be consistent with the Collaborative Style, the only justification for *unplanned* intervention in the clinical session would be a situation in which the client's welfare was in serious jeopardy. This might include an accident warranting assistance, an emotional crisis, or a major error by the clinician which might have severe irreversible repercussions in the client's learning. This is a particularly cogent issue in settings where clients are paying fees for a session that takes a negative turn in relation to learning. The client's right to high quality service must be considered; at the same time, supervisors must be sure that their judgments about the negative features of the session are accurate and not merely from their own "square boxes." In other words, the techniques may be different from those the supervisor would use. The issue at stake here is the learning that is taking place.

A special situation is probably presented in the case of observation of assessment sessions, especially if it is a one-visit evaluation where there will be no other opportunity to obtain reliable data. Incorrect administration of test instruments or errors in the use of certain assessment techniques may then warrant interruption by the supervisor. However, adequate planning and preparation may prevent such problems, or at least alleviate some of the defensiveness that may be engendered.

Rassi (1978) described a supervisory procedure in audiology assessment in which the supervisor demonstrates for the student, explains rationale between questions of the patient, and then has the student perform the activities while the supervisor is still in the room. The supervisor then listens in an adjacent room and "if deemed necessary and/or appropriate, supervisor may intervene to assist student or give him suggestions" (p. 46). Rassi stressed the dangers of dependence on the supervisor and said, "Beware of transforming the student into a robot" (p. 47). Oratio (1977) called a similar approach a "supervisor-centered process" (p. 14), as opposed to a clinician- or client-centered process.

When there is no observation room, a totally different situation is created. In some settings, supervisors may have to sit in the room where the session is being conducted. Intervention in such cases might be planned in such a way that the supervisee could request the supervisor to join in the session or to demonstrate a specific activity without intruding in the clinician-client relationship. In some situations, supervisors and supervisees may work cooperatively with the clients on a more or less regular basis, thus giving the supervisor a natural opportunity to demonstrate. Sensitivity and planning are as important here as in the prior example. It is probably safe to say that here, too, in terms of the Collaborative Style, *unplanned* intervention should not take place unless a critical problem occurs in the clinical session.

Live Supervision

The term *live supervision*, referred to briefly in the discussion of observation, has developed in the training of professionals in the specific practice of marital and family therapy (Goodman, 1985) and has real applicability for speech-language pathology and audiology. Byng-Hall and Whiffen (1982) stated the dilemma of the beginning family therapist who must remain in charge of the session or "be swallowed up by the family system"; therefore, supervisory techniques are required which are "swift enough" to intervene within the same time scale as the family interactions. The trend in this type of therapy has been "to close the gap between the supervisor and his trainee and to move ever closer to where the action is" (p. 3). These writers traced the evolution of family therapy supervision from case discussions, audiotapes, role playing, exploring the therapist's own family, and videotapes, methods that only allow a retrospective view of the therapy activities. As supervisors in that discipline have tried to have more immediate contact with the trainee, they have developed various techniques—consultation behind a screen with the supervisor at a prearranged time, a telephone into the therapy room, the earphone or "bug-in-the-ear," and finally, supervisors joining therapists in the therapy room with the family. This model of training may also be applied to individual therapy (Goodman, 1985).

Kaslow (1977) said that the traditional model of one-to-one supervision in psychotherapy, characterized by a conference between supervisor and supervisee, had an indirect quality based on "recall, subjective reporting, and selective remembering" (p. 223). In the live supervision approach, the supervisor plays the role of *co-therapist*. Kaslow stated that there are many advantages in this model, where "the student can be exposed to intensive learning by direct observation and participation with the supervisor. Such experiences can be exhilarating and highly productive" (p. 224). This type of supervision also has its disadvantages, according to Kaslow—the possible assertiveness of the supervisor, the modeling that may take place, and the repression of the supervisee's spontaneity in favor of the supervisor's action. It is hoped that, for supervisees, "the supervisor will help them maintain their individualities, find their own styles, trust their hunches, and gradually feel free to move in more rapidly, so that ultimately the teams will be well balanced" (p. 225).

Does this methodology have application in speech-language pathology and audiology? Discussion with supervisors has identified instances where such a procedure is used, but there is nothing in the literature, except Rassi's approach to audiology supervision, that describes it. The writer has frequently seen this model in operation in off-campus settings where supervisor or supervisee "work together" with the client. The procedure deserves investigation. Although it may appear to be the antithesis of the proposal made here, the method may be particularly suited to interactions at either end of the continuum. At the early stages, there may be a need for modeling, demonstrating, immediate intervention, or reinforcement of the beginning clinicians to give them skills that will move them out of the first stages. The methodology may also be viable with the so-called marginal student, who has remained at the Evaluation-Feedback Stage and is having difficulty moving along the continuum. At the last stage of the continuum, it may be the ideal way for peers to work together in solving certain problems or for the experienced clinician to receive consultative assistance.

As with other procedures, it must be planned rationally on the basis of supervisees' needs and their ability to accept it. Its regular use might be questioned on the basis of the dependency of the supervisee. It may be difficult for supervisees to develop their own professional image if such a procedure is continued for too long. It may also interfere with the clinician/client relationship. On the other hand, it may be a productive approach if true collaboration can be achieved. For the Consultative Style, it is particularly appropriate—two colleagues working together to solve a problem.

Supervision by Earphone

A form of live supervision that has been given some attention in the literature is that of the bug-in-the-ear technique. This method utilizes electronic equipment such as an FM transmitter and receiver, allowing the supervisor to communicate directly with the clinician in such a manner that the client is not privy to the conversation.

The bug-in-the-ear appears to have been a popular device for supervision in certain disciplines (Boylston & Tuma, 1972; Montalvo, 1973; Ward, 1960). Called the most intrusive device in use in supervision, both cognitively and emotionally, by Loewenstein and Reder (1982), it has apparently been used for many years in social work and psychotherapy (Kadushin, 1976).

Byng-Hall (1982) listed the advantages and disadvantages of this methodology. The immediate effect of the intervention, the quicker way of learning techniques, and the intensity of the intervention are cited as advantages. The fact that it is a tool that lends itself to the supervisor taking over the therapy is discussed as a disadvantage. "He knows that he is breaking the first golden rule which is that supervision is teaching the trainee, not treating the family. If he wants to do that he can walk into the room and take over" (p. 48). Byng-Hall also cited the difficulty for the trainee whose autonomy is invaded.

The speech-language pathology literature contains a few references to the bug-in-the-ear procedure, although there is no documentation of the frequency of its use. Brooks and Hannah (1966) reported it as a supervisory tool, but warned that the supervisor must avoid dominating the instruction and "causing the student to become a voice-operated automaton." They also indicated that it is sometimes difficult for the supervisor "to hold himself in check in this regard" (p. 386) and cited dependency of students as one of the dangers of such a system. A similar procedure was described by Starkweather (1974) for use in behavior modification training of clinicians, but he warned, "The whole procedure rests on the assumption that the supervisor's judgment is perfect, which is obviously unrealistic" (p. 610) and followed that with the cogent statement that the same problem exists in traditional training, but that the degree of independence of the student in the traditional "may enable the excellent student to overcome some of the shortcomings of his mentor" (p. 610). Hagler (1986) utilized this method in a study of the supervisory process, which will be reported later.

Other Structures for Feedback

Before moving into a detailed discussion of the structured conference, probably the most common vehicle for feedback, others that might be utilized in speech-language pathology or audiology should be mentioned.

The microteaching and video confrontation methodologies described in the observation chapter utilize feedback, often from peers, and often immediately. Case presentations and discussion provide opportunity for feedback, usually on the client, in some settings. The case presentation, or staffing, rather than the conference, has been the classical means of supervising the clinical years of students in psychiatric education. With this method, the trainee evaluates a case, presents it to his or her supervisor and a group of peers, or conducts an interview before a group. The trainee's performance is then discussed by the supervisor and the group (Kagan & Werner, 1977). This format has also been used in speech-language pathology but, like other procedures, there is nothing in the literature about its advantages or disadvantages. Group conferences are a commonly used opportunity for sharing feedback and will be given more detailed treatment later. Demonstration therapy can also be a form of feedback.

SCHEDULED CONFERENCES

The conference appears to have become the most commonly used structure for communicating feedback in all the helping professions where there is applied training—education, social work, counseling, psychotherapy, and certainly in speech-language pathology and audiology. Geoffrey (1973) reported that 96 percent of the 111 facilities responding to her survey utilized regularly scheduled conferences. Of the 501 supervisors studied by Schubert and Aitchison (1975), 98 percent reported the use of posttherapy conferences.

Reference to the conference in the literature from the helping professions consists of a broad range of theoretical statements, descriptive information, perceptions, recommendations, guidelines, or personal preferences. Much of the descriptive literature on the conference has come from education, and because this literature has probably most directly influenced the writer, as well as others in speech-language pathology and audiology, some of it is presented as a background for the discussion of the conference in speech-language pathology and audiology.

Descriptive Studies of the Conference in Education

Dussault (1970) maintained that supervision in education is at the stage of natural history in the development of a science, a stage at which the entities, phenomena, and relations of a field of inquiry are inventoried, named and described, and classified in orderly systems. The stage of theory, he said, then goes beyond these realities of what is and seeks to discover why reality is what it is. With this in mind, the descriptive information about the conference is presented. This literature has been referred to throughout the book as it pertained to a specific topic but has not been presented in its entirety.

Description of conference interaction received considerable attention in the 1960s. The pioneering work of Blumberg and his associates has been very important to students of the supervisory process (Blumberg, 1974; Blumberg & Amidon, 1965; Blumberg & Cusick, 1970; Blumberg & Weber, 1968). Departing from the nature of the previous educational literature on supervision, which dealt mainly with organizational and curricular concerns, he and his associates addressed the nature of the human relationships between supervisor and teacher, the place where Blumberg believed that most of the problems in supervision arose. The main point of interaction of such relationships is in the conference; it was to that experience that Blumberg turned his attention.

The trend toward analysis of the conference began with Blumberg and Cusick (1970), when they developed an interaction analysis system, *A System for Analyzing Supervisor-Teacher Interaction*, and used it to analyze 50 conferences between supervisors and teachers. The results of analysis of these conferences provided the first published view of what actually was happening in supervisory conferences and the first use of the terms *direct* and *indirect* to describe supervisory behavior. In their analysis, Blumberg and Cusick found that supervisors talked slightly less than the teachers (45 percent of the time for supervisors, 53 percent of the time for teachers, with 2 percent silence and confusion). What is more interesting than the amount of time, however, is the type of verbal interaction. While the supervisors were talking, they were about 33 percent more direct than indirect (that is, they were giving information, telling or suggesting to teachers what they should do, giving opinions, criticizing). They gave information five times as often as they asked for it. Supervisor talk was heavily weighted toward telling, as compared to asking, in both problem solving and task-oriented behaviors. They spent about seven times as much time telling their supervisees what to do as they did in asking teachers for their ideas or their suggestions. Supervisors asked opinions of teachers about one and one-half times more often than they gave opinions, and this behavior was interpreted by teachers as an attempt to trap them or "box them into a corner" (Blumberg, 1974, p. 109). Supervisors spent less than one percent of their time asking teachers for suggestions; teachers asked very few questions.

Further discussion of the results includes the interpretation that the supervisors did not deal directly with teachers' negative feelings in a way that helped the teachers. Interaction was mainly instruction from the supervisors. Teachers did not perceive supervision as being helpful, which was probably the reason they asked so few questions.

During the time that supervisors were engaged in accepting and clarifying teachers' ideas, 90 percent of the time was spent in giving short responses such as "I see," "Uh huh." Very little time was spent in clarifying the supervisees' remarks. When teachers did evidence negative social-emotional behaviors, the responses of the supervisors were not "therapeutic" but tended to be hostile and defensive. In trying to create a positive social-emotional climate, supervisors often used brief praising or evaluative comments such as "good" or "I like that."

In another discussion of this study, Blumberg (1974) proposed that the behavior of supervisors was antithetical to the accumulated knowledge about helping relationships. Certainly the supervisors Blumberg studied did not maintain a collaborative, problem-centered relationship with their teachers. This is particularly significant since they are talking about employed professionals—not inexperienced students where a teacher-student or supervisor-subordinate relationship might have been expected.

Although their analysis system focuses only on behavior, not content, Blumberg and Cusick (1970) discussed their impressions from the study and stated that supervisors tended not to deal directly with complaints from teachers; that when supervisors gave advice and information, teachers did not question or ask for a rationale; and that the bulk of discussion revolved around "maintenance procedures" such as schedules, movement of children in the room, and so forth. Further, supervisors backed away from dealing with teachers' defensiveness and Blumberg and Cusick perceived the whole process as a rather stereotyped, role playing process. Very little of the behavior was related to action or problem solving, resulting in conferences in which the interaction was not related to critical problems in the classroom, nor was it collaborative.

Other studies of the content of supervisory conferences in education at that time reported similar data (Heidelbach, 1967; Lindsey, 1969; Link, 1971; Michalak, 1969; Pittenger, 1972). Weller (1969), whose interaction analysis system will be encountered in the next chapter, found in a study of conferences that over 93 percent of the conference time was spent in analysis of instruction. Items related to this analysis were evenly divided between methods and materials (37.3 percent) and instruction and interactions (35.9 percent), while objectives and content received only 20 percent of the attention. Planning conferences concentrated mainly on objectives and methodology and this discussion was not extended, in other words, little time was spent on each interchange. Over two-thirds of the conference content was cognitive, rather than affective or social-disciplinary, although the affective increased in later conferences.

These early descriptive studies of the conference in teacher education formed an important foundation for the study of the conference in speech-language pathology and audiology. There has been substantial evidence that conferences in speech-language pathology and audiology are very similar to those described in education.

Studies of the Conference in Speech-Language Pathology and Audiology

Several descriptive studies of conferences are available from the speech-language pathology literature. Although generalization to audiology or assessment conferences may be made from the studies reported here, it should be remembered that the descriptive data has been based mainly on conferences related to speech-language therapy. It seems reasonable to assume, however, that the process, if not the content, of supervisory conferences is similar across areas.

A pioneer work by Hatten (1966) was the forerunner of several studies of the conference. Interestingly enough, this unpublished study, completed long before the current interest in supervision, stood alone until the mid-1970s. Hatten reported descriptive data concerning the temporal, topical content, and social-emotional characteristics of 40 mid-semester supervisory conferences in a university educational program. Supervisors talked approximately 60 percent of the time in the conference, with supervisees speaking 35 percent of the time. Supervisees spoke more often, giving short responses, which were most frequently agreement or "Uh huh." Mean length of the conference was approximately 16 minutes, and the range of topics discussed was from 4 to 10, with a mean of 6.55 topics. The number of topic changes within a conference, including returns to a previous topic, ranged from 5 to 49, with a mean of 24. Topics of discussion, in order of the time spent on each, were therapy techniques (41.97 percent), client's qualities (21.86 percent), therapist's qualities (13.87 percent), motivation (7.54 percent), clinical clerical (4.21 percent), social (2.86 percent), parents (2.74 percent), interpersonal (2.58 percent), theory (1.70 percent), and equipment (0.64 percent). Thus, the first three topics accounted for approximately 78 percent of the conference time. Only one content category (client's qualities) was present in all conferences. Hatten suggested that these percentages might change according to the time of the semester the conference was held.

In a later study of the supervisory conference in speech-language pathology, Underwood (1973) utilized the *System for Analyzing Supervisor-Teacher Interaction* (Blumberg & Cusick, 1970) to investigate several variables in the conference and reported results similar to those of Blumberg and Cusick. She found that supervisory conferences with students in speech-language pathology were longer than those with teachers—a 24-minute average for speech-language pathology as compared to 13 minutes in education. The least-used supervisory behavior was Supervisor asks for suggestions, as in Blumberg and Cusick's study. Least-used behavior for clinicians was Negative social emotional behavior.

Another view of the supervisory conference in speech-language pathology comes from a study of the interaction of 10 supervisor-clinician pairs over a 12-week period (Culatta & Seltzer, 1976). Some of these data have been referred to throughout other chapters. As a group, the trend was for the supervisees to provide raw data about the sessions; supervisors then used the data to suggest strategy for the next session. Sixty-one percent of all strategy statements were made by supervisors, who also asked about 70 percent of the questions, although the types of questions asked were not indicated. Supervisors spoke 55 percent of the time. There were no conferences in which clinicians made more statements than supervisors. Culatta and Seltzer noted the absence of evaluation statements by the supervisor or self-evaluation by the supervisee. Only nine percent of all responses tabulated were evaluative; two-thirds of them were made by supervisors. Few evaluative guidelines were provided by supervisors, and supervisees were not involved in self-analysis or self-evaluation. In addition, Culatta and Seltzer's data reveal that, even though supervisors thought they changed their behaviors during the 12-week term, there was virtually no change in the relative proportion of responses of supervisors and clinicians, time spent talking, and the categories of response. A follow-up study by Culatta and Seltzer (1977) found approximately the same proportion of behavior occurring in conferences and confirmed the fact that supervisors did not change, even on self-selected behaviors.

Similar data on conferences were provided by Schubert and Nelson (1976), who used the *Underwood Category System for Analyzing Supervisor-Clinician Behavior* to analyze nine supervisory conferences. Behavior used most frequently was clinician positive social behavior, including such responses as "mmhm" and "O.K." (21.4 percent). Next most frequent behavior was supervisors providing opinions/suggestions (20.6 percent). Supervisor talk consistently accounted for a larger part of the conferences (65 percent) than supervisee talk. Of the total amount of supervisor talk, the most frequent behavior was providing opinions/suggestions (42 percent) and providing factual information (32 percent). Schubert and Nelson also found no supervisor criticism or negative social behavior from clinicians.

Irwin (1975, 1976) studied supervisory behavior during conferences that followed microtherapy sessions (use of videotape) and also found that the direct style (instruction, modeling, negative reinforcement) was used significantly more than the indirect style (asking questions, positive reinforcement), with supervisees responding to supervisors, not initiating.

Similar behavior was cited by Roberts and Smith (1982), who described behavior of supervisors and supervisees over a six-week period based on analysis with the *Multidimensional Observational System for the Analysis of Interactions in Clinical Supervision* (MOSAICS) (Weller, 1971). Supervisors, they said, assumed the initiatory role by structuring and soliciting responses and by contributing more pedagogical moves (uninterrupted verbal utterances). Supervisees assumed a predominately reflexive role, that is, they responded and reacted to the supervisors and participated less. Supervisors set the content and interaction patterns and directed the dialogue, thereby affecting and controlling the remainder of the conference. Supervisors talked less about previous behavior and more about what should be done in future sessions. As in the Culatta and Seltzer study, supervisees appeared to present data about the session; supervisors focused on prescribing what supervisees should do and also gave opinions and suggestions for future sessions. Supervisors provided more facts, experiences, and observations than evaluative statements, again in agreement with Culatta and Seltzer. Both supervisor and supervisee used simplistic rather than complex statements, meaning there was little explanation, justification, or rationalization of statements from either party in the conference. Behavior did not change over time.

A content analysis system was developed by Tufts (1984) to quantify the topical content of supervisory conferences. Tufts found data similar to the other studies. About half of the time in the conferences was spent on two categories of behavior—clinical procedures (techniques, materials, client management) and lesson analysis (discussion of what the client did). When the category Client Information (general comments about the client not related specifically to the observed session) was added, the allotted time rose to approximately 70 percent. Less emphasis was placed on client information, nonjudgmental focus on the supervisor and supervisee, and planning for future therapy sessions. Minimal attention (less than 10 percent) was allotted to the supervisor giving information of an academic nature about disorders and their management, judgmental statements about the supervisee or supervisor, discussion of general professional items, and nonprofessional/social comments.

Tufts looked at differences in conference content related to supervisee experience and found no major differences between three experience levels, except in lesson planning. In this category, supervisees with the most experience spent much more time in planning and assumed more responsibility for planning than did those with less experience. Tufts's study also supported other findings that supervisees spend more time providing observation/information than their supervisors.

Descriptive information resulted from Shapiro's (1985) study of commitments made in the supervisory conference. Forty-seven percent of the total commitments made were in the areas of planning, analysis, and evaluation of the clinical process, with particular focus on the behavior of the client. Second most frequent commitments (39 percent) addressed implementation of treatment or assessment techniques for the client. Only eight percent of the commitments included planning, analysis, or evaluation of supervisee behaviour, and only four percent addressed implementation of supervisee behavior. Academic commitments were made least often (two percent). These findings reinforce the impression of conferences focused on client rather than clinician or supervisee behavior.

Two studies in speech-language pathology have focused entirely on the interpersonal aspects of the conference. McCrea (1980) adapted scales developed by Gazda (1974) for measuring the supervisor facilitative behaviors of Empathic Understanding, Respect, Facilitative Genuineness, and Concreteness as well as the ability of the supervisee to self-explore, all concepts from Rogerian theoretical positions (Carkhuff, 1967, 1969a,b; Carkhuff & Berenson, 1967; Carkhuff & Truax, 1964; Rogers, 1951, 1957, 1961, 1962). After modification of the scales, she analyzed 28 conferences. Respect, Facilitative Genuineness, and Concreteness were demonstrated only at minimal levels and Empathic Understanding and Supervisee Self-exploration were not identified often enough to be utilized in statistical analysis. Two shortcomings of this study were that audiotapes of conferences were utilized, thereby eliminating the nonverbal behavior through which much of the affect is carried, and that the identification of behaviors was done by trained raters and did not reflect the perceptions of the supervisees. Despite this, it appears very clear that the emphasis in these conferences, too, was not on clinician affect nor behavior, but on such cognitive content as client problems, discussion of activities, planning strategies, and procedural matters.

A very different methodology was used in the other study of the interpersonal aspects of the conference by Pickering (1979). A descriptive, naturalistic approach was utilized to examine interpersonal communication in 40 samples each of therapy sessions and supervisory conferences. The findings will not come as a surprise to the reader at this point. The supervisors' communication in the conferences was predominantly instructional, giving suggestions, advice, opinions, directives, and questions. Supervisors seemed to have an individual style which they maintained. Emphasis was on resolving issues regarding clients, not supervisees; content was cognitive and analytical. Supervisors shared few feelings, they were sympathetic and supportive and reinforcing when supervisees expressed feelings and concerns, but did not aid supervisees in expanding those feelings or expressing their own. Supervisors frequently failed to attend to supervisees' expressions of feeling associated with therapy, often asking a cognitive question to turn the conversation back to the solution of client problems. The supervisors and supervisees rarely discussed the supervisory relationship or their feelings about each other. At the same time, supervisors were keeping journals in which they indicated the importance of the students' feelings in the therapeutic relationship with the client. Supervisees, too, focused on cognitive issues, shared feelings more frequently than the supervisors, but they were frequently vague and reflected past feelings rather than current (probably because the discussion was the typical recounting of the clinical session).

Group Conferences

Although one-to-one supervisory conferences seem to be the traditional method in speech-language pathology and audiology, group or team conferences are apparently used frequently. Supervisors may be motivated to use group conferences simply because their work loads prevent individual scheduling or they may have strong beliefs in the value of group interaction in the learning process.

As with any other methodology, group supervision has its advantages and disadvantages. Economy of time and effort while communicating about matters of common concern, sharing experiences and problem solving, emotional support, comfortable learning environment due to safety in numbers, specialization of function, and peer influence are among the advantages in social work supervision listed by Kadushin (1976). Some disadvantages, as he saw them, are the fact that it is difficult to attend to individuals needs, some individuals may be uncomfortable in the group situation, supervisees in the group may abdicate to other members responsibilities that they might have to accept in individual interaction with the supervisor, and group members may not be compatible or cohesive.

Hart (1982) stated that, so far as skill development is concerned, group supervision exposes supervisees in counseling to a wider variety of cases than their own case load and aids in generating a variety of techniques and strategies from which supervisees can choose. There is opportunity for different points of view in feedback. "When the group is the only mode of supervision, however, each supervisee gets little individual attention" (p. 84).

Dowling (1979a) has been the main proponent of group methodology for supervision in speech-language pathology and audiology in the form of a procedure called the *Teaching Clinic*. Developed for teacher training, the Teaching Clinic is a specifically structured peer-group form of supervision. As described by Dowling (1979a), the Teaching Clinic consists of six sequential phases: (1) review of the previous teaching clinic, (2) planning, (3) observation, (4) critique preparation, (5) critique and strategy development, and (6) clinic review. The group consists of a demonstration clinician who contributes a videotape of a clinical session, and a clinic leader, who serves as facilitator. Although usually the supervisor, this role may later be assumed by a group member. Other participants are a group monitor (a peer), who observes the group process to see if roles are being fulfilled and ground rules followed, and peers of the demonstration clinician.

The script of the Teaching Clinic is as follows: The previous clinic is reviewed to maintain continuity. The demonstration clinician discusses the results of implementing the suggestions made in the previous clinic. Ground rules or problems in previous clinics are discussed by the group monitor. During the planning session, the demonstration clinician presents his or her therapy objectives and plans, and requests certain data she or he would like to have collected. The clinic leader then discusses data collection tasks to be carried out by the peers.

The team members, including the demonstration clinician, view the videotape (10 to 15 minutes). The demonstration clinician leaves the room to analyze the collected data independently and the clinic leader and peers analyze their data, problem-solve, and determine how to provide feedback in the most supportive manner. The demonstration clinician returns to room, presents his or her self-analysis, followed by group feedback, problem solving, and generation of strategies for the next clinical session. The final phase is the clinic review, in which the group monitor reviews the effectiveness of group interactions.

The Teaching Clinic has been compared to conventional supervision by Dowling and Shank (1981), using Culatta and Seltzer's (1976) *Content and Sequence Analysis System* for analysis, but no differences in talk behavior were identified. The teaching clinic appeared to be comparable to the conventional model of supervision. Since Dowling and colleagues (1982) later determined that the Culatta and Seltzer system was neither reliable nor valid for research purposes, the results of the Dowling and Shank study must be questioned. On the basis of a later analysis, Dowling (1983a), utilizing the MOSAICS System (Weller, 1971), concluded that conventional supervision contained more indirect behavior than the teaching clinic and, thus, was more conducive to the development of self-supervisory skills.

Johnson and Fey (1983) compared the relative effects of individual and teaching clinic (group) conferencing methods on students' attitudes toward therapy and their clinical effectiveness and found no differences between treatment groups. Given the complexity of comparing these types of supervision, there are still many questions to be asked and answered.

Individuals who wish to utilize group conferences should be sensitive to the needs of supervisees. Many students prefer to have some opportunity for individual contact with the supervisor along with the group interaction. Certain aspects of the Collaborative Style lend themselves to a group methodology. For example, much of the introductory aspects of the first component, Understanding the Supervisory Process, could be done in a group, not only to save time, but to allow supervisees to share insights and experiences. Teaching supervisees the techniques of data collection and analysis, as well as demonstrating certain clinical techniques, are other subjects for group situations.

Kadushin (1976) stated that research in social work has not indicated significant differences between the two methods and, because both have certain strengths and weaknesses and are appropriate to different needs and situations "it is desirable to employ them as planned, complementary procedures" (p. 335). This is relevant for speech-language pathology and audiology, and consistent with the Collaborative Style, should be a part of the overall planning.

For the Consultative Style, the group conference may be especially appropriate. Self-supervising clinicians have much to share with each other and such conferences could be an effective means of promoting professional growth, whatever the setting.

One issue in the utilization of group supervision in speech-language pathology and audiology is the extent of the preparation of supervisors in group processes. There is an analogy to be found in group therapy. Most supervisors have observed so-called group therapy, which was simply a few minutes of individual therapy for each client who happened to be sitting in the group. Among the reasons for this are the fact that the group has been defined on the basis of scheduling convenience rather than on common goals or problems or the ability to work together, and their needs are so varied that even the most skillful group leader would have difficulty utilizing the time appropriately. Another reason is the lack of preparation, experience, or insight of the clinician about group processes, which results in ineffective use of group time. Clinicians become supervisors and their lack of skill in this area may be carried over into the supervisory process. Although group supervision is thought by many to be valuable, it is highly dependent upon how it is carried out by the supervisor. "Group supervision often comes about through default, rather than design. . . . Any structuring of supervision should be based on the needs of the practitioners. Group supervision should not be entered into simply to relieve time pressures of the supervisor" (Munson, 1983, p. 131). Supervisees, too, often need help to adjust to the group situation. Any supervisor who wishes to utilize group supervision would do well to investigate the vast literature available on group processes. Lack of preparation or insufficient information about dealing with groups should not be a permanent condition.

Varying Perceptions of Conferences

There is evidence that supervisees and supervisors in speech-language pathology and audiology perceive the activities within conferences differently. This fact, coupled with the data that indicate the supervisory process is not discussed, increases the opportunity for misunderstanding and frustration (Culatta et al., 1975; McCrea, 1980; Pickering, 1984; Roberts & Smith, 1982; Shapiro, 1985; Tufts, 1984).

Culatta and colleagues (1975) found that supervisees and supervisors frequently reported "completely contradictory interpretations of the same event" (p. 152). The discrepancies in relation to lesson planning have been reported in the chapter on planning. Other areas where discrepancies existed are relevant to this component. For example, supervisors said they believed it was important to have supervisees review the client's case history and confer with the supervisor before client contact. Seventy percent of the supervisees, however, reported that supervisors did not attend these conferences, resulting in disappointment and confusion on the part of the supervisees. Supervisors felt positively about reviewing videotapes, supervisees did not. There were differing views about the value of various types of reports and of the supervisory conference. Most important, the areas of difference were never discussed during conferences.

Similar results have been reported by others. Russell (1976) also found differences between competencies valued by supervisees in their supervisors and what they perceived their supervisors actually did, as did Anderson and Milisen (1965).

Such differences in perceptions are illustrated by the following situation. An off-campus supervisor says to the university supervisor, "I wish the student would use more of her own ideas and not do just what I do," while the supervisee says, "I feel that I have to do therapy the way she does it. That is what she wants." And, as in the study by Culatta and colleagues (1975), they seldom discuss these differences except with the university supervisor. In fact, this may become a major function of the university supervisor of the off-campus practicum—bridging the "communication gap."

In an extensive study of the conference, Smith (1978) and Smith and Anderson (1982b) found that supervisors, supervisees, and trained raters each perceived different effectiveness variables in the conference content. Such differences of perception are not surprising. What is significant in relation to these differences, however, is the previously mentioned lack of discussion in conferences. It might be assumed that such differences between expectations and reality would be clarified at some time, but such does not seem to be the case. Relevant to this fact is the recommendation made by Smith and Anderson (1982a) "that supervisors and supervisees should keep their self-perceptions of the conference at a conscious level, investigating them at frequent intervals to determine if their perceptions are similar. A lack of information regarding the convergence or divergence of perceptions of those involved in conference interactions, if allowed to exist over time, may greatly diminish the effectiveness of the conference" (p. 258). Going back, then, to the Understanding component, there should be discussion both before and during the supervisory interaction.

A word must be said about this mass of descriptive data on the conference and the consistency of the findings that supervisor behavior does not change over time or according to the supervisee's experience. There are, admittedly, weaknesses in some of the studies. Change has been measured over a short time, possibly not sufficient to expect change. The questions asked, the settings in which the research was conducted, the instruments used, and the preciseness of the methodology used in the studies vary greatly. It must be assumed that they do not describe every supervisory conference. Yet, the results are so similar in the various studies that they must be given credence. Further, they are supported on a subjective basis by experience in viewing hundreds of videotapes of conferences and reading the results of student self-studies. The knowledge that supervisors' perceptions of their own behavior and its change are not accurate cannot give much comfort to the supervisor who says, "But my conferences are not like that. I do alter my behavior according to the needs of the supervisee." This statement may be true, but no one can say that with any certainty until they have engaged in some type of objective study of their conferences.

WHAT'S A SUPERVISOR TO DO?

What do all these studies and all this discussion tell the supervisor about the provision of feedback or the supervisory conferences? Except for general knowledge about learning, motivation, communication, interpersonal interaction, leadership, and other relevant topics, there is not enough specific information to support the merits of any method of feedback or any particular type of conference. This allows the writer the freedom to speculate that professional growth, including specific behavior change in supervisees, will or will not take place mainly as a result of the interaction in the conference. It is the thesis of this book, then, that the conference, while only one of several types of interaction between supervisor and supervisee, is probably the most important. This belief comes not only from the fact that it appears to be the most commonly used occasion for communication, but because of the sheer dynamics of this interpersonal "happening"—this event that can be so important to its participants. Further, there is an assumption that it is through the intensive study of the conference that the positives and negatives of the supervisory process will begin to unravel.

What *is* known about the conference, as described, is that it is consistent with the Direct-Active Style appropriate to the Evaluation-Feedback Stage, not with the Collaborative Style nor with the Consultative Style. If the continuum and the styles appropriate to its different points are accepted, conference behavior can be measured against that standard.

Conferences Using the Collaborative Style

An alternative to the Direct-Active Style is the Collaborative Style, which has been alluded to, but not described specifically. Some of the characteristics of such a style are listed here. The items are not all-inclusive—there are many other behaviors—but these are considered important. They are not necessarily in order of importance, nor is it implied that any one conference will include all components. Content will be determined by individual needs, place on the supervisory continuum, current objectives, and other factors.

■ The conference will include some evidence that it has been planned. This planning may be the setting of agenda items at the beginning of the conference or it may be a carry-over from planning done in a previous conference.

■ There will be evidence that both long-range and short-range goals and objectives have been set for all participants— client, clinician, supervisee, and supervisor.

■ There will be evidence of data collection on both client and clinician behaviors by both supervisor and supervisee.

■ The data will be presented in an organized manner which gives some evidence of planning the data collection. For example, it will be obvious that data are related to previously stated objectives. Not only will it be obvious that planning took place to determine what data would be collected, how and by whom, but how it will be presented in the conference.

■ There will be emphasis on analysis of the data related to the relationship between client and clinician behavior, not the single-minded attention to the client behavior as seen in so much of the data on conferences. Inferences will be drawn from the data about the relationship between the clinician and the client.

■ Analysis will be related to goals and objectives.

■ There will be data collection, analysis, and discussion of goals and objectives for supervisee and supervisor, that is, the supervisory process will be studied to determine if appropriate learning is taking place.

■ There will be a mixture of direct and indirect supervisor behaviors and active and passive supervisee behaviors. The balance will be determined by the place on the continuum.

A similar classification of supervision styles was recently presented by Farmer and Farmer (1986), which utilizes the terms *unilateral* and *bilateral* and that is useful in understanding the combination of styles that may exist in conferences. Unilateral conferences are supervisor-dominated; bilateral conferences involve joint participation by both supervisor and supervisee. Farmer and Farmer described behaviors for Unilateral-Dyadic, Unilateral-Group, Bilateral-Dyadic, and Bilateral-Group Conferences.

■ Topics other than data from the clinical session will include procedural or administrative issues, academic topics, personal or affective concerns, professional issues, unexpected events, and other items as they arise.

■ Although the emphasis will be on analysis, particularly self-analysis by the supervisee, leading to self-evaluation, there is a time and place for varying degrees of evaluative feedback and information-giving by the supervisor.

■ The supervisor will assume the responsibility for structuring opportunities for joint problem solving through open, thought-provoking questions, appropriate responses to the supervisee, type of objectives set, and other techniques. In turn, the supervisee will accept his or her responsibility for participating in problem solving.

■ Part of the learning process will be the expansion of verbal statements by supervisor and supervisee—explanations, justifications, rationale for opinions and suggestions, questioning each other for such expansion if it is not there. This is not to suggest that a conference should become a sparring contest to force justification of every statement. However, the data are clear that, traditionally, utterances are simple and short, rather than leading to in-depth discussion and information exchange. This probably does not lead to optimum learning. More discussion of options, justification, and explanations of suggestions by supervisors, and expansion of ideas should lead to more learning and more generalization to other situations. Without such interchange, much learning may be lost.

■ The interpersonal interaction in the conference will be supportive and facilitative, with both participants being sensitive to the needs and feelings of the other.

■ Supervisor and supervisee will review periodically their own objectives for the supervisory process, compare their perceptions of whether or not these objectives are being met, and make appropriate adjustments.

The Consultative Style

The Consultative Style, appropriate to the Self-Supervision Stage, is not as clear-cut as the other two styles. It may include behaviors from each of the other styles, but the supervisor and supervisee will maintain a different type of relationship. Referred to rather commonly in the literature in other helping professions, consultation is not so frequently discussed in speech-language pathology and audiology. Flower (1984) stated that consultation is "the most frequently overlooked" (p. 12) component of education and training in speech-language pathology and audiology.

According to Hart (1982), consultation in counseling is "an informal educational experience usually used in place of supervision" (p. 12). Kurpius and Robinson (1978) called the consultant a "collaborator who forms egalitarian relationships with the consultees to bring about change. In this collegial relationship, there is a joint diagnosis with emphasis on the consultees finding their own solution to their problems. The consultant serves as a catalyst or facilitator for the problem-solving process" (p. 322). Kurpius and colleagues (1977) said that consultation is a frequently employed approach to supervision and that it "implies shared problem definition, problem solving, and evaluation between supervisor and supervisee. . . .There is a suggestion in the literature that consultation becomes a more dominant mode of supervision as the trainee becomes increasingly able and professional in his performance" (p. 228).

Consultation in speech-language pathology and audiology is often thought of as a process in which an outside professional is employed to advise about certain aspects of the work of an agency or an organization (Bess, 1987; Flower, 1984; Griffith, 1987). Others have written of the consultative role of the speech-language pathologist or audiologist in working with classroom teachers or physicians within the organizations in which they work (Flower, 1984; Frassinelli, Superior, & Meyer, 1983; Freeman, 1982). Flower (1984) contended that the consultant role of speech-language pathologists and audiologists is currently being expanded beyond health and education to the place where they are now being asked to consult on legal matters, to offer expert testimony about relationships between communication disorders and medical or vocational situations, and to provide consultative services to business and industry.

Reviewing the definition of the Consultative Style of supervision given in Chapter 4, it is a style that results from the need to solve a problem. The Consultative Style has a voluntary, and possibly an intermittent or temporary, component not found in the other styles. The supervisee is perceived as identifying the area of need; the supervisor as helping the supervisee solve the problem, utilizing his or her own knowledge, skill, and expertise to the greatest possible extent. The supervisor offers input, direct or indirect, as appropriate. The needs of each situation may require different roles and skills for each participant. The *process* of problem solving must never be forgotten in the Consultative Style, even though there are times when the focus is on content through providing information, knowledge, rationale, or other content. Such emphasis on problem solving will enare able the supervisee to function more adequately in the future (Brasseur, 1978).

This definition may seem little different from the definition of the Collaborative Style. Actually, the difference is a matter of degree. Consultation is an expansion of the Collaborative Style to meet the needs of supervisees who have truly reached the point where they are capable of self-supervision, are able to analyze their clinical work, and can identify their own needs. The time at which the supervisee reaches this stage will vary, as suggested by Figure 4-3. If it is reached during the educational program, the supervisor may become a monitor, may help supervisees expand their clinical activities, or may assist them in spending more time in analysis of the supervisory process. If it is reached during the off-campus practicum or the *Clinical Fellowship Year* (CFY), supervisors may need to adjust their expectations and their behaviors to truly operate as a consultant, that is, to assist supervisees to use their own knowledge and skills in problem solving. In the service delivery setting, where supervisor and supervisee are both fully qualified professionals, the interactions will vary even more. Conference content between supervisor and supervisee will be determined not only by the nature of the problem to be solved but by the frequency with which the supervisor is able to interact with the supervisee in the work setting. Despite the efforts of the profession to establish standards, one cannot assume that every professional in the work force has the ability to be self-supervising in every situation. The supervisee may reach the Self-Supervision Stage in one area of clinical expertise and not in others. And, herein, lie the hazards in the use of the Consultative Style in any setting—the possible inaccurate perception of supervisees of their own ability, either positive or negative, or the inability of the supervisor to accurately determine the true nature of the supervisee's skills in relation to the Consultative Style. The suggestions from the chapter on planning for determining the appropriate point on the continuum are relevant here. Beyond that, it may be necessary to problem-solve with the supervisee for a period of time to determine his or her skill level.

This is the stage at which it is most important for the supervisor to discard the Direct-Active Style, to recognize the educational background and experience of supervisees, to exercise the professional control advocated by Cogan (1973), and to perform a facilitating role in the problem solving necessary to assist supervisees in achieving change. The writer recalls a personal supervisory experience that occurred far too long ago to be so well remembered. Having completed several years of experience in three different school systems, the semiannual visit of a "supervisor" came during a session with a young, very severe stutterer with whom the writer had been working for a long period of time. Activities over that time period had included frequent discussions with parents, teachers, and others in the child's environment; direct therapy; referral to a university clinic for consultation; and whatever other activities were in her clinical repertoire at the time. After the child left the room the "supervisor," asking no questions about what had been done, said, "I think you should have a conference with the parents." If this appears to be a caricature of a supervisor, be assured that the incident did happen. Its clarity in the writer's memory after all these years might provide encouragement for all supervisors to consider the import of their remarks to supervisees, particularly at the Self-Supervision Stage.

This event certainly characterizes the superior-subordinate relationship so soundly rejected by Cogan (1973), who suggested that the supervisor who performs in this manner psychologically diminishes the supervisee by placing her or him in an inferior role, that of a person with less competence who needs the direction of the supervisor. Cogan then slyly suggested that, in a discussion of the "superior-subordinate" relationship, perhaps no one has ever wondered if "superior" refers to the teacher or the supervisor! The reality is, in this time of proliferating knowledge, that supervisors at any stage will do themselves and their supervisees a favor by learning what supervisees actually do know before providing advice.

Flower (1984) summed it up when he stated "Good consultation resembles any other professional service; it is valuable only if offered in a way that is useful to the recipient" (p. 12). Consultation, he said, will be helpful only when it is sensitive to the recipients' needs and is "relevant, practical, and applicable" (p. 13).

COMMUNICATION IN THE CONFERENCE

The implementation of the continuum of supervision is dependent upon the communication skills of both supervisor and supervisee. The ability to be clear, specific, and concrete is essential to sharing perceptions, expectations, planning, discussion of data, and to determining the effectiveness of the supervisory interaction. Further, the supervisor's ability to encourage appropriate participation by the supervisee in the problem solving that takes place in the conference is essential to movement along the continuum. Supervisors whose verbal behavior dominates the conference do not increase supervisee input or opportunity to problem-solve. On the other hand, supervisees' verbal behavior is often too extensive, not well-planned, and not clear or focused. This, too, may need attention in relation to effective communication.

Clarity in Communication

Nothing is more discouraging or distressing to speakers than to see their verbal behaviors written in script form. Even some of the most proficient users of the language are horrified by their excessive and irrelevant fillers—"O.K.," "you know," "um," "uh,"—the redundancies, the fragmented sentences, the tortured syntax. Consider the following excerpt from a transcript of a supervisee's actual utterance in a conference: "Um, I think that—I guess that some or a lot of—well, you know—I think a lot of the words we've worked on—not, you know—I think it's near the, it's the same type of sound that we've been working on—you know—the voiceless—well, it's not a stop plosive, you know—um—the other sounds we um—you know—worked on were stop plosives but the poorer articulation was—you know—would be /s/—you know—pretty much the same. I think—." This was in response to a supervisor question about four utterances back, which had asked where they needed to go now with the client. This type of utterance may be the result of several conditions—the supervisee's natural lack of facility with the language, anxiety, lack of preparation, poorly stated objectives, and other reasons.

Supervisors are not immune to such cluttered and imprecise verbalizations. For example, the following supervisor's utterance is from another conference. After lengthy planning for the client, the supervisor says, "Well, let's see. I also want to—we need to—you know—discuss the supervisory session—the supervisory process. You know—we need to talk about what we do, how we spend our time—how we manipulate our time in the conference because—well, we need to spend some of the time talking about you as a clinician instead of, you know, all the time about the client. We need to do that especially now, you know, when we are doing the diagnostic report and analyzing the data on therapy—that's important, but we also need to spend some time with that and then, like what we've been doing here, you know, um, we need to talk about supervision, you know, the actual supervisory relationship between ourselves, between us, you know, how to think about this, about how to handle these issues in the future. They are important, you know." To which the supervisee responded, "Was there anything else you wanted to say about the transcript (of the session)?" Such interactions when multiplied through a total conference or a whole semester are inefficient, time-wasting, and nonproductive.

Listening to an audiotape or viewing a videotape of a conference early in the interaction will probably reveal many types of behaviors that are obvious targets for objectives for supervisors or supervisees. The basis of such scattered, unclear communication may be in the planning and analysis components. If the agenda is planned carefully and the plan followed, there may be less "rambling." If that planning is combined with skill in analysis, the data can be presented clearly and concisely.

One role of supervisors is to improve the communication behavior of their supervisees and themselves. Not only can improvement in verbal and nonverbal skills increase the efficiency and effectiveness of the conference, it should carry over to the clinical process. The supervisee who cannot clarify issues in the supervisory conference probably cannot give clear, precise directions to clients either, and may fill clinical sessions with unnecessary verbiage.

Strategies for this task must be carefully planned. Supervisees may perceive their verbal style as a personal characteristic that no one has a right to change. That may be true in terms of the individual's private life; when it becomes an issue in terms of professional interactions, it is another story. Several years ago, a student enrolled in a supervision practicum with the writer demonstrated a voice and manner of speaking that was coy, passive, flirtatious, and that conveyed an attitude of dependence and immaturity. In actuality, she was a highly intelligent, mature, capable professional. These behaviors were identified easily in the practicum by both participants and objectives were set for modifying them, mainly through intensive observations of videotape and tallying occurrences of contributing actions. The student was highly motivated and was able to make extensive changes. In fact, her comment in the final conference was, "My friends tell me I don't sound like a little girl anymore." Not all behaviors would be changed so readily and the writer is well aware of the emotional and psychological components that might be involved in similar situations. Nevertheless, professional communication styles remain a concern.

One method for approaching the verbosity of supervisee or supervisor is to include in the planning a procedure whereby the verbatim utterances from a portion of a tape are transcribed and then rewritten in a clear, concise manner. The individual who is redundant *ad nauseum* soon becomes conscious of the behavior in subsequent conversations. Such verbal activity is easily tallied and charted so that progress is seen, or not seen, as the case may be.

From the counseling literature (Carkhuff & Truax, 1964), four facilitative dimensions in interpersonal interaction have been identified. These have been adapted by McCrea (1980) for use in analyzing supervisors' behavior in speech-language pathology and audiology (see Appendix G). One of these dimensions is *concreteness*, and it is relevant to the issue of clarity discussed here. Concreteness means being specific, and the scale used for its measurement ranges from the lowest Level 1—Supervisor statement which is extremely vague, causes confusion and greatly detracts from the flow of the discussion—to the highest Level 7—Supervisor statements must be specific with an example and a rationale. Roberts and Smith (1982) indicated that supervisors do not give rationale and justification for their statements, and McCrea (1980) found that concreteness in supervisor behavior in the conferences she studied occurred below the minimally facilitative level of functioning described by Carkhuff (1969, a,b). Because examples and rationale clarify topics being discussed, the findings of these studies suggest that supervisors need to examine their own conferences in this regard. Supervisors interested in this dimension of their conferences could use the McCrea scale to gain insight and set objectives for themselves. They could also have their supervisees or another person rate them to check the reliability of the self-ratings. Although not validated on supervisees, the rating scale could, however, be used for self-study by supervisees.

SKILLS FOR FACILITATING COMMUNICATION IN THE CONFERENCE

Any of a multitude of books on counseling, the helping relationship, and interviewing contain descriptions of skills that facilitate communication (Benjamin, 1969; Brammer, 1985; Condon, 1977; Hackney & Nye, 1973; Knapp, 1972; Luft, 1969; Luterman, 1979, 1984; Molyneux & Lane, 1982). Such information may be familiar to many supervisors, having been a part of their basic training as clinicians. In recent years, however, it appears that the study of basic communication theory has not been such a recognized need for clinicians as it once was. Nevertheless, it is an area where supervisees and supervisors can easily upgrade their skills through reading and continuing study.

Listening Skills

The importance of listening skills is well known in counseling, therapy, and conversation with friends. In general, people do not appear to be good listeners, a fact well described by Kagan (1970), when he said, "We don't really listen to each other. I tell you about how much I hurt and you're just waiting for me to finish so you can tell me how much you hurt" (p. 95). The desire of supervisees to be listened to, to have supervisors pay attention to them, and to take them seriously surfaces frequently in the literature on expectations. In addition, if supervisors wish to have supervisees participate in the conference, it is not enough just to reduce their own verbal behavior by listening; they must do something to encourage supervisee input. This means really *attending* to what supervisees say, accepting it, but more than that, building upon what supervisees have said. The impact of the "Yes, but—" statement is well known. In the supervisory process it may shut off problem-solving as quickly as anything a supervisor can do. One of the categories of Blumberg and Cusick's (1970) interaction analysis system is Accepts or uses teacher's ideas, and is defined as statements that clarify, build on, or develop ideas or suggestions by teachers. This is an activity extremely important to both the Collaborative and Consultative Styles. Thus, listening is more than just hearing what the supervisee has said. It is responding it to the input, rephrasing it to test understanding, clarifying it, restating it to better interpret what the supervisee has said, focusing the discussion, checking to see that perceptions are accurate. There is a danger, however, in the concept of using the supervisee's ideas. If supervisors use supervisees' ideas as their own, it is not conducive to the encouragement of additional ideas. Listening, then, is more than just hearing. It is an active process and its extension—responding, amplifying, clarifying, building upon ideas—contributes to joint participation in conferences.

Listening is not a one-way street in which supervisors must assume all responsibility. Supervisors can help supervisees become aware of their own listening patterns. A brief look at a videotape of a conference will reveal very quickly what is happening between the two participants. Listening is a skill that is also important in the clinical process. If the supervisee is not utilizing it in the conference, he or she may not be using good listening skills in the clinical session, either. Stating listening skill as a supervisory objective and working on it in the supervisory process should facilitate generalization to the clinical process.

Carl Rogers (1980), in a retrospective discussion of the development of his theories about dealing with people, related that in his early years as a therapist he discovered that simply listening to clients was important in being helpful. "So, when I was in doubt as to what I should do in some active way, I listened. It seemed surprising to me that such a passive kind of interaction could be so useful" (p. 137). Perhaps this is a thought that supervisors need to contemplate seriously.

Questioning Skills

The ability to ask good questions may be the most important skill in the supervisor's repertoire—questions that generate thinking by the supervisee, questions that do not already contain the answer desired by the supervisor, questions that have a purpose and are carefully thought out before they are uttered. In fact, it is possible that the type of questions asked by supervisors may, in many instances, be the determining factor in whether or not supervisees move along the continuum. Their impact may be either positive or negative.

Carin and Sund (1971), Cunningham (1971), and Davies (1981) suggested that learning in the classroom is determined largely through questioning techniques. Carin and Sund (1971) amplified this further when they said, "Involved in any deep communication between persons is the ability to ask appropriate questions and to listen. This is the genius of communication. To listen and question at just the right place and degree delineates the truly brilliant instructor from the average. An insightful question appropriately delivered may stimulate the individual to reach a new level of mental mediation. We learn to think only by thinking. We become creative only by having opportunities to be creative. A properly phrased question often is the necessary 'input' needed to ignite the student's thinking and creative process" (p. 2).

The use of questions in the classroom has received extensive coverage in the education literature. Questioning is the most frequently used utterance of teachers, but questions are least commonly used to stimulate thinking. Rather, teachers use questions in giving directions, managing the classroom, initiating activities, and in other learning situations. Critical thinking, however, seems not to be stimulated by teachers through questioning (Cunningham, 1971). Is this true of supervisors?

Questioning has many purposes—to obtain feedback or responses, to get data, to encourage thinking, to promote problem solving, to evaluate the student's preparation or participation in planned activities, to determine strengths and weaknesses, to review or summarize, to help the student recall, understand, synthesize, or apply, and to focus. (Carin & Sund, 1971; Cunningham, 1971; Davies, 1981; Whiteside, 1981)

There is an assumption that high levels of questioning behavior raise the cognitive level of students, forcing them to reflect, refocus, clarify, expand, and be more creative in their thinking, although the research is somewhat contradictory. Nevertheless, many systems for classifying and studying questions have been proposed and they are worthy of attention in the self-study of verbal behaviors in the conference. Sanders (1966) used seven categories: memory, translation, interpretation, application, analysis, synthesis, and evaluation. Davies (1981) classified questions as open or closed. Wittmer and Myrick (1974) divided them into least person-centered and most person-centered. Lowery (1970) suggested three broad categories: broad, narrow, and miscellaneous, with broad questions subcategorized into open-ended and valuing, narrow into direct information and focusing.

Probably the most useful category system for questioning is presented by Cunningham (1971). He divided questions into narrow and broad categories which he then broke down further. The narrow category includes cognitive memory questions (recall, identify- observe, yes or no, define, name, designate) and convergent questions (explain, state relationships, compare and contrast). The broad category includes divergent questions (predict, hypothesize, infer, reconstruct) and evaluative questions (judge, value, defend, justified choice). It is easy to see the increasing complexity of these classifications of questions.

Recognition of the importance of these levels of questioning in encouraging thinking and problem solving by supervisees is an important part of any supervisor's approach to supervision.

Questioning in Speech-Language Pathology and Audiology

Interest in questioning by speech-language pathologists has increased with the profession's involvement with the language-disordered child and the emphasis on the study of children's questions and answers (Ervin-Tripp, 1970; James & Seebach, 1982; Leach, 1972; Tyack & Ingram, 1977). More recent interest in discourse analysis has further focused attention on questions in relation to language development (Gallagher & Prutting, 1983). Although questioning has always been a tool of the clinician and, thus, a concern of supervisors, there is no indication of it having been a major topic of study as related to clinician behavior.

Questioning in the Supervisory Conference

Questioning in the supervisory conference was an important issue to Blumberg and Cusick (1970) in the development of their interactional analysis system for studying the supervisory process, as noted by their inclusion for both participants of items related to requesting information, opinions, and suggestions. Their analysis of conferences revealed certain information related to questioning which has already been discussed—less asking for ideas and suggestions than telling by supervisors, less asking of opinions than giving of opinions. In fact, asking for suggestions was the least-used supervisory behavior, and teachers never asked "Why?" when given advice. Thus, they said, teachers are not involved in problem solving about conditions they face in their classrooms. The interaction is *not* collaborative. Additionally, teachers reacted most negatively to supervisors asking for information, assuming that they were being "trapped." Blumberg and Cusick did not analyze the type of questions being asked but, if they had, they might have found a clue to the hostility engendered by such question asking.

Blumberg and Cusick also reported that conferences rated High Direct, High Indirect and those rated Low Direct, High Indirect were perceived as more productive than the High Direct, Low Indirect and the Low Direct, Low Indirect. The reader will recall from a previous chapter that the High Direct, High Indirect would include both telling, suggesting, giving information, criticizing, as well as reflecting and *asking* for information and suggestions. The Low Direct, High Indirect would contain less telling and more reflecting and asking. It is not known, of course, from Blumberg and Cusick's data if the conferences *were* more effective, only that the teachers perceived them in that way. Thus, although there was a preference in terms of productivity or effectiveness for both kinds of behavior, there was a stronger emphasis on the asking and reflecting behaviors.

Smith and Anderson (1982b) also found questioning behaviors of supervisors and supervisees to be related to the perceived effectiveness components (direct and indirect supervisory behaviors) of the conference. Smith (1979), in another study, provided an extensive description of questions used in supervisory conferences in speech-language pathology and audiology. Questions were usually cognitive and dealt with objectives or methods and materials. They asked primarily for factual information such as "What did Mary do when you asked her. . ." and "What are John's objectives?" (p. 11). Thus, they would be found in Cunningham's (1971) narrow category, and probably in the cognitive-memory subcategories. It was shown that supervisors asked 81 percent of the questions. The only difference in type of questions was that supervisees asked more opinion questions than supervisors. It did appear that supervisors varied their types of questions on the basis of such supervisee variables as experience and grade point average. Smith concluded that supervisors are dominating the questioning process and, by asking for the type of factual information indicated in this study, they are depriving supervisees of a vital opportunity for problem solving. She reflected, "If, as clinical supervisors, we intend to relinquish power and authority and utilize the clinical supervision model while training supervisees to problem-solve, self-analyze, and self-direct their own behavior, we *must* critically analyze and change, if necessary, our use of questions during conference interactions" (p. 9).

The way in which questions are stated will determine not only the answer but the type of thought that must go into the answer. In addition to the classifications just discussed, there are other types of questions familiar to everyone. The "yes-no" question in treatment sessions where clinicians are attempting to encourage the client to talk are well known to any supervisor. One of the first lessons the inexperienced clinician may learn is to avoid such questions; yet it is easy to do, even with experience, unless there is constant monitoring and planning of new behaviors. The same can be said of supervisor utterances. "Do you think it would be better if he wrote it out?" is deceptive. It may appear to request an opinion, but to the supervisee, if the supervisor suggested it, the answer may automatically become a *yes*.

In addition to "yes-no" questions, Cunningham (1971) listed several other problem questions. The ambiguous question does not include enough criteria to enable the answerer to define a good response. 'What about the session?" may appear to be a broad question to the supervisor, but the supervisee may feel that he or she must play a guessing game to find out what the supervisor wants to hear.

Another type of problem question is the "spoon-feeding" question, sometimes called leading or rhetorical, where the answer is embedded in the question. This type of question ranges from simple to complex. From transcripts of tapes of conferences, the following stand out as spoon-feeding: "That's more appropriate, isn't it?" "That was mostly nonverbal, wasn't it?"

Confusing questions, according to Cunningham (1971), include too many factors for the answerer to consider at one time. Consider this example from a tape of a conference: "What would you say—how high a success rate? Have you noticed, like, if he is succeeding at 60 or 70 percent of the time, is he usually O.K. versus 20 percent of the time if he's getting one out of five right? Does that make a big change in behavior for you, in your situation or not? Or have you been able to determine any of that? What do you think?" The obvious answer is "I think this is a very confusing question," but most supervisees would not have the courage to answer that way. This supervisee countered with "What do you mean? In the group?"

Whiteside (1981) reported on "tugging questions" such as "Well, come on, you know that" or "What did you do? Come on, now you can tell me about that. What did you do?" These are perhaps more commonly used by clinicians in attempts to get a response from a nonresponding client. Molyneux and Lane (1982) included in their categories of behavior in the interview a similar type of question which they called "bombardment"—an utterance that contains three or more questions of any type. Other question types listed by Molyneux and Lane (1982) are indirect, direct (two types), leading, double question (two types) for the interviewer and request for information only by the interviewee.

The Answers

The importance of listening has been stressed earlier. Acceptance of answers to questions and the responses to them are important in future participation and problem solving. Responses to incorrect or inaccurate answers require diplomacy, involving response, redirecting, helping the respondent move closer to a better answer, not blocking communication by responding negatively (Carin & Sund, 1971). In the supervisory conferences there are often answers that are neither right nor wrong and appropriate responses will encourage further discussion.

Responses are important, but frequently silence is just as important. Silence may mean resistance or simply mean that the responder is engaged in exploring the issue (Brammer, 1985). Wait time between questions and answers has been a popular area for study in education. Carin and Sund (1971) reported on a study that found the teacher's wait time was one second. When the wait time was extended, it resulted in longer student responses, less "I-don't-know" answers and more whole sentences, increased speculative thinking, more questions from children, revised teacher expectations of children, and a wider variety of questions asked by the teacher. Supervisors, too, need to learn to tolerate silence. Some people need more time to get their thoughts together than others, and the wait may result in a better answer.

INTERPERSONAL ASPECTS OF THE CONFERENCE

It was stated earlier that the interpersonal aspects of the supervisory process would not be treated extensively in this book. Yet it must be clear to the reader that the approach presented here is based on an assumption of attitudes of respect, empathic understanding, facilitative genuineness, concreteness of expression, unconditionality of regard, congruence, and self-exploration—all the interpersonal qualities proposed by Rogers (1957, 1961), Carkhuff (1969 a,b),

Carkhuff and Berenson (1967), and the many others who followed them. Obviously, it is not because of the writer's disregard for its significance that the specifics of interpersonal communication are not included. Rather, it is because of the volume of available material, the pursuit of which would have extended the writing of this book into the twenty-first century and would have expanded its size beyond the capacity of most book shelves. Further, this aspect of the supervisory process has been receiving an increasing amount of attention by other writers in recent years. All readers are encouraged, indeed implored, to make themselves familiar with this literature. Some of the many sources from the counseling and communication literature are Brammer (1985), Danish and Kagan (1971), Deetz and Stevenson (1986), George and Cristiani (1981), Luft (1969), and Smith and Williamson (1985).

Although Pickering (1986) recently stated that the profession of speech-language pathology has *not* been exemplary in "probing aspects of interpersonal communications in its helping, clinical relationships" (p. 16), it is encouraging that there has been some focus in recent years on the interpersonal communication aspects of the supervisory process. The research of Pickering (1979, 1984) and McCrea (1980) were discussed earlier. Others who have studied this area are Caracciolo (1977), Caracciolo and colleagues (1978a, 1978b), Klevans, Volz, and Friedman (1981); Volz (1976); Volz, Klevans, Norton, and Putens (1978); Oratio (1977), and Oratio and colleagues (1981). More recently, Pickering (1987a, 1987b), Crago (1987), and McCready and colleagues (1987) have addressed in depth the intricacies of interpersonal communication in the supervisory process.

The supervisory relationship may be one of the most intense interpersonal experiences in which a person can engage. The emotional dimensions of this vital relationship may influence both participants in ways that have not even begun to be identified. Mosher and Purpel (1972), in discussing the personal development of prospective teachers during the student teaching experience, asserted that not only does learning to teach require the student to change what she or he does, it also requires "that he change what he is" (p. 115). They stressed the need to assist the student in his or her process of changing from a *person* to a *professional person* and offered suggestions for supervisors to deal with this critical period in the student's life. Pickering (1984) and McCrea (1980) found only minimal evidence of facilitative interpersonal interaction between supervisor and supervisee in speech-language pathology and audiology. Is this the state of the art today? Perhaps supervisors have focused on teaching and instruction to the neglect of attending to the interpersonal needs of their supervisees.

Ward and Webster (1965a, 1965b), over twenty years ago, expressed their concern about personal needs of students in their growth and development as clinicians. Pickering (1977) stressed the importance for supervisors of an understanding of four concepts of human relationships—authenticity, dialogue, risk taking, and conflict. In a later report of her research, Pickering (1984) contended that neither students nor supervisors appear to know "how to analyze the interpersonal dimensions of therapeutic relationships" (p. 194).

Much of the counseling literature reflects the need of counselors to help counselees express themselves about their feelings, their concerns, their anxieties. Although supervisors are not counselors and a line must be drawn between the two roles which is analogous to the line between clinical work and counseling, supervisors will find times when they need to reflect the supervisee's words and focus on their feelings. Indeed, supervisors cannot escape situations where they must deal with the supervisee's feelings.

There are signs that the profession is turning its attention to this area of study. If it is as important as it seems to be, then every supervisor in her or his role as facilitator of the supervisory process should become familiar with the literature and assist supervisees in learning about it. More than that, however, they need to study their own interpersonal interaction to determine its possible impact upon the supervisory process.

SUMMARY

The last component to be discussed, Integrating, is also the beginning. It is the place where everything that has happened in the other components comes together and the future is determined. Each of the other components feeds into this component.

Because the other components have been discussed individually, this chapter focuses on the communication that takes place between supervisor and supervisee. The conference is discussed at some length because this is the usual place where communication between supervisor and supervisee occurs.

This chapter includes extensive discussion of feedback, which is defined as interaction between all participants about all components of the process, *not* as just the traditional reporting on observation. This component, then, becomes the culmination of all the effort and time that have gone into the supervisory process.

Studying the Supervisory Process

Systematic study and investigation of the supervisory process is seen as necessary to expansion of the data base from which increased knowledge about supervision and the supervisory process will emerge.

ASHA Committee on Supervision (1985b, p. 60)

A basic principle underlying the proposal made here for the supervisory process is that the interaction between supervisor and supervisee must be studied. Once the entry point on the continuum has been determined, there must be monitoring of the interaction to determine if the style is appropriate and if the style changes as the supervisee operates more independently. This, then, enables new objectives to be set and new procedures to be planned.

This process parallels the study of the clinical interaction and has the same purpose—optimal growth for the participants. In other words, the study of the supervisory interaction is simply an extension of the study of the clinical interaction. Questions to be answered change from, Is the client making progress? to, Is the supervisee making progress in her or his efforts to develop independence, self-analysis, and self-evaluation? And is the supervisor making progress in developing those behaviors that will facilitate these qualities in the supervisee?

Many supervisors are currently indicating an interest in knowing more about supervisory procedures. They are asking questions about the validity of their procedures and ways to improve their techniques. There are few general answers for them at this point. There are probably specific answers to their own questions about their own behaviors in the self-study of the conference. This is consistent with the four-fold planning discussed earlier—one cannot plan for clients in the absence of information about what they *can* do and what they *are* doing. Neither can one plan for the supervisee or the supervisor without similar information.

Any supervisor or supervisee who is serious about learning about the process in an effort to obtain maximum levels of productivity cannot wait for researchers to deliver neatly packaged directions for "what to do when." They must start with self-study—individual supervisors and supervisees looking at their own behavior.

That self-study will be the focus of this chapter. Most of the discussion of self-study will focus on observation and analysis of the conference, not because it is the most important component, but because it is where all components of the process are usually planned or discussed. But study of every component should be included.

IMPORTANCE OF SELF-STUDY

Traditionally, supervisors have not been accustomed to studying their own behavior. Although supervisees are repeatedly required, especially when they are students in educational programs, to audiotape and videotape their clinical sessions for future observation and analysis, it is rare to find a supervisor who has made either kind of record of a conference and viewed it, much less subjected it to analysis. Yet, if Blumberg (1980) is right, this point of interaction is where the problems arise. Taking a more positive approach, it might also be said that it is at the conference level where learning takes place or where the learning from the other components of the process is integrated and change projected.

Several items of rationale for studying the conference present themselves. The analogy to the clinical process is relevant. Clinicians are not expected to become effective in the clinical process without study, yet the same need has not been assumed in supervision. Self-study is particularly important to the proposal presented here, which suggests that supervisees and supervisors move along the continuum from Evaluation-Feedback through other stages. If it is through the Collaborative Style that this progression is accomplished, then it is essential for both supervisors and supervisees to have objective, reliable data about the amount and types of participation of each person as they work together.

Further, if supervisors are to implement the first component—discussion and interpretation of the supervisory process—with their supervisees, it follows that both must understand what is actually happening in their interactions. If they wish to strengthen their skills as supervisors they must first have an understanding of what they are doing.

It has also been seen that perceptions of supervisors and supervisees about the conference are neither accurate nor in agreement (Blumberg, 1980; Blumberg et al., 1967; Culatta & Seltzer, 1976, 1977; Link, 1971; Smith, 1978). If congruence between perceptions is important to the interaction, it can only be attained on the basis of actual, objective knowledge of what happened. The supervisory procedures recommended in this book clearly and simply cannot become reality without such knowledge.

PLANNING FOR SELF-STUDY

One of the many analogies that exist between the clinical and the supervisory processes is planning—setting objectives and planning the procedures to meet them. The concept of four-fold planning was introduced in a previous chapter—planning for the supervisor and the supervisee—that is, for the supervisory process as well as the clinical process. Planning for the study of the supervisory process mandates the collection of some type of data on what is actually occurring and whether or not objectives are being met, just as in the clinical process. It requires that the supervisor and supervisee observe audio- or videotapes of their interaction, collect data on behaviors, analyze those data, and form hypotheses. From this information comes the content of the joint planning for both supervisor and supervisee. Data are collected on supervisee behaviors as well as on supervisor behaviors for the same reason that data are collected on both clients and clinicians—because the *interaction* between the two is as important, possibly more important, than individual behaviors.

OBSERVATION OF SUPERVISION

Principles and methodologies of observation and analysis of the clinical session were covered in previous chapters. Virtually everything stated there applies to observation and analysis of the supervisory conference. To review, observation and analysis of the conference must have a purpose. It must be objective and scientific. It must be perceived as the collection and analysis of data on behaviors, not evaluation. Its primary focus should be gathering data to determine if objectives have been met. It should obtain data that show if change is needed and, if so, if it takes place. It should be planned cooperatively by supervisor and supervisee.

Differences between studying the clinical and supervisory processes will be found in the questions to be answered, the types of behavior to be observed, the data to be recorded, the method of observation, the observation instruments used, the method of discussion with the supervisee, and the implementations of change. Otherwise, the basic principles for objective, scientific observation and analysis of the clinical session apply. The reader is urged to review the chapters on observation and analysis of the clinical session before continuing with this chapter.

STEPS IN SELF-STUDY

Self-study of the supervisory process will include all or some of the following steps:

■ The task of learning about what actually occurs in the interaction may begin with unstructured, open-ended listening to an audiotape or viewing of a videotape. Since most supervisors and supervisees have never done this, they may find themselves in the same place as beginning clinicians who are told to observe a tape or a live clinical session without guidelines. What do they do?— they probably see a mass of behavior for which they have no labels or categories.

Repeated experiences in such unstructured observations, however, may make it possible for both supervisees and supervisors to become more objective and to begin to see types of behavior that are repeated, certain responses to each other that stand out, or even behaviors that are missing. It may be very easy for them to see who dominated the discussion, what topics were discussed most frequently or at greatest length, whether or not supervisees were involved in problem solving, and many other kinds of behavior. This first step should be unstructured, with the viewers remaining as open and nonjudgmental as possible. The temptation will be, as it is in viewing the clinical session, to make immediate judgments—"instant evaluations." This is no more profitable in most cases than it is in the clinical session.

■ The next step is analogous to screening in the clinical process—objective identification of certain behaviors, to which further, more specific attention will be given. For instance, the broad look at the conference may make certain behaviors very apparent to the viewers. The supervisee may be contributing very little to the conference even though it has been determined in the planning stage that he or she is well advanced along the continuum. The supervisor may interrupt the supervisee frequently. The supervisee may engage in very long utterances. The supervisor may ask many questions or may ignore the supervisee's utterances. The supervisee may appear to not be answering the supervisor's questions. From these behaviors, then, selections can be made for further in-depth observation and analysis.

Another way to obtain this early information about the conference is to use as a screening device one of the interaction analysis systems that will be described subsequently. Certain systems are better for this purpose than others and will be so identified. As a result of their use, some patterns may emerge that might not be noticed through the unstructured observation or that might be misperceived or misinterpreted during the subjective observation.

■ Once patterns to be further studied have been identified, the interaction can be observed in greater depth. The student of the conference has the same choices for data collection that are available in the clinical process—individually devised tally systems, verbatim or selective verbatim recordings, anecdotal reports, checklists, or interaction analysis systems. The type of behavior, the availability of appropriate systems, the goal of the observation, and the complexity of the interaction will determine the methodology.

■ After the data are collected they will be subjected to the same type of analysis suggested for clinical data. Behaviors will be categorized, sequences identified, inferences proposed, hypotheses stated.

■ Objectives will then be set for further study, for behavior change in both supervisor and supervisee, and for subsequent data collection on the planned modifications of the behaviors.

OBTAINING FEEDBACK ABOUT THE SUPERVISORY PROCESS

If the supervisory process is to be discussed and analyzed by supervisor and supervisee, information must be gathered to form the nucleus of this discussion. Attitudes, perceptions, actual behaviors, needs—all go into the analysis.

In addition to the objective data obtained by the observation systems to be discussed next, there is a need to obtain subjective feedback about the conference. Rosenshine (1971) and Rosenshine and Furst (1973) have strongly urged the use of high-inference ratings (subjective ratings) along with low-inference category counts, which are more objective, as have Ingrisano and Boyle (1973) and Smith and Anderson (1982a). "Low-inference systems are classification systems which code specific, notable supervisor and supervisee behaviors and require few inferences on the part of the coder who is analyzing one event at a time. High-inference systems are classifications which rate general supervisor and supervisee behaviors and require inferences on the part of the rater who is analyzing a series of events" (Smith & Anderson, 1982a, p. 243).

Goldhammer and colleagues (1980) identified the post-conference analysis as the final stage of their model of supervision and said that it is "clinical supervision's superego—conscience" (p. 43). This is when the supervisor's behavior is examined with all the rigor with which the teacher's behavior is analyzed and for basically the same purposes. 'In both instances our principal rationale is that examined professional behavior is more likely to be useful—for everyone—than unexamined behavior" (p. 43). Goldhammer (1969) nicknamed this analysis the "post-mortem" (p. 57).

How is this feedback obtained? Three methods are useful to varying degrees for this purpose: (1) general discussion with the supervisee, (2) the use of rating scales or evaluation forms, and (3) the collection of objective behavioral data through the use of interaction analysis systems.

General Discussion

Discussion about the supervisory process was presented as a part of the first component—Understanding the Supervisory Process. Such discussion continues throughout the entire interaction. What are supervisees' perceptions of whether or not their anticipations, needs, and goals are being met? Objectives for the supervisory process, set during the planning stage, should be reviewed periodically. New impressions of the supervisory process, gained through experiences, should be expressed.

One drawback of attempting to obtain feedback directly from the student is that it may be difficult, if not impossible, to obtain honest feedback from supervisees, especially if it is negative. Supervisors *do* give grades to supervisees, or write recommendations or evaluations. A supervisee recently said of her supervisor, "I want to tell her that I don't like it because she is always late and because she spends time talking about irrelevant issues during our conferences. I want to be assertive but I know I won't be. I can't bring myself to tell her that."

There are other kinds of behaviors that may be even more difficult to discuss with the supervisor. How do student clinicians tell supervisors that they talk too much? That they don't give the supervisees a chance to use their own ideas? That they always tell them about the negative aspects of their clinical work, not the positive? Or a host of other complaints one hears from supervisees—some justified, some not?

Supervisors, too, may find it difficult to engage in this general discussion of supervisees' activities. They may not have any better understanding of the components of the supervisory process than the supervisees, and therefore may not know how to structure such a conversation. They may also not be able to deal face-to-face with their supervisees on sensitive issues.

The success of analysis of the conference depends upon the individual situation. The manner in which the supervisory process is presented at the beginning of the interaction will influence the ongoing discussion. Without adequate information about the components of supervision, supervisees may not even know what they wish to discuss. This discussion may come more easily as they progress along the continuum. The interpersonal skills of the supervisor will make a difference in the supervisees' ability and willingness to be open and frank. The specificity of the objectives set for the supervisory process may determine the productivity of the discussion. For example, if an objective has been to increase the amount of talk by the supervisee in the conference and, if data are available to quantify this talk, it will be easier for both.

The direction of such discussion will need to be considered carefully by the supervisor at first. While it should be encouraged, it may come easily only after experience with the types of feedback to be discussed next, or from a very experienced or secure supervisee. It is also important to deal with this feedback as *perceptions*, which may or may not be accurate. Their validity can be tested through the collection of data, but until that point, they must be dealt with as reality, at least for the perceiver.

Rating Scales

Rating scales or evaluation forms are high-inference scales that are a slightly more objective way of obtaining feedback about the supervisory interaction than general discussion. Such forms may be developed and used by the agency or supervisors may develop their own. In the chapter on interpreting the supervisory process, it was suggested that such rating forms as those developed by Powell (1987) (Appendix B) and Smith and Anderson (1982a) (Appendix C) are a good basis for the early discussion of the process and in setting objectives for supervisor and supervisee. They are also valuable guides for ongoing discussion.

Interaction Analysis Systems

Although there is a place for the high-inference methods just reviewed, they cannot be considered objective measures of what happened in the conference. The use of interaction analysis systems for observation and data collection of behaviors in the supervisory conference is perhaps more important than it is in the clinical session (Anderson et al., 1979). Although subjectivity is never completely eliminated, the use of such systems in conjunction with the other methods is necessary for study of the conference. From the collected data, inferences can be made and compared with the results of ratings. This is particularly important for the conference where there is so little information about variables that are effective.

Interaction analysis systems for the clinical process were discussed in the chapter on observation. Those systems were an outgrowth of similar systems for recording interaction in the classroom, based on the idea that a better understanding of what happens in the classroom will help teachers do a better job. This concept has been transferred now to supervisory activity. "Any situation in which people are interacting is amenable to behavioral analysis by categories appropriate to it. Once the goals of the projected interaction are stated, it should be possible to deduce the kinds of information needed to understand it better" (Blumberg, 1980, p. 114).

To review what was said about the clinical session, interaction analysis systems are not evaluations. They are low inference instruments for collecting data on behaviors within the conference, which can then be examined, analyzed, and categorized, so that inferences can be drawn about the interaction of the participants and its effects on their learning.

Systems from the education literature and from speech-language pathology for analyzing the supervisory process will be discussed here in relation to their objectives, content, usefulness, methodology, strengths and weaknesses, validity and reliability, and how closely they meet the criteria for interactional analysis systems proposed by Herbert and Attridge (1978), as discussed in Chapter 8.

A System for Analyzing Supervisor-Teacher Interaction (Blumberg)

Originally printed in *Mirrors on Behavior* (Simon & Boyer, 1970a,b, 1974), this system was developed to quantify supervisor/teacher interaction. It was used in Blumberg's studies of the supervisory conference (Blumberg, 1974, 1980). Based on analysis instruments for use in the classroom (Bales, 1951; Flanders, 1967, 1969), the basic assumption of the system is that learning in the conference and satisfaction with the supervisory process are directly related to the supervisee's level of independence and ability to participate in the conference. The system is designed to help supervisors get some insight into their behavior and its effect on the course of their interaction with teachers. Underwood (1973) indicated that it is equally appropriate for speech-language pathology supervisors.

The system is time-based, that is, behaviors are recorded every three seconds and/or when a change of behavior occurs within the three-second interval. It is a single-scoring system, meaning that only one category number is applied to a verbal behavior.

The system includes 10 categories for supervisors, four for supervisees, and one that applies to both. Supervisor behaviors are (1) Support-inducing communication behavior, (2) Praise, (3) Accepts or uses teacher's ideas, (4) Asks for information, (5) Gives information, (6) Asks for opinions, (7) Asks for suggestions, (8) Gives opinions, (9) Gives suggestions, and (10) Criticism. Supervisee behaviors are (1) Asks for information, opinion, or suggestions,

(2) Gives information, (3) Positive social emotional behavior, and (4) Negative social-emotional behavior. The final category, Silence or confusion, applies to both participants.

Blumberg justified the unequal number of categories in his system by referring to Flanders's seven categories for teachers and two for pupils. Since it is the behavior of the supervisor that is responsible for setting the tone and atmosphere in the conference, he says, it is more important to learn about the supervisor's behavior.

The Blumberg system is easily learned and used. The directions are clear and specific and include a description of each category and a form for collecting data from a tape recording. He also included a unique method for transferring recorded data to a matrix, which makes it possible to analyze the data both qualitatively and quantitatively.

Data obtained from use of the system are interpreted in view of each act as a response to the last act of the other person in the interaction or in anticipation of the next act of the other. Blumberg made this important point because he views behaviors as sequentially related, rather than isolated. He also views the system as recording interaction from the point of view of the receiver of the behavior, not the giver; in other words, the effects, not the intention of the behavior.

Blumberg did not present reliability and validity data, but addressed reliability of observation by providing what he called "ground rules," which are helpful in training for reliability in recording (Blumberg, 1980). Brasseur (1980a,b), who used the system in a study, stated: "The amount of training needed to use the Blumberg system depends upon the user's objective—self-study or research. For personal self-study, the categories are easy to learn and it is rather easy to establish consistency with oneself in assigning behaviors to given categories. Learning to tally every three seconds on a time-based system is sometimes difficult but can be dealt with by using a tape containing a series of beeps at three-second intervals and by lengthening the time interval or coding all behaviors during the learning process. For research purposes the time required for training would depend upon the number of coders and the percentage of agreement to be obtained" (Brasseur, 1980b, p. 72).

The system relates exclusively to cognitive behaviors. It is possible, however, to make assumptions about the affective from certain of the categories and especially from the use of the matrix which identifies what Blumberg calls "steady state" areas of behavior such as "building and maintaining interpersonal relationships."

The content of the conference behaviors is not identified by the system; therefore, significance of behaviors cannot be fully interpreted. There are, however, many questions that can be answered which relate particularly to the questions of the balance of active/passive behaviors. It is possible, through analyzing the collected data, to determine the most frequently used behaviors and the ratios of various behaviors to each other. For example, how talking time is used—asking, telling, criticizing, what behaviors follow other behaviors, and to identify other categories which then allow for inference making, interpretation, and value judgment.

Certain strengths and weaknesses are found in this system, as in all of the systems to be described here. Reliability and validity data are not given. Categories are not exhaustive, that is, do not cover all possible behaviors, nor are they mutually exclusive (although Blumberg addressed the latter dilemma in his ground rules). Items are quite general, lacking in the specificity that would make them useful in analyzing some specific aspects of the conference.

The emphasis on supervisory behavior and the grouping of three behaviors for supervisees into one item, although justified by Blumberg, limits its value in studying the styles of supervision proposed here where the behavior of the supervisee is deemed equally important to that of the supervisor. If used for the purpose of determining behaviors of both parties to the conference, the supervisee categories should be divided into three separate ones. For example, the item Asks for information, opinion, or suggestions should become (1) Asks for information, (2) Asks for opinions, (3) Asks for suggestions.

The system also has many strengths, one being the matrix, which provides a method of analyzing data. This makes it possible then to make inferences and value judgments which can lead to planning modifications of behavior. Another strength is its relative simplicity and ease of learning when compared to some of the other systems to be discussed. Its focus on direct-indirect (active/passive) behavior makes a real contribution to the study of the collaborative methodology presented here.

The system is not to be construed as an evaluation, but is recommended for self-analysis by supervisor and supervisee, peer analysis, or research. Its use will, in Blumberg's (1980) words, "help a supervisor see, to some extent, the flexibility of his behavior and would also give him some understanding of the predominant ways he makes use of self" (p. 124).

Underwood Category System for Analyzing Supervision-Clinician

Underwood (1979), after utilizing Blumberg's system in a dissertation study (Underwood, 1973), modified the system. The final version includes the following categories for supervisor behavior: (1) Supportive, (2) Praise, (3) Identifies problem, (4) Uses clinician's idea, (5) Requests factual information, (6) Provides factual information, (7) Requests opinions/suggestions, (8) Provides opinions/ suggestions, (9) Criticism. For supervisees, behaviors include: (10) Identifies problem, (11) Requests factual information, (12) Provides factual information, (13) Requests opinions/suggestions, (14) Provides opinions/suggestions, (15) Positive social behavior, (16) Negative social behavior. Underwood then includes category (17) Silence or confusion as Other Behavior, which applies to both participants. The system contains a fairly detailed description of each category and some ground rules for making certain decisions about categories, a scoring sheet and two analysis sheets to assist in interpretation of the data. The first,

Supervision-Clinician Conference Analysis, provides a form for summarizing the behavioral counts and establishing percentages for the data, and a formula for what she calls Factual Information Exchange and Problem Solving Behavior. The second analysis sheet, *Supervision-Clinician Conference Analysis of Behavior Change Over Time*, provides space for recording the summarized data over time.

Purposes, procedures, uses, and strengths and weaknesses are similar to those of the Blumberg system, since it so closely parallels it. Her items are, in several instances, more specific than Blumberg's and she does include more categories for supervisees. Her items for both supervisors and supervisees combine opinions/suggestions, and it might be questioned if the dynamics of these two categories are not different enough in the perception of the supervisee to be quantified separately. She does not utilize the matrix, which is so useful in interpreting the data from the Blumberg system, although she does provide an analysis form.

The system is relatively simple and easy to learn and interpretations can be made regarding the active-passive component of supervision. Like the Blumberg system, however, it relates to behavior rather than content, to the cognitive rather than the affective, although again, it is possible to make inferences and assumptions about the affective from the data. She did not attend to the sequencing of behavior as Blumberg did; rather, she summarized her data as percentages similar to the summary sheet used by Boone and Prescott (1972).

The major weakness of the revised system is that no information has been provided in the unpublished document that describes (1) the development and modification of the revised system, and (2) reliability and validity (Brasseur, 1980c). Despite this, the Underwood system is an interesting and useful tool which could be very well utilized, particularly in self-study. Its use in research is questionable at this point until reliability and validity data are available. The system deserves further study.

Content and Sequence Analysis System of the Supervisory Session

This system, developed by Culatta and Seltzer (1977), was the first published system for studying the supervisory process in speech-language pathology and has been used in several research studies. The authors perceived the importance of isolating the interaction variables in the supervisory conference and grouping them into manageable categories. To do this, they modified the Boone-Prescott *Content and Sequence Analysis System* for recording clinician-client behavior (1972). The theoretical base for both systems is behavior theory (Roberts, 1980).

The *Content and Sequence Analysis System* provides for recording behavior on one dimension only and in the cognitive domain only. It is a frequency-based system, recording all verbal behaviors as they occur. The authors gave directions, defined the categories, and gave an example of each. Despite the title, users can record only the type of behavior, not the content of the interaction. Categories are divided equally and include, for supervisors: Good Evaluation, Bad Evaluation, Question, Strategy, Observation, Information, and Irrelevant.

Categories for supervisees include: Good Self-evaluation, Bad Self-evaluation, Question, Strategy, Observation, Information, and Irrelevant. A chart is provided for marking the behaviors and then connecting the marks so that a type of graph is produced.

In addition, although this is a frequency-based system, Culatta and Seltzer presented a unique methodology for changing from the time-free analysis, which may produce misleading information, to a graph that also charts the number of seconds spent in each behavior. They presented an example of the way in which the two methodologies may provide entirely different pictures of what actually happened. For example, the time-free analysis may show a relatively equal interchange between supervisor and supervisee while the addition of the time component may reveal that the supervisor used long verbal statements while the supervisee only responded with "Uh-huh."

The system's main strength is its practicality, its simplicity, and its clarity. It can be learned easily and a large amount of valuable data can be collected rather quickly. It is particularly useful as an early introduction to isolating behavior in the conference. It can serve as a screening instrument to identify behaviors which may be studied in greater length (Roberts, 1980). The data collected can be used to answer many questions: Most frequent categories used? Ratios of the behaviors? Balance of input (using the time-based methodology)? Sequence of behavior?

The system has several weaknesses, despite its usefulness. Its theoretical bias may not be congruent with all approaches to supervision. Therefore, it may not measure all appropriate behaviors (Roberts, 1980). Categories are broad and undimensional. For example, the number of questions asked by each participant can be identified. This information is of relatively little use in interpretation, however, unless there is more specific information, such as the type or content of the question or the supervisees' reaction to it. The same can be said for the strategy category. Categories do not describe all components of the conference or represent all possible interactions. Some are not mutually exclusive—one sample of behavior might be coded as a question, a strategy, or an evaluation. The authors give no ground rules for coding when confusion exists between categories. They also do not include a method for analysis of data, as in Blumberg's or Underwood's systems. The method of recording also makes it impossible to determine when a new sequence of behavior begins (Roberts, 1980). The method could be altered to accomplish this by the use of certain symbols.

Major weakness is that the authors presented no reliability or validity information, nor information about the development of the system, except that it was based on the Boone-Prescott system. A study by Dowling and colleagues (1982) questioned the reliability and validity of the system and stated that it has serious limitations as a research tool. However, because of its ease of learning and the fact that it identifies the occurrence and sequence of process variables in the conference, they suggested that it is an appropriate tool for supervisors with limited time who wish to objectify their own supervisory behavior.

Although it is clear that the system should not be used for research purposes and that the findings of several studies that have used it are somewhat suspect, the system has merit, as indicated. It must also be said that the authors made a major contribution by calling attention to the need to subject the supervisory conference in speech-language pathology to analytical study.

McCrea's Adapted Scales

None of the previous systems provide for the recording of data in the affective or interpersonal domain. The *McCrea Adapted Scales for the Assessment of Interpersonal Functioning in Speech-Language Pathology Supervisory Conferences* addresses this complex issue (McCrea, 1980) (Appendix G).

Developed from the work of Carkhuff (1969a,b) and Gazda (1974), these scales are based on the work of Carl Rogers (1957) and test his theories, which stated that, if certain core facilitative conditions are present within a clinical relationship and are perceived by the client, the client will experience positive change. The original concepts were developed for use in mental health, but workers in other helping professions have assumed that these constructs are applicable, not only to psychotherapy, but to other interpersonal situations such as parent-child, student-teacher, and supervisor-supervisee interactions (McCrea, 1980).

The *McCrea Adapted Scales* provide data about the presence or absence of four interpersonal categories of supervisor behavior: Empathic Understanding, Respect, Facilitative Genuineness, and Concreteness, and one category of supervisee behavior: Self-exploration, which is assumed to be analogous to self-supervision.

The system is frequency based as well as rating based, that is, the presence or absence of the behaviors is noted and then the behavior is rated according to its degree of facilitativeness on a scale of 1 to 7, with the higher ratings being facilitating and the lower nonfacilitating.

The categories are clearly described, as are each of the seven points on each rating scale. Very specific ground rules and procedures are given for use of the scale. Score sheets and an analysis sheet are included. The system is easily used and it is not difficult to learn. McCrea (1980) estimated 5 to 7 hours of training to use the system in self-study, more to obtain agreement for a research project.

Although the reliability study for this scale appears to indicate that it can be used to observe and analyze interpersonal processes in supervision in speech-language pathology, reliability was demonstrated only for Respect, Facilitative Genuineness, and Concreteness. Because of the infrequent occurrence of Empathic Understanding and Self-exploration, reliability was not shown. The author, however, indicated the likelihood that reliability could be obtained if those behaviors were present in greater numbers (McCrea, 1980).

The system can be used in self-study or research to obtain baseline levels of interpersonal functioning and to measure attempts to modify behavior in the interpersonal processes within supervision.

Weaknesses of the system are in the ambiguity and subjectivity of the scales on which the system was based (Gazda, 1974; Carkhuff, 1969a,b). Because of the system's base in Rogerian theory, the only supervisee behavior identified is Self-exploration, defined as the ability to talk objectively about personal behavior and its consequences. This is an important behavior, however, in the facilitation of the continuum described here because self-supervision is perceived as a natural consequence of the ability to self-explore (McCrea, 1980).

Another weakness in the system is that it does not identify or categorize nonverbal behavior. A major portion of affect is carried through the nonverbal; therefore, data obtained from this scale can be assumed to be incomplete.

Despite these major weaknesses, the system has strengths. It is the first system in speech-language pathology to record and analyze interpersonal behavior. It has a strong theoretical base in the works of Rogers and Carkhuff and an operational base from Gazda.

Oratio Transactional System

This system is based on the author's belief that supervision is a transactive action which includes "both cognitive and conative learning" (Oratio, 1977, p. 131).

The *Oratio Transactional System* is both qualitative and quantitative and codes both affective and cognitive behaviors in the conference. It includes 12 categories, seven for supervisors, five for clinicians. The author stated that these categories are adaptations of the research of Carkhuff and his colleagues (1969a,b) in counselor education and of Culatta and Seltzer (1977), both discussed previously in this chapter. Four of the supervisor categories—Conveys Empathy, Conveys Positive Regard, Demonstrates Genuineness, and Functions Concretely, and the clinician category of Clinical Self-exploration are from the Carkhuff scales (1969a,b). The categories: Provides or Requests Observation/Information and Provides or Requests Strategy for both supervisor and clinician are similar to two of the Culatta and Seltzer categories. Problem identification, however, is similar to a category in the Underwood system (1979) (Andersen, 1980a).

The system lists the categories and describes three levels under each category. Behaviors, then, are recorded in two ways. A frequency measure is taken every three seconds or whenever a change occurs during the three-second period, as in several other time-based systems described. In addition, each behavior is rated at one of three levels, which are described in some detail and an example given for Level 1 and Level 3. Procedures for recording and scoring the behaviors on a graph similar to that used by Culatta and Seltzer (1977) are provided. An analysis sheet is also included for collection of data into four "category clusters": Conference Climate, Clinician Introspection, Growth Facilitation, and Strategy Intervention. Frequency data on the behaviors can be obtained from the system as well as some qualitative information resulting from the three level ratings.

Despite a commendable recognition of the fact that both cognitive and affective components are important, this system has major weaknesses all similar to the systems from which it is adapted. Oratio suggested as delimitations the subjectivity of the user, the identification of only verbal transactions by the system, and the limits of the behavior which can be identified. In addition, as in the Culatta and Seltzer system, categories are not mutually exclusive, that is, behavior can be coded in more than one category. This fault is in fact exacerbated by the combination of the cognitive and affective components into one system. A behavior, for example, might be scored as Provides or Requests Observation/Information and also as Functions Concretely. A decision would have to be made by the coder on each behavior as to the component in which it would be placed. Data would then be lost from the other component.

Categories are also not exhaustive—other behaviors can take place in the conference. Each category is broad. Provides or Requests Observation/Information could include so many types of behaviors that reasonable inferences from the data would be impossible (Andersen, 1980a).

Many of the definitions of the levels in each category are difficult to operationalize and reliability probably could not be obtained with the three levels of ratings. Additionally, the analysis sheet has many problems. The author presents no reliability, validity, or agreement data on any aspect of the system nor a description of the procedures for developing it, other than citing the works from which it is adapted (Andersen, 1980a). In view of more recent work which questions the reliability and validity of the Culatta and Seltzer system (Dowling et al., 1982) and McCrea's (1980) finding that self-exploration and empathic understanding did not occur in conference at significant levels to establish reliability, the combination of these components is extremely questionable, especially for research purposes.

Despite these problems in the system, it provides an original approach in the summary sheet that accompanies it. Oratio has attempted to combine the data and develop a formula for determining effectiveness of the conference. This methodology for determining the formula may be questioned. It does, nevertheless, indicate a need for a measure of effectiveness which should be pursued. Such a measure must be theoretically based; and, at this point, information about supervisory variables is too limited to submit to the temptation of equating summary data with evaluations of effectiveness.

The main strength of the system is in the recognition of the two dimensions of the supervisory conference and the attempt to break down their components, even though the system needs much refinement in delineating those behaviors. If the system could be modified and validated it might combine the two types of analysis, high- and low-inference instruments, suggested by Rosenshine and Furst (1971). Until this is done, the system could be utilized for self-study for some behaviors but should not be used for research.

Smith's Adaptation of the Multidimensional Observational System for the Analysis of Interactions in Clinical Supervision (MOSAICS)

Smith (1978) adapted and validated the *Multidimensional Observational System for the Analysis of Interactions in Clinical Supervision* (MOSAICS) for use in speech-language pathology. The system provides an analysis of both content and process of the interaction in individual or group supervision (Appendix H).

The system is multidimensional, each unit of discourse (pedagogical move) being scored in six different dimensions. For example, each move is scored as follows: (1) according to the person doing the speaking—supervisor, supervisee, or observer, (2) according to type—structuring, soliciting, responding, reacting, or summarizing, (3) according to topic, which is in turn broken down into instructional and related.

If the move is instructional, a decision is made under the heading of generality—Is it general or specific? Then the focus of the discussion is coded—objectives, methods and materials, or execution. The third decision made is whether the move is in the domain of cognitive, affective, or disciplinary/ social interaction. If the move is not instructional, it is coded under related areas, and here the choices are subject matter, supervision, general topics related to speech-language pathology or not related to speech-language pathology. The final category is the logical analysis area or substantive logical meanings. The move is again coded to analyze the instructional process and there are ten choices: defining, interpreting, fact stating, explanation, evaluation, justification, suggestion, explanation of suggestion, opinion, and justification of opinion (Smith, 1980). Weller (1971) included more categories in the original system, but they were not used in the Smith adaptation.

Although the system appears somewhat formidable, Weller (1971) provided extensive procedures and definitions for its use. Smith (1978), in her adaptation, rewrote certain definitions to fit speech-language pathology, clarified some of the rules for scoring the system, and developed a score sheet for recording the behaviors.

Extensive suggestions were given by Weller (1971) about the interpretation of the data that can be gathered with the system. The most useful are the analysis of the teaching cycles or the sequence of the pedagogical moves and the critical ratios produced by manipulating certain data. The analysis procedures counteract what is probably the main weakness of the system—the massive amount of data obtained. Another weakness of the system is its complexity, which makes it appear to be difficult to learn, and for research purposes, to obtain agreement among coders.

The strengths of the system are so great, however, that the weaknesses are almost inconsequential in a consideration of its use. Of all the systems presented here, it comes closest to meeting the standards set by Herbert and Attridge (1975). It is the only one, other than the next one to be discussed (Tufts, 1984), which addresses content, and its multidimensional nature provides in-depth information. Categories are clearly described, exhaustive, and for the most part, mutually exclusive. Directions for use and analysis are clear. No transcript is needed for coding, that is, it can be coded directly from audio- or videotape. Weller's suggestions for data reduction through critical ratios and teaching cycle analysis make it possible to manipulate the data for in-depth interpretations.

The MOSAICS can be used for self-analysis, peer analysis, joint analysis with supervisees, and for individuals or groups. Its great advantage, however, is in its appropriateness for research. No other system described here approaches it in terms of its support as a research tool or its multidimensional nature. Data from the system can be used in correlational, descriptive, or experimental research and a computer program is available for analysis of the data (Smith, 1980).

Tufts Content Analysis System

A content analysis system developed by Tufts (1984) for use in a dissertation identifies the topical content of the supervisory conference. Categories included are (1) Clinical Procedures, (2) Teaching Function (Academic Information), (3) Client Information, (4) Lesson Analysis, (5) Supervisor-Supervisee Clinical Analysis (Nonjudgmental), (6) Supervisor-Supervisee Clinical Evaluation (Judgmental), (7) Lesson Planning, (8) Professional, (9) Nonprofessional/Social.

This is the only system that looks solely at the content of the conference. The categories in this system are mutually exclusive. All utterances are coded and timed. Reliability is high. The author suggested that the topical categories are broad and that further research is needed to break down certain categories into subdivisions, for example, Clinical Procedures, Client Information, Lesson Analysis, and Supervisor-Supervisee Clinical Analysis (Nonjudgmental).

The system was not validated for use in diagnostic conferences, only those covering ongoing therapy. It has not yet been used in other studies, but appears to be easily learned. It would provide interesting and useful information, especially if used in conjunction with other systems such as Blumberg's or Underwood's, which are not content oriented.

Use of Interaction Analysis Systems

In discussing the use of interaction analysis systems in the clinical session, it has been stated that there is still uncertainty about the sampling process in studying the clinical process. With this statement as a background, what then of the supervisory conference? This question is as important to the study of supervision as it is to the study of the clinical process. Some attempts have been made to determine whether or not sampling of supervisory conferences is adequate to represent the entire conference.

Underwood (1973) stated that 5-minute segments using the Blumberg system are representative of the total conference. Culatta and Seltzer (1977) utilized a 5-minute segment of their system to analyze 10 conferences and gave as their support for this sampling the work of Boone and Goldberg (1969), Boone and Prescott (1972), and Schubert and Laird (1975). This support is highly questionable, however, since those are all systems for the clinical session, not the supervisory conference.

Oratio (1977) suggested a randomly selected 5-minute excerpt from the middle of the conference for scoring his *Transactional System*, but said initial and final 5-minute segments should not be selected for analysis. This makes sense because it seems reasonable that these segments will be different, but he gave no data to support his statement.

Against this background of assertions and contradictions, Casey (1980) used *McCrea's Adapted System* for analyzing supervisor interpersonal interaction and supervisee self-exploration to ask what portions of the conference, if any, can be considered representative of the entire conference. Findings were that "scores derived for respect, facilitative genuineness, and concreteness [the only categories that occurred frequently enough to be analyzed by McCrea (1980)] during (1) the beginning 5-minute segment, (2) the ending 5-minutes, (3) a random 5-minute segment from the middle of the conference, and (4) two random 2-and-1/2-minute segments from the middle of the segment are representative of scores derived by coding the entire conference with *McCrea's Adapted System* (Casey, 1980, p. 65)." No such conclusions can be drawn for empathic understanding or self-exploration because of their infrequent occurrence.

Casey further stated that it is possible to generalize the results of her investigation to all systems used for supervisory conference analysis. This statement is based solely on the fact that all these systems are frequency based, not on the fact that they are all equally adequate instruments for analyzing conferences. Generalization cannot be made to clinician-client interaction from this study.

Further, Casey cautioned that the time segments would not be valid for categories of behaviors which have a minimal frequency of occurrence during the segment. Minimal frequency is defined as between 20 percent and 25 percent of behaviors in the segment. This is an important point in view of the fact that some analysis systems include categories that have been found to occur infrequently in conferences, that is, questions, empathy, and others identified in the various descriptive studies of the conference. Valuable guidelines for researchers and practitioners for use of interaction analysis systems concluded Casey's report.

Hagler and Fahey (1987) investigated the use of short-segment samples of supervisory conferences with the MOSAICS system (Weller, 1971) and found 5-minute samples to be generally valid representations of events of the entire conference. All of these studies contain some problems, which result in a reluctance to wholeheartedly recommend small-segment sampling for study. More work is needed in this area. Certainly it would further the study of the process if the supervisor could assume the representative nature of the small sample. Questions must be asked about the purpose of the study and the content and variability within the conference before depending upon small samples.

REALITIES OF STUDYING THE CONFERENCE

The discussion of these methodologies for studying the supervisory process may seem overwhelming and impossible. They are neither. For purposes of self-study, they may be used to whatever degree is possible in terms of time and interest. If the only thing supervisors and supervisees can do to gain some insight about their interaction is to listen to audiotape and gain a subjective impression of their behaviors—that is better than nothing.

For those who profess an interest in learning about themselves as supervisors, however, there is no better way at the present time than the methods suggested here. Those who wish more information are encouraged to start slowly, to use the simpler systems first to gain some insights, and then to devise a plan for ongoing study. Even studying one behavior will raise the consciousness level about what actually happens in the conference and this is *where the action is*!

SUMMARY

The position has been taken in this chapter that the study of the supervisory process is as important as the study of the clinical process. Methodologies for such studies have been given but there is need to develop better approaches. In the earlier discussion of observation and data collection in the clinical process, it was stated that new clinical methods, and consequently, new approaches to data collection on clients could influence the study of clinician behavior as well. Similarly, such developments may influence the supervisory process. For example, discourse analysis offers vast possibilities for the study of the supervisory process. Those who are interested in studying this process should utilize all possible avenues to further develop reliable and valid techniques.

*P*reparation for the Supervisory Process

Supervision, as a field of study, is filled with myths, unclear definitions and distinctions, and untrained supervisors who operate with good intentions as their main resource.

(Hart, 1982, p. 5)

Preparation for supervisors? Unnecessary in the opinion of some, crucially needed in the opinion of others. Speech-language pathologists and audiologists are expected to have extensive preparation to become professionals. Psychologists, social workers, teachers, doctors, counselors—all the helping professions—have varying amounts of education to prepare them for their professional roles. Much of the preparation of such professionals—the applied aspect of it—is provided by supervisors. Yet it has been generally assumed in most of those disciplines, certainly in speech-language pathology and audiology, that preparation of those supervisors who provide a critical part of the education of practitioners is not necessary.

Education has for many years recognized the need for preparation and special certification for supervisors. Yet, as one reads the literature in that area, the focus, as Blumberg (1980) pointed out, has not been on the specific interaction between supervisor and supervisee but on more general topics. Boyd (1978) called for an increase in supervision preparation, leading to more effective supervisory practice in counseling. Hart (1982) said that supervision is considered by most supervisors in counseling in only "the most visceral way" (p. 44) because most of them have had no preparation—formal, informal, or in-service training—in supervision. Kadushin (1976) said that studies in social work have shown that supervisors with formal education in supervision do a better job. He proposed that social work needs to seriously consider "a more active program of explicit, formal training for social work supervision in order to increase the number of better supervisors doing better supervision" (p. 450).

In many disciplines, the apprentice model has been the prevalent model in transferring skills from one professional generation to another, "learning by doing" (p. 242) or copying a master practitioner (Kurpius et al., 1977). In discussing clinical practice, Ventry and Schiavetti (1980) said, "The student depends, to a very large extent, on the knowledge, the wisdom, and the experience of the mentor. Ideally, the mentor provides the framework and the tools that enable the students to arrive at independent decisions once they become practicing clinicians. How successful the process is depends not only on the skills and talents of the professional but on the skills and talents of the students" (p. 15). The hazards of the apprentice model, or mentoring, with all its advantages, have been noted previously.

AMOUNT OF PREPARATION IN VARIOUS DISCIPLINES

Data are hard to come by on the number of supervisors in the various disciplines who are working with or without preparation. Munson (1983) reported that over 60 percent of supervisors in a survey in social work had no formal academic education in supervision. Only 13 percent of graduate schools required a course in supervision, 28 percent had no course, and 58 percent offered one as an elective. Loganbill and Hardy (1983) reported on a survey of 55 programs in clinical psychology, only 10 of which had formal course work in supervision, while 19 had no method of preparing supervisors. In another discussion of training of supervisors in psychotherapy and counseling, Hess (1986) summarized several studies and reported that more time is spent on supervision by clinical psychologists than other tasks such as group psychotherapy, behavior modification, and research. Virtually all graduate school curricula feature these topics, but supervisory training is offered in only 14 percent of graduate psychology programs. Hess and Hess (1983) reported that only one-third of clinical psychology internships offer education in supervision and that one-third of the facilities they surveyed had their interns providing supervision to others with no one supervising their supervision. (This is comparable to the situation that was prevalent at one time in educational programs in speech-language pathology and audiology—graduate students with little or no clinical experience, and certainly no experience in supervision, supervising other students without guidance from anyone. As ASHA requirements have changed to require supervision in educational programs only by holders of the CCC, it is hoped that at least that requirement is met. It is still true, however, that doctoral students with the CCC are assigned to supervise with little or no assistance from anyone.)

Hess (1986) said, "The assumption is alive and well that it takes a therapist to be a supervisor, but training in supervision is second in importance. The assumption is unfairly made, too, since it requires the supervisor to capitalize on various and incidental learning processes as the major modality by which supervision is learned" (p. 58).

The picture in speech-language pathology is similar. Several early surveys showed that few supervisors had any preparation. Only 10 percent of school program supervisors had preparation in supervision directly related to speech and hearing, although some had general or special education administration or business management course work (Anderson, 1972). When these supervisors were asked if supervisors of speech and hearing programs in the schools needed preparation, 92 percent of full-time and 81 percent of part-time supervisors answered in the affirmative and provided a total of 454 suggestions about what should be included in an educational program for supervisors. Of 157 university supervisors of off-campus school practicum responding to another survey, 51 percent had no preparation and 53 percent of the programs reported they provided no in-service offerings for the clinicians in the schools who supervised their students in the off-campus practicum (Anderson, 1973a). Schubert and Aitchison (1975) found that 64 percent of clinic supervisors who responded to their questionnaire had no preparation in supervision; 18 percent had 1 to 3 semester hours. Eighty-three percent indicated that they thought academic course work in supervision would be important for someone preparing to be a supervisor, 13 percent did not. Fifty-two percent of the respondents had been supervising over 4 years, 29 percent over 6 years with no preparation. Further, their clinical experience was limited, 73 percent of them having had less than 5 years' experience as clinicians prior to becoming supervisors.

Wilson-Vlotman and Blair (1986) reported that educational audiologists in the schools occasionally take on the role of supervisor. They do not feel that they have been prepared to supervise others, and therefore, their supervision focuses on technical skill rather than wider supportive dimensions.

A survey of private speech & hearing centers (Stace and Drexler, 1969) found similar data. Only 30 percent of the 57 agencies with student trainees in practicum reported that someone in the agency had received any special preparation in supervision. They also reveal an intriguing attitude. Of those agencies reporting supervisors *with* special preparation, 94 percent thought it was necessary; in agencies in which no special preparation was reported only 46 percent considered it necessary. Stace and Drexler said, "This inverse relationship might suggest that, initially, supervision is not conceived as being an unusual kind of interaction. However, after exposure to some kinds of special preparation, supervisors begin to see the supervisory process as a more complex phenomenon, or at least one about which they feel a need to know more. Colloquially speaking, they might begin 'to know what they don't know'. But it appears that for supervisors without special preparation, 'ignorance is bliss'" (p. 319). This is a very important statement in relation to preparation in the supervisory process. The writer's own experience supports this. Before beginning an extensive study of the supervisory process, it seemed rather clear-cut and simple. The more it has been studied, the more complex it has become. Students have expressed the same thought, "I never thought supervision was so complicated until I studied it" or from experienced supervisors, "I thought I had all the answers about supervision until I took this course!" These statements are not made to "scare off" any potential students of supervision. Rather, they epitomize more than anything the fascination and challenge of studying the process.

PREPARATION IN SUPERVISION IN SPEECH-LANGUAGE PATHOLOGY AND AUDIOLOGY

Acceptance of the need for preparing supervisors in speech-language pathology and audiology has come slowly, although it has increased rapidly in the past few years. Yet, there is still resistance. The idea that *anyone* can supervise is firmly entrenched. Various reasons are given. "We've supervised for all these years and we are doing O.K. Why do we need to train our supervisors?" "We have no data to prove that training makes supervisors any more effective." "We don't know enough about the supervisory process yet to begin training programs." "We can't afford to add another course to our curriculum." Such statements usually do not come from supervisors themselves, who generally express a great need for more information about what they are doing.

Some programs verbally support the concept of preparation; in reality, however, they may provide a token course or an occasional 3-hour workshop and feel that they have fulfilled their obligation. This, of course, may be better than nothing, although that thought may be challenged. Certainly it cannot be assumed to be adequate.

There is no refuting the point that there are no substantial data for the profession to show that supervisors who have taken course work or practicum in supervision obtain better results than those who have not. Neither are there data to support the fact that any one kind of supervision makes any greater difference than another in the preparation of clinicians, yet it has been a pervasive and expensive part of college and university programs and service delivery settings since the very beginning of the profession, just as it has been in all the helping professions. Rejection of preparation for supervisors on the basis of lack of information about the process has its humorous aspects, however, for a profession whose members have worked with many types of disorders long before there was much information available about the appropriate clinical procedure for the disorder. How much data did the early clinicians have about stuttering when they began working with stutterers? How much data do clinicians have now about the effectiveness of procedures for some of the disorder areas with which they have recently begun to work? Yet, professionals continue to do clinical work and research in tandem, refining methodologies as they go along.

In an earlier article (Anderson, 1974), the writer stated, "Training programs for such supervisors cannot wait until all aspects of the role have been defined and all the necessary competencies identified. They must be established concurrently with research efforts directed toward defining the role, the necessary competencies, and the best methods of preparing supervisors for the job they must do" (p. 10). The matter of cost of increasing educational requirements or adding faculty to teach such coursework must be taken seriously in the days of reduced budgets, but perhaps it becomes a matter of establishing priorities. Culatta and colleagues (1975) treated the issue of cost in relation to time spent in supervision in a statement that is relevant to the cost of preparation for supervisors. "The implicit suggestion is that we re-examine our educational priorities to redetermine how critical a factor adequate supervision is in the training of new professionals. Although the knowledgeable administrator will quickly point out the cost of clinical supervision, with its necessarily low student-faculty ratio, one can scarcely venture a guess as to how many poorly trained students, economically produced, equal one expensively well-trained professional successfully meeting the needs of her or his clients" (p. 155). Similarly, efficiency and effectiveness of well-prepared supervisors may eventually balance out additional costs accrued in their education and produce better clinicians in the bargain. The argument that supervisors have been preparing clinicians successfully without preparation in supervision will be treated in greater depth in the chapter on accountability, but it can be said here that support for that statement is negligible.

It has been heartening recently to see two strong statements about preparation in supervision in the literature. O'Neil (1985), in an article that provides strong support for the importance of supervision in the profession, stated that, since 300 clock hours of supervised practicum are required in a master's degree program, "clinical supervision and the qualifications of the supervisors should be of major importance" (p. 23). In another source, Hardick and Oyer (1987) said:

> Increasing attention has been directed toward the preparation of trained clinical supervisors and the identification of desirable characteristics of supervisors and the supervisory process. Research in supervision and the teaching of this content are legitimate components of the educational process.... The expanding literature on the subject also makes it feasible for university clinics to offer in-service training for staff supervisors, including faculty members who participate in supervision. The administration of a university speech and hearing clinic should provide encouragement and support for staff participation in workshops, courses, or less formal activities designed to improve the supervisory process and individual skills. (p. 49)

Development of Preparation for Supervision

Although there had been a limited amount of preparation in the 1960s, it was not until the decade of the 1970s that the profession saw the real beginning of formal educational programs in the supervisory process. A few colleges and universities began to provide course work, practicum, or in-service offerings. In 1975, however, a survey of university clinics (Schubert & Aitchison, 1975) found that 82 percent of the accredited programs and 83 percent of the unaccredited programs still offered no course work in the supervisory process.

A survey done by the ASHA Committee on Supervision revealed that such educational offerings were sparse (ASHA, 1978a). Of the 279 programs responding to the survey, 41.5 percent reported some form of preparation in the supervisory process. When analyzed, the data revealed that 25 percent of the programs included the content in other courses, 40 percent offered one course,

8 percent offered more than one course, 41 percent offered a practicum, 19 percent an internship, and 27 percent individual study. These were offered intermittently by 29 percent of the programs, as requested by 47 percent, every semester by 61 percent, and yearly by 50 percent. Since a total of only 2,776 students were reported to have been enrolled in all these offerings in the 5 years preceding the survey, the data can hardly be interpreted as indicating a stampede toward educational offerings in the supervisory process.

Content of the offerings was not clearly identifiable, and often seemed to be more related to administrative aspects of the supervisory role, that is, program management rather than clinical teaching, as defined by the ASHA Committee on Supervision (ASHA, 1978a). Much of the preparation still appeared to be offered through the format of workshops or institutes and these, too, frequently seemed to focus on administrative aspects, often in school settings.

Current data on the extent or type of education in the supervisory process are not available. It appears that there has been a continuation of in-service offerings as well as course work and other types of instruction, although that fact is not documented. Pickering (1985) reported that she knew of 35 universities where regular courses in supervision are taught and she assumed that there are more. Currently, the ASHA Committee on Supervision, the Council of University Supervisors of Practicum in Speech-Language Pathology and Audiology, and the Council of Graduate Programs in Communication Sciences and Disorders are cooperating on a project to identify types of educational programs and the places where they are being conducted.

A major boost has been given to preparation in the supervisory process by the list of tasks and competencies for supervisors adopted by ASHA (ASHA, 1985b). The first draft of this document included a recommendation for minimum qualification for supervisors "to achieve the skills necessary for effective supervision" (ASHA, 1982a, p. 339). These included, in addition to the master's degree and the CCC in the area supervised (speech-language pathology or audiology) and two years of professional experience, the following requirements: coursework in supervision consisting of six semester credit hours or nine Continuing Education Units applicable to the supervisory process, of which at least one-half must be specific to the supervisory process in speech-language pathology or audiology, and a practicum in supervision in which at least fifty clock hours of supervision would be supervised through a variety of procedures listed in the document. Suggestions were made for interim fulfillment of requirements until such time as the practicum could be supervised by someone who had already been through the process.

When the total document was submitted to the membership, the tasks and competencies received positive reaction, albeit some justified concern about their validity. More concern was expressed about the requirements for preparation. Arguments ranged from stated opinions that supervisors do not need preparation to concern about a lack of information regarding methodologies and a lack of courses currently available for individuals to meet the requirements. A more valid concern, in the opinion of the writer, should have been, Who will teach such courses or supervise such practicum, since so few supervisors have had course work themselves? Thus, what would be the content of such courses? This is not to suggest that courses cannot be developed—they can. But the mandate at that time perhaps *was* premature for this reason. At any rate, the suggested tasks and competencies were published again in a later issue (1982b) along with some of the letters of reaction to the original document. Further modification was made of the total document; it was adopted by the ASHA Legislative Council in November 1984, and subsequently published (ASHA, 1985b).

Despite the rejection of the educational requirements, the 1982 document served a purpose. It did attract the attention of many individuals and, for probably the first time, created dialogue in the profession about the possibility of preparation for supervisors.

The revised document (ASHA, 1985b) includes a section on preparation of supervisors that makes suggestions about ways in which special preparation can be obtained to acquire the skills and competencies listed in the document. These include pre-service instruction, continuing education, academic offerings and practicum at universities, and self-study. Thus, the requirement for preparation was deleted, but the Committee endorses the concept and addresses the availability of opportunities for such study. "The steadily increasing numbers of publications concerning supervision and the supervisory process indicate that basic information concerning supervision now is becoming more accessible in print to all speech-language pathologists and audiologists, regardless of geographical location and personal circumstances" (p. 60). The Committee further states that course work and continuing education on the supervisory process are becoming steadily more available in speech-language pathology and audiology and that there are commonalities in the principles of supervision across other disciplines. Thus, there is little reason for supervisors not to avail themselves of some opportunities for becoming more knowledgeable about the supervisory process.

Impetus for preparation, besides self-motivation, may come from several sources. Some individuals may take courses or workshops in supervision to obtain ASHA Continuing Education Units (CEUs) or for some recognition from their own organizations for continuing education. Some states have special certification requirements for program supervisors in the schools which include course work in the supervisory process as it pertains to speech-language pathology and audiology. A few states or universities have recently begun to require at least a course in supervision for school supervisors of all student-teaching experiences, including speech-language pathology and audiology. And, some employers are beginning to look for preparation, rather than experience alone, as a part of the credentials of people they wish to hire as supervisors.

Content of Supervisory Preparation

It is important that supervisors remain current in the disorder areas in which they are supervising. For supervisors in educational programs who are also teachers in the disorder areas, the study of the disorder areas will be assumed. For full-time supervisors in college and university programs, it is essential that they be knowledgeable about what is being taught in the academic course work in the program. For supervisors outside of an educational program, such as off-campus, CFY, or service delivery settings, the need to maintain current information is just as essential.

It is contended here and by the ASHA documents just cited that that is not enough—that there are certain types of information and certain skills related to the supervisory process that supervisors must attain. The question about the content of such preparation is not what it *should* be, but what can be *selected* from the vast array of knowledge important to the supervisor.

Some suggestions for content of preparation have come from supervisors themselves. The 454 suggestions provided by the school supervisors in Anderson's (1972) survey fall into five categories: supervision techniques, business management, further course work in speech pathology and audiology, school administration, and research techniques. Stace and Drexler's (1969) respondents' suggestions were in three categories: additional course work in speech pathology and audiology, development of management skills, and human relations. Schubert (1974) listed 200 clock hours of supervision practicum and six hours of academic course work in supervision as minimal requirements for preparation of supervisors.

Content will vary, depending upon the orientation of the program and the instructor's philosophy. This book presents an approach which is based on, though not the same as, the clinical supervision model of Cogan (1973), Goldhammer (1969), and Goldhammer and colleagues (1980). It has never been assumed by the writer that this is the only way to supervise. There are other approaches that have been referred to throughout the chapters. What *is* assumed to be absolutely essential is that those who supervise or those who teach others about the supervisory process have some model, some theoretical base, some solid foundation upon which they can build their procedures, form their hypotheses, develop their plans. Too much supervision, and presumably the teaching of it, is not rationally and logically planned on such a foundation. Thus, it may become fragmented, inconsistent, lacking in direction and focus, with no rationale and justification.

Anyone who plans to teach a course in the supervisory process will need to read widely, not only in the speech-language pathology and audiology literature, but in the literature in the many other areas touched upon here. Knowledge from many disciplines bears upon the study of supervision. Yet, all this information is manageable and can be sifted out by each person into a format that is useful. Students of the supervisory process should be prepared for the fact that one or two books are just enough to "whet the appetite." Shapiro (1986) called supervision a "process in progress" (p. 89), a phrase that captures the state of on-going efforts to learn more about its many facets.

Models for Preparation in the Supervisory Process

There are many ways in which preparation in the supervisory process can be implemented. The models that will be discussed here range from inclusion of information in early clinical management courses to preparation at the doctoral level. At each level there are different purposes and different procedures.

Inclusion in Clinical Management Courses

Clinical management procedures are part of the educational requirements for ASHA certification. They are taught in college and university programs, either in separate courses or as sections of other courses. It is highly recommended, as discussed in the chapter on Understanding the Supervisory Process, that basic information about the supervisory process be included in such course content. A basic introduction to the supervisory process at this point makes it easier for individual supervisor/supervisee dyads to begin a discussion of their own individual interaction. The purpose at this level is to assist supervisees in learning about what to expect of supervision, what their rights and responsibilities are as supervisees, and what they can do to obtain the most benefit from this experience in which they will be involved for the rest of their professional careers.

McCrea (1985), in describing a component on supervision in an undergraduate clinical management class, listed the objectives as (1) to encourage undergraduate students to view the clinical and supervisory processes as complementary and interactive, (2) to introduce undergraduate students to the participants and their primary roles and responsibilities within both processes, and (3) to introduce undergraduate students to problem-solving strategies to enhance both processes. McCrea then made the point that each part of the clinical process has its counterpart in the supervisory process and that they can be taught in such a way that the complementary and interactive nature of the two processes is emphasized. For example, evaluation and goal setting for the client have their counterparts in goal setting for the clinician's development, as do observation, data collection, and data analysis. These are all points made consistently throughout this book. Because time may be limited in such courses for inclusion of teaching about the supervisory process, the instructor must be knowledgeable about the process and able to distill the information into meaningful concepts appropriate to the particular level of the students. Such content should be extended beyond undergraduate-level courses to all levels of student clinical experience. Even advanced graduate students will profit from opportunities to discuss their changing roles as supervisees. McCrea (1985) suggested such procedures as lecture, problem-solving, and in-class discussion, as well as "'hands on' experiences. . .through the presentation of actual examples of supervisory problems, experience with observation tools, and viewing and analysis of videotaped samples of supervisory conference behavior" (p. 3).

Another area tangentially related to the supervisory process that should be addressed at some point, probably in clinical courses as well as by individual supervisors, is the interaction between the student clinician assigned to a client and inexperienced students who are completing their observation and participation requirement prior to beginning their own clinical work, as specified by ASHA requirements. Student clinicians have expressed concern about their role in this interaction. Are they to assume any type of supervisory role, or does their supervisor maintain the supervisory responsibility with the participant? This is an excellent opportunity for the supervisor to present some basic supervisory concepts to the advanced student clinician, and to provide them with opportunities to "try-on" the supervisory role with the assistance of the supervisor, in order to learn something about the dynamics of the process at an early stage in their careers.

Basic Course in Supervision

Course work in supervision is provided for master's- or doctoral-level students in some colleges and universities. It is often taken also by professionals in the field who are supervising or preparing to do so. The wisdom of providing a course in supervision as part of the master's degree curriculum is seen in the fact that the demographic data indicate that the major portion of the supervision being performed is done by professionals who hold master's degrees, most of them without preparation or even much clinical experience (Anderson, 1972, 1973a,b; Schubert & Aitchison, 1975; Stace & Drexler, 1969). Additionally, there is a feeling, totally undocumented but nevertheless a reasonable assumption, that students and professionals who have the opportunity to take a course in supervision become better supervisees. Knowledge of the process seems to give them more confidence about their own participation and what they can expect to gain from supervision.

The ASHA report on tasks and competencies for supervisors (ASHA, 1985b) listed many ways that individuals can obtain information and course work about supervision. It is a fact, however, that there is little encouragement or reward, much less requirement, in most organizations for supervisors to obtain such preparation. It is usually self-motivation that leads supervisors to such additional work. A course during the master's-degree program may be the only opportunity that some professionals will have, or will take, to study the supervisory process. Remembering the attitudes reflected in the Stace and Drexler (1969) study, the completion of one course in supervision, however, may help professionals realize its complexities and encourage them to seek further information when they do become supervisors.

The wisdom of such a course for doctoral-level students is similar. Most of them intend to obtain positions in college or university programs where their responsibilities are very apt to include supervision of students preparing to become clinicians, or they may become supervisors in other settings. Further, if they are the holders of the CCC, they may be engaged in supervision as doctoral students at the time they are taking the courses.

Professionals who take such a course may be supervisors in the program in which the course is taught, supervisors in nearby programs, or, very importantly for the training program, may be serving as supervisors of the off-campus practicum. They may be participating in a supervised supervision practicum at the time they are enrolled in the class or at a later time. The practicum will be described later.

Such a course should include at least the following topics: relevant information on supervision from other disciplines; preparation for the role of supervisor; professional/political issues in supervision in speech-language pathology and audiology; the planning, observation, and analysis role of the supervisor in relation to the clinical process; the planning, observation, and analysis of the supervisory process; supervisory techniques; interpersonal aspects of the supervisory process; variations in supervision across sites; accountability and evaluation in the supervisory process; preparing supervisees for the process; and research in supervision. Assignments should include extensive reading from the speech-language literature as well as other disciplines, viewing of videotapes of conferences, a self-study of students' interaction in taped conferences, whether they are supervisors or supervisees, a research proposal or review of literature on a specific topic, or other assignments as they meet individual needs and interests. The course should be oriented in such a way that it could be taken by both speech-language pathologists and audiologists.

Such courses and their content were discussed at an ASHA convention by Rassi (1985), Laccinole (1985), Casey (1985a), Brasseur (1985), and Ganz and Hunt-Thompson (1985) in a seminar moderated by Smith (1985). Rassi described an introductory course in supervision for "advanced clinical students in the audiology graduate program (at Northwestern University) who aspire to supervisory positions and/or have an interest in formal study of the supervisory process" (p. 1). Rassi stated that this course provides opportunity for potential supervisors to study the process as they are experiencing it. Content includes, among other topics, an examination of supervision research, methodology, and theory in communication sciences and allied professions, clinical decision making, competency-based instruction, supervisory competencies, leadership and supervisory styles, data collection, conference analysis, interpersonal relationships, observation, attribution and judgment, and evaluation and self-evaluation. Activities include participation in laboratory experiences or practicum which is monitored by a regular staff supervisor, listening to conference tapes, preparing a journal based on involvement in the supervisory process, and role-playing in a laboratory session. Rassi's program is also extended to on-campus and off-campus supervisors affiliated with the audiology department.

Course work described by Casey (1985b) at the University of Wisconsin-Whitewater has a content and requirements similar to Rassi's, but based more specifically on the ASHA-adopted tasks and competencies (ASHA, 1985b), which provide the focus for the course objectives, content, and requirements. Course content is appropriate to master's level, doctoral level, or post-degree levels and is adjusted according to need. It includes a practicum experience, a conference analysis, and the use of self-assessment instruments related to the ASHA list of competencies. Casey noted that the material in the course not only prepares people to supervise, but also enhances the student's performance as a supervisee.

A transdisciplinary approach in a graduate course on the supervisory process stresses models of supervision from various disciplines and the functioning of speech-language pathology and audiology in relation to related professions (Laccinole, 1985). Content includes planning, organizing, staffing, directing, evaluating, and representing. More program management topics appear to be included in this course than in the others described here. Activities include lecture, discussion, role playing with videotaping which is similar to the microteaching discussed briefly in an earlier chapter (Irwin, 1972, 1975, 1976, 1981a,b), practicum, planning and analysis of conferences, peer supervision, and evaluation.

Practicum Experiences in Supervision

Each of the courses described has included a very important laboratory or practicum component. Just as clinicians need practice in gaining clinical skills, supervisors also need opportunities to try out the skills they are learning about. The ASHA competency list has provided a guide for such practice.

The practicum experience as a part of a doctoral-level preparation program has been described previously (Anderson, 1981) as probably the most significant component of the program. 'This experience is a necessary step in gaining insight about the supervisory process, in the modification of the supervisory behavior of the trainees, and in defining the questions that lead to research in the supervisory process" (p. 80).

Procedures for the doctoral-level practicum in supervision as conducted by the writer are dependent upon need. Some doctoral students have had experience in supervision, all have had clinical experience and hold the CCC. They are assigned a certain number of student clinicians to supervise. The trainee (doctoral student) plans, observes, and analyzes the clinical work and holds conferences with the students. Similarly, the trainee's work is planned, observed, analyzed, and discussed in conference with the senior supervisor. Extensive use of audio- and videotape and interaction analysis systems form the basis of the conference between the trainee and the senior supervisor. Additionally, their conferences may be studied much as the conferences between the trainee and the student clinician are studied.

Practicum or laboratory experience for master's-level students must be handled differently since they will not have the CCC and, therefore, cannot be independently responsible for supervising student clinicians. Thus, they should be assigned to a clinical supervisor and involved *with* the supervisor at whatever level is appropriate. At the beginning of the experience, the clinical supervisor, the master's-level student, and the student clinician who is to be supervised discuss the purpose of the experience, set objectives, and develop a plan for the semester. This plan includes the master's-level student's role in observation, data collection, and analysis of the clinical sessions. It also includes procedures for observation, data collection, and analysis of conferences between the supervisor and the student clinician or the master's-level student and the supervisor. The plan will specify procedures to be used—use of certain observation systems or other data collection methods, journal writing, observation of other clinicians or supervisors, methods of analysis and reporting in the conference, and other suitable activities. Depending upon the dynamics of the situation, the student may participate to some degree in the conference when appropriate. If this is done, the student then will have opportunity for self-analysis of his or her interaction in a conference situation. The student will also have weekly conferences with the supervisor to discuss his or her progress toward the objectives that were set.

Combined Practicum and Academic Work

Although each of the courses described has a very important laboratory or practicum component or accompaniment to the course, the following program is described by its instructors in a slightly different way. Conducted at Western Washington University, it is called the Speech-Language Pathology Intern Supervisor Training Program (Ganz & Hunt-Thompson, 1985). Developed out of concern for a competency-based program for prospective clinical supervisors, it too is based on the ASHA list of tasks and competencies. Participants include the intern (student) supervisor, senior supervisor, student clinician, client, and course instructor. The student intern's supervisor level is determined on an *Intern Supervisor Level Assignment* instrument which is similar to the W-PACC (Shriberg et al., 1974) system for determining clinician level. An entry-level self-evaluation is completed on a form based specifically on the ASHA list of competencies, which serves as a baseline. Midterm and exit evaluations are completed by the senior supervisor. The intern makes individual contact with the senior supervisor at least once a week and participates in a weekly discussion with the total intern group. At the same time, the intern participates in a one-hour weekly academic seminar, the content of which appears to be similar to the other courses described, but with reports of the intern's performance providing a focus for the discussion. Upon completion of this basic experience, students are encouraged to participate in other supervisory experiences such as additional seminars or practica or research. (The description is not clear on this point, but it is assumed that the senior supervisor is involved in the practicum to an extent that meets ASHA requirements, since the intern may not have the CCC.)

Preparation for Off-Campus Supervisors

Supervisors of off-campus practicum are very influential in the development of clinical skills by students. If preparation can make a difference in the effectiveness of supervisors, as has been assumed in all the programs described, it should be extended to off-campus sites.

Many programs provide educational offerings for their off-campus supervisors in the form of a regular credit course or in-service offerings. One of the roles of the university supervisor of the off-campus practicum may also be seen as assisting site supervisors to develop their supervisory skills.

In the short-course presented at ASHA, a program for this purpose, funded by the U. S. Office of Education, was described (Brasseur, 1985). The objective of the program is to improve the performance of first-year professional clinicians through improving the supervision they receive during their school practicum experience. Thus, the target population of the program is clinicians working in the schools who are serving as supervisors or who wish to serve as supervisors of students from one university program (California State University-Chico). After the first year of the program, which has just been completed, graduate students will be incoporated into the program for two reasons—(1) it will help them to be more participative, analytical supervisees, and (2) there is a high probability that they will become supervisors at some time during their careers.

In order to achieve the competencies for supervisors, a program was developed to include an introductory seminar, practicum, and advanced seminar for off-campus supervisors, first within the county and later to be extended to graduate students and to supervisors in a larger geographical area. Part of the training is offered via Instructional Television Fixed Services (ITFS), a closed-circuit microwave television system.

The supervisory practicum, a minimum of 50 clock hours of experience, uses a variety of formats: direct on-site observation by the university professor who directs the program, audio- and videotapes of interactions between the student and the supervisor-in-training, individual conferences between the supervisor-in-training and the university professor, and group discussions with all the trainees. Just as the supervisor and student plan, observe, analyze, and discuss the clinical work, so the work of the supervisor-in-training is planned, observed, analyzed, and discussed with the university professor who observes and holds a conference once every two weeks with each trainee. Once a month, all trainees meet on campus for three hours to view and analyze videotapes, discuss problems, and plan objectives and strategies for achieving the competencies.

A final component of the program is an advanced seminar. In this seminar, students study the existing research in supervision, and the focus changes to prepare the supervisors-in-training to function as consultants for other supervisors of students in the school practicum in their own setting. Thus, the results of the program are extended beyond the original students.

This type of program has many possibilities. It could be extended to supervisors in other settings. Additionally, graduate students may be inspired to take more than the beginning course after they obtain their CCC.

Other types of offerings are provided for off-campus supervisors by other educational programs. Every effort should be made to improve communication between participants in off-campus practica and to provide preparation for supervisors.

Doctoral-Level Preparation

It appears that preparation in the supervisory process at the doctoral level has been available in several forms for some time but, as with so much of the information, it is not clear how much or in what form. Course work, practicum, independent study, and internships have been provided to some extent at this level as a part of some traditional doctoral programs. Beginning in 1972, however, a doctoral-level program, in which the main emphasis of the program was preparation in the supervisory process, was funded by the U. S. Office of Education at Indiana University with the writer as the director of the program (Anderson, 1981, 1985). The program was funded for 10 years and has been subsequently continued by the university. Since 1972, 14 dissertations on the supervisory process have been completed and one is currently in progress. Other research has also been conducted. The program has been refined so that the following guidelines can be presented for others who are interested in developing a similar program:

■ The objectives of a doctoral-level program should be (a) to prepare personnel who can teach other supervisors, and (b) to prepare researchers in the supervisory process.

■ The core content of a program in the supervisory process for the doctoral student should include at least the following: an introductory course that introduces the student to the literature in speech-language pathology and audiology as described earlier; an advanced seminar in which research in the supervisory process is studied intensively (this must include the 23 dissertations that have been identified in speech-language pathology as well as other relevant research); practicum experiences directed toward the development of the competencies listed by ASHA (1985b); independent study as needed to fill in areas not covered in course work and practicum; research experiences; and dissertation.

■ Programs for doctoral students should be individually planned, based on students' experience and needs. In addition to course work, practicum, and research experience in supervision, each program should include a concentration in another area of speech-language pathology and audiology that the student will be able to teach in a university once they attain their degree. This is important, because the reality is that most university programs are not currently able to employ a person to teach *only* supervision courses. Although many programs desire someone who has had preparation in supervision, their budgets require that they find prospective employees who can teach in more than one area.

■ The supervised practicum requirement, as described earlier, should be considered an essential part of the program. It is here where skill training takes place and where important research questions are identified.

■ Programs should include a strong research emphasis, both academic and experiential, because of the great need for research about the supervisory process.

■ Programs should meet all the basic requirements of the regular doctoral program in the university—research, dissertation, qualifying examinations.

■ Whenever possible, courses from other departments of the university that are relevant to students' goals should be included in their program, for example, from business management, counseling, education, higher education, special education, psychology, sociology, computer science.

■ Since most doctoral students are preparing themselves to teach in universities, they should have an opportunity for teaching experience. This experience should be supervised by a faculty member.

■ All of the competencies adopted by ASHA are relevant to students of the supervisory process at the doctoral level. In addition, competencies in teaching and research should be identified and attained by each student.

■ A minor concentration consisting of coursework and practicum should be provided for doctoral students who prefer to concentrate in another area but wish to obtain some information and experience in the supervisory process.

Continuing Education

Another form of disseminating information that may be more common and more accessible than the others discussed here is continuing education. Participants in this type of instruction will usually, but not always, be at a post-master's level and may vary greatly in terms of experience and knowledge; therefore, objectives may be different for each situation. Ulrich (1985) suggested that the purposes of continuing education in the supervisory process may be to either increase knowledge or to develop skills in the task of supervision and that it is important for the leader to differentiate between the two objectives. The ASHA list of competencies may also be utilized as a foundation for continuing education. Formats range from lectures and panel discussions, peer interaction, and contemporary paradigms for distance learning such as teleconferences and directed independent study.

Continuing education takes place at conventions, conferences, seminars, special organizations of supervisors, and within organizations. Some college or university programs provide such opportunities for the off-campus supervisors who work with their students. A group of supervisors in an organization can gain a great deal from group study of the process. Because of the granting of Continuing Education Units (CEU) by ASHA, many people will continue to be interested in continuing education as a source of information.

Implications of Adult Learning Styles

The extensive literature on adult learning or adult education has been neglected, if not ignored, by most speech-language pathologists and audiology supervisors and the people they supervise. At the most basic level, supervisors frequently observe clinicians attempting to utilize with adolescents, or even adults, virtually the same techniques they use with children. Perhaps this same lack of attention to changing stages of development is what makes it difficult for some supervisors to develop a collaborative approach to supervision. Shapiro (1985) reported total rejection of the concept of colleagueship by a supervisor—"Like hell I'll consider a student a colleague" (p. 104). This reaction is antithetical to the proposals made in the adult education literature, but it must be taken seriously in relation to the teaching of the supervisory process.

In the adult education literature, Knowles (1984) differentiated between *pedagogy*, the teaching of children, and *andragogy*, "any intentional and professionally guided activity that aims at a change in adult persons" (p. 50). The two are seen as somewhat similar to the continuum presented here, moving from dependency of the learner in pedagogy to self-directiveness in andragogy. Knowles suggested that an andragogical model of learning is based on several assumptions: (1) adults need to know why they need to learn something before they begin the process; (2) adults have a concept of being responsible for their own decisions which may lead to resistance to certain types of educational experiences; (3) because adults bring more experience to a learning situation, not only is there a greater need for individualization in teaching but often the "richest resources for learning reside in the adult learners themselves" (p. 57), providing educators can open up their minds to new approaches; (4) readiness to learn is as important to adults as to children; (5) orientation to learning in adults is life-centered, that is, task-centered or problem-centered, not subject-centered (in other words, adults learn best when they can perceive application of the learning to their daily life); and (6) although adults respond to some external motivators like money and promotions, the most potent motivation for learning is from internal pressures (increased job satisfaction, self-esteem, quality of life). Knowles advocated such methods as organizing adult learning around needs and interests, life situations (not subjects), analysis of experience, mutual inquiry, and allowing for differences in style, time, place, and pace of learning. In fact, the points he made are compatible with the continuum of supervision. Thus, the continuum is as relevant for the supervisor-in-training as it is for the clinician-in-training.

Knowledge of adult stages of development are also relevant to preparation of supervisors. Individual differences and needs are factors that should be known. Adult learners are often voluntary participants, which implies sacrifices of time and money (Haverkamp, 1983). On the other hand, they may be meeting mandatory requirements of an organization or a degree requirement, which leads to different attitudes.

Although group activities are recommended, if small-group techniques are used to involve learners more directly in their own learning, it must be realized that "few learners are adequately prepared to function in group learning efforts" (p. 8). Therefore, an orientation to group participation is often a useful tool if the instructor intends to use this methodology. Additionally, many individuals who attempt to lead groups are not very skillful, a point that has been discussed previously (Haverkamp, 1983).

Is Education in Supervision Effective?

As preparation in the supervisory process continues, as it undoubtedly will, the profession will need to ask itself some searching questions. Any kind of educational program, pre-service or continuing education, costs time and money and effort on the part of the teacher and the learner. The effectiveness of any kind of preparation for supervisors obviously needs to be demonstrated. But, more than that, the wide variety of possible approaches must be investigated.

The profession must know if pre-service preparation is effective—in other words, if education at this level carries over to the somewhat distant future when the supervisee becomes a supervisor. There is also a need to know if continuing education can be designed to meet the needs of adult professionals in a skill area such as supervision.

Particularly important at the present time, because many of the offerings appear to be continuing education, are certain questions about its effectiveness:

1. What is the effect of convention presentations, with their wide variety from scientific reports to didactic, tutorial sessions?

2. What is the value of a three-hour lecture or a six-hour workshop that may include a period of group dicussion or experiential activities in changing attitudes, helping listeners develop a philosophy about supervision, or identifying and modifying skills?

3. What is the impact of a college professor who, in addition to an already overloaded schedule of teaching, supervision, and research at the university, drives across the state one night a week to teach a course to professionals who have also worked a full day?

4. What is learned by the professional who has supervised for years, whose habits are firmly established, and who is taking a course merely to meet a certification or organizational credit?

5. Is the use of television and other new communication systems more effective than face-to-face lectures?

Need for Research on Preparation of Supervisors

The need for preparation of supervisors for their roles now seems to have been accepted officially by the profession of speech-language pathology and audiology with the adoption of the position paper of the Committee on Supervision (ASHA, 1985b). Now the need is for research, not only to validate the tasks and competencies included in that document, but to determine how to prepare supervisors so that they can effectively perform those tasks.

Dowling (1986) analyzed the task behavior in conferences of two supervisors enrolled in a doctoral program with emphasis on the clinical supervision approach advocated by Cogan (1973) and Goldhammer (1969). She found the task behavior of these supervisors to be different from that of supervisors in other descriptive studies of the conference (Culatta & Seltzer, 1976, 1977; Roberts & Smith, 1982; Smith, 1979). Conferences included more equality in the relationship, supervisors did not dominate and supervisees were not passive as indicated in the other studies. Further, conference behavior varied from one supervisee to another, a finding also different from the other descriptive studies. Whether or not these differences can be attributed to the academic and practicum work in which the supervisors were involved cannot be determined from this study. More research to determine the impact of such training must be undertaken by the profession.

One study (Hagler, 1986) that used the "bug-in-the-ear" technique described earlier attempted to modify the amount of verbal behavior of supervisors during the conference by providing feedback through an electronic device which delivered immediate feedback to subjects. The findings show that supervisors were able to reduce their verbal behavior as a result of a verbal directive to "try to talk less," which was delivered via the bug-in-the-ear at two-minute intervals. Data provided to the subjects about the amount of verbal behavior and contingent social praise delivered in the same manner did not produce change. Generalization to other behaviors cannot be supported without further research, but as the author states, the study does constitute a "first step toward systematic modification of a supervisor conferencing behavior, which may lead someday to strategies for teaching supervisory styles" (p. 67).

Another study in progress (Strike & Anderson, in progress) is attempting to modify supervisor behavior over a longer time period. Methodology is the presentation of analyzed data and discussion of the desired changes with the supervisor.

Such research must continue. A subsequent chapter will offer suggestions about research methodologies that seem particularly applicable to supervisory research.

SUMMARY

Preparation in the supervisory process has not been considered necessary, nor has it been available to many supervisors in the past. That situation has been changing and the recent recognition of the tasks performed by supervisors and the competencies necessary to carry them out gives further impetus to the development of preparation programs in the supervisory process. A variety of preparation models are available. They should be developed in conjunction with research that will determine their effectiveness.

Accountability

Supervision may well be the oldest, most traditional approach to quality assurance.

Flower (1984, p. 297)

The growth of the profession of speech-language pathology and audiology has been characterized by a constant effort to provide better services for clients and better preparation for those who are planning to become speech-language pathologists or audiologists. There is ample evidence of this in what has become a rather vast literature for a relatively young profession. There is further evidence in the continually increasing standards set by the professional organization for certification of programs or individuals and the development of a variety of approaches to what has come to be known as "quality assurance"—how to assure that the clients served by the profession receive the best possible service.

As the profession has continued its concern for clinical accountability, certain formalized systems have been developed through ASHA or other agencies or organizations. Such ASHA publications as the *Child Service Review Manual* (1982c), the *Patient Care Audit Manual* (1978b) and the standards for accreditation of training programs (Educational Standards Board) and clinical programs (Professional Services Board) and for continuing education (Continuing Education Board) are all part of the accountability of the profession. These and other accountability procedures are well covered by others (Adair, 1983; Battin, 1983; Bloom & Fischer, 1982; Diggs, 1983; Douglas, 1983; Flower, 1983, 1984; Kent, 1985; Mowrer, 1972; Pendergast, 1983; Siegel, 1975; Vetter, 1985; Wisconsin Speech-Language-Hearing Association, 1980). More recently, ASHA has developed the Program Evaluation System (1986), a detailed procedure for assuring quality across all work settings and areas of practice.

Suggestions in the writings cited are directed toward quality assurance for clinical services through such processes as accreditation, peer review, record systems, and audits. They also focus on accountability of individuals through self-assessment, continuing education, and the use of single-subject approaches for determining effectiveness of procedures. Most of these proposals are compatible with suggestions made in this book for a scientific approach to the clinical and supervisory processes as a means of documenting effectiveness. Interestingly enough, however, only two of these sources give much attention to the role of the supervisor in accountability (Flower, 1984; Pendergast, 1983), even though all the systems described might be coordinated by supervisors. However, if as Kent (1985) said, "Assessment and management have an essential underpinning of empirical observation and systematic analysis" (p. 11) and the practitioner is responsible for developing and maintaining that underpinning to demonstrate accountability, does the supervisor not have at least equal responsibility to that of the clinician?

In actuality, supervisors have enormous responsibilities for accountability. Many professional obligations fall to them. In educational programs they are, in many ways, the "gatekeepers" of the profession. In addition to questions about what is happening to the clients served by their programs, they must also ensure that the clinicians are adequately prepared to leave the educational program and fulfill their responsibilities to clients in the off-campus, CFY, or service delivery setting.

Most of the important decisions in the profession are made, in large part, by supervisors—continuation in practicum, grading, references, continuation in the profession, promotions, more responsible assignments, and many others. If they do not perform these responsibilities professionally and appropriately, problems often result or are compounded. For example, the ineffective student allowed into the off-campus practicum, the CFY, or the service delivery world because of inadequate accountability systems in the educational program creates difficult situations for others.

This chapter will assume two types of accountability in which the supervisor will be involved: clinical and supervisory. What has been said by others about the procedures and processes of clinical accountability will not be repeated. Only the role of the supervisor in clinical accountability will be discussed. The issue of supervisory accountability has not been a topic of discussion in other sources and it, too, will be presented here.

CLINICAL ACCOUNTABILITY

Supervisors have important roles in clinical accountability to the client and to the clinician. This dual responsibility often leads to conflict that is difficult to resolve. The dilemma for the supervisor is how to balance student and client needs so that both achieve the maximum from the situation while still meeting the goals of the organization.

Accountability for Clients

Part of the supervisor's role in terms of clinical accountability should be seen as determining if client needs are being met by clinicians. Many of the procedures discussed in the literature cited would be helpful to supervisors in this activity. Some organizations have instituted their own accountability systems as a part of the larger program, that is, the school, hospital, or other agency. ASHA has just developed a software system, the Program Evaluation System (PES), for documenting quality of services (Larkins, 1987). It will provide data rather than just opinions about the quality of services being provided. The supervisor will play a major role in implementing such programs.

Vetter (1985) captured the essence of clinical accountability in an excellent article in which she pointed out the need for "systematic accounting of the effects of treatment" (p. 55) and the importance of a scientific approach to clinical intervention. She offered many suggestions for clinicians to use in determining the success or failure of the treatment they have used for each client. The procedures she advocated are not new to many professionals, but they *are* important. They involve establishing baseline measures, planning, predicting criterion behaviors, and utilizing "a mechanism for ethical and accountable behavior management" (p. 64). The article would be a valuable reading assignment for beginning clinicians and an excellent reminder of some significant procedures for other clinicians and supervisors.

A part of the implementation of client accountability by supervisors is a teaching process. Students in the educational program need to learn (1) to read and write reports accurately, (2) to collect data, (3) to check their own effectiveness, and (4) all the other aspects of accountability. This will be learned mainly through the supervisory process. In the settings where supervisees already have earned entry-level credentials, supervisors may implement and monitor clinical accountability programs but may find that they need also to teach the principles and procedures of such activities to clinicians who have not learned such skills adequately or who are unfamiliar with the structure of the program.

Accountability for Clinicians

The other part of the clinical accountability role of supervisors, in addition to determing client results, is determining clinician effectiveness and ongoing development. Are clinicians' skills appropriate so that clients receive the services they need? Are clinicians growing and developing professionally?

The entire plan for supervision presented here has been directed toward accountability—preparing clinicians to observe, analyze, and evaluate their own work. This must be seen as the very essence of supervision. Supervisors must teach clinicians to be accountable for their own activities.

What Ever Happened to Evaluation?

The use of the word *evaluation* has been avoided assiduously as one of the factors in the supervisory process. It has been mentioned as a chracteristic of the early stage of the continuum and one which is to be left behind as soon as possible in favor of analysis and self-evaluation. Evaluation is discussed briefly in the chapter on Analyzing and presented as the very antithesis of the analysis component. This has been done mainly to deemphasize the subjective aspect of supervision and to emphasize the analytical approach which is perceived as such an important part of the teaching/learning process. Therefore, it is interesting to note that the literature cited here about quality assurance systems rarely uses the word, either. Rather, the authors talk about establishing criteria, setting objectives, self-assessment, peer review, and other forms of accountability, not subjective judgments.

The thrust of this entire book has been on supervisors as facilitators of objective supervisee self-analysis or on joint analysis as a teaching process which enables the participants to make changes in behavior to better meet objectives that have been set. It is contended that this is a learning process that will result in greater generalization by the supervisee than if the supervisor makes all the evaluations and suggestions. It is also an accountability procedure. Clinicians become self-analytical, able to measure their own progress, and therefore, accountable.

But how does this fit the realities of life for supervisors? At some point in most supervisory experiences, the time comes for a product called *evaluation*. Whether to fulfill a grading requirement or a recommendation, or whatever the reason, the organization will probably demand some type of formal evaluation.

What, then, of the evaluation that traditionally has been perceived as the role of the supervisor? Evaluation forms are found in every organization and maintained for various reasons. Supervisees expect to receive a critique of their work, to learn about their strengths and weaknesses, as reported earlier. Is evaluation part of the role of the supervisor? And how does it mesh with the total accountability process?

It has been reported that the descriptive literature on supervisory conferences reveals little evaluative behavior by supervisors (Culatta & Selzer, 1976; Roberts & Smith, 1982). This finding may be spurious. The behaviors in the conferences from which these data were taken were categorized by someone other than the participants. It is not known if supervisees themselves might perceive the behaviors directed at them differently than someone not involved in the conference. For example, the response "Why don't you try. . ." after a supervisee's recounting of what he or she had done might be scored on some systems or interpreted by an observer as a question or a suggestion. To supervisees, however, it may communicate that what they did up to that point was wrong and should be modified, thus taking on the connotation of an evaluation. One doctoral student who worked with the writer found, in fact, that student raters of conference behaviors of others rated the most casual observations or the giving of information by supervisors as a suggestion more often than other raters did. In other words, from the perspective of the supervisee, if the supervisor said it, it must be a suggestion for what to do. Thus, perhaps the validity of the statements that supervisors do not evaluate must be questioned unless it is known how the statements were perceived by the listener. Roberts and Smith (1982) suggested that evaluation may be avoided by supervisors because it may be perceived as threatening and might lead to confrontation or negative social reactions from the supervisee. Supervisors may, for this reason, couch their evaluations in less punitive terms, which do not appear to raters to be evaluative. Additionally, the absence of evaluation or a nonverbal behavior may be interpreted either positively or negatively by a supervisee as an evaluation, even when not intended as such by the supervisor. This is just one of the many reasons for supervisors to monitor their verbal behaviors carefully. This is not to say that supervisors should never make an evaluative statement, but that its intent should be clear and its rationale sound. Further, it would seem to be important for a supervisee to know when a statement was intended to be evaluative.

Whether or not evaluative statements are made as a part of ongoing conferences, it is known that some type of formal evaluation is usually made at some point. How these judgments are made is an important point. Roberts and Naremore (1983) applied attribution theory to supervision in speech-language pathology to determine how supervisors make decisions. Based on a paper and pencil task in response to a request to imagine a hypothetical session going well or poorly, they found considerable agreement among supervisors about why therapy sessions go well or poorly. Outcomes of sessions were attributed to clinician factors such as strategies used in session planning and instruction, rather than client characteristics or clinician personal or interpersonal behaviors. The authors suggested that this may be because planning and instructional behaviors are more readily observable and more easily documented. Information that the session was going well or poorly did influence the reactions of the subjects. Thus, the authors suggested that supervisors approach clinical sessions with preconceived beliefs that influence the way in which they attribute causes for the outcome. This lack of objectivity, if it exists in the general population of supervisors, does not bode well for unbiased decision making.

Russell and Halfond (1985) interviewed both supervisees and supervisors about the evaluative component of supervision. Supervisees saw clinical grades as subjective, as anxiety producing and based on academic as well as interpersonal factors, as nonnegotiable, final assessments, and as based on inconsistent standards from one student to another and from one supervisor to another. Supervisors saw grades as not only based on observation, but as reflecting the supervisee's potential, past experience, and the complexity of the client. They were also perceived by supervisors as inconsistent and anxiety producing and the most difficult aspect of clinical instruction. Clinic grades were perceived as based on less consistent criteria and as less precise than course grades because it is too painful to give poor clinical grades and too difficult to determine subtle differences. Nonetheless, clinical grades were seen by both groups to be necessary, inevitable, and a symbol that is ultimately meaningful and useful. In a later study, Halfond and Russell (1986) obtained reactions to written evaluations. The major finding was that all written comments should be accompanied by oral discussion to be of maximum benefit. Such discussion clarifies issues, resolves disagreements, embellishes ideas, and helps negotiate final evaluation. These few attempts in the literature to clarify the complexities of the evaluative process only expose the tip of the iceberg. It is, certainly, an iceberg that needs further exploration.

The trend throughout this book has been to down play the subjective evaluation in favor of the objective, analytical joint- and self-analysis. This trend is also found in the literature on accountability, which emphasizes the scientific measurement of effectiveness against specific objectives, a systematic approach by individuals for their own accountability in each situation. If personal objectives are set and joint-analysis is conducted continuously and objectively throughout the total supervisory sequence, both supervisor and supervisee should find the formal evaluation coming out of that analysis. It should be a natural development after continued analysis for supervisors to encourage self-evaluation by the supervisee or to provide their own evaluation, when appropriate, based on data. Such an evaluation should be more palatable to both supervisor and supervisee than judgments from the supervisor alone. There should be no surprises in the evaluation for the supervisee if such a process of supervision has been instituted, because they will have been aware of their place on the continuum throughout the entire procedure. It is clear from the current literature on accountability and leadership that the totally subjective evaluation made by the supervisor is no longer acceptable.

The Marginal Clinician

Does this mean that supervisors should never have a negative thought or utter a negative statement? Certainly not! The collected data and the analysis of the clinician's performance may make it necessary for supervisors to take a negative stance about the supervisee if they are to fulfill their professional responsibilities. In this case, the formal requirement for an evaluation may be an unpleasant experience, but the deemphasis on evaluation in no way is intended to negate the need for accountability on the part of the supervisor. Supervisors do have certain responsibilities. If supervisees do not have the ability to make appropriate progress along the continuum toward independence, the grim fact is that it is the professional duty of supervisors to react to this situation directly, honestly, and professionally. In the educational program, this may mean terminating the student's program. It may mean that the student will be required to repeat certain clinical experiences. It may mean delaying an off-campus assignment until the student has developed more skills and is able to work more independently. It may call for more intensive supervision or peer assistance. In the service delivery setting, it may result in more supervision and assistance from supervisors or peers or in termination of employment.

Unfortunately, this is not as easy as it sounds. Because of differences in perceptions of clinical competencies, evaluation decisions become very difficult and are subject to great variability across supervisors. This fact provides even greater support for a scientific, data-based methodology for supervision. Yet, even that may not be sufficient in some instances. Some supervisees may be unable to understand or participate in the analysis or may refuse to hear what they do not wish to hear. Many supervisors and most educational programs bear the scars of unpleasant experiences at some time in their history from their attempts to terminate a student who was not performing adequately in her or his clinic work and who refused to accept dismissal from the program, sometimes to the point of legal action.

Similar experiences are not unknown in the off-campus assignment, the CFY, or in the service delivery setting, despite the efforts of educational programs to prepare their students in the best possible way. Students who perform well in the relative security of the college or university program may not be able to cope with other situations, and in these cases, supervisors are again challenged. Any organization that has had the experience of dealing with an inadequately performing clinician will understand—if they didn't before—the importance of data in documenting problem areas and supporting action that may need to be taken—in other words, accountability.

Educational programs need to have an established procedure for dealing with such students, and many do. At an ASHA miniseminar (Pappas, 1983), several different proposals were presented for dealing with the student identified as having clinical problems. Procedures included some method of identifying competencies that are not being met, setting specific behavioral objectives, and establishing time limits for their accomplishment, followed by further review. Such procedures frequently utilize team supervision as well as input from the clinic coordinator in making a final decision about continuation or dismissal. The program in which the writer works has developed a highly structured plan for dealing with the student who is having major problems in clinical interaction. The clinic coordinator, at least one supervisor, and the student's academic advisor form a team to identify specific problems. They then, with the supervisee, develop an individual plan that includes objectives, procedures, criteria, and time limits, and specifies the type and amount of supportive data to be collected by supervisors during the period of probation. One type of data to be collected is a videotape of a supervisory conference. The interaction in the conference often reveals as much or more, both positive and negative, about the student's basic understanding and application of the principles of the clinical process as does a videotape of a clinical session. Thus, it provides valuable data for making decisions about marginal students.

Plans such as this must be structured very carefully to protect the rights of the student. They must assure that the university has provided every opportunity for the student to achieve, while still protecting itself and the profession.

Accountability in the Service Delivery Setting

There are special issues in terms of accountability once the student leaves the educational program. Pendergast (1983) detailed the accountability responsibilities of the supervisor in school programs and Adair (1983) stated that hospitals provide accountability through management and professional supervision. In service delivery settings, supervisors are ultimately responsible for the quality of services. Many supervisors in such settings are responsible for so many supervisees that they have only brief, occasional interaction with each one. Many of the supervisors' responsibilities in such cases are related to program management activities, rather than supervision, as defined earlier. More significantly, many speech-language pathologists and audiologists have supervisors who are not prepared in the profession—school administrators, doctors, business managers. Since many such administrators tend to evaluate on items not related to client progress or clinician growth, that is, personality characteristics, general ability to interact with others, or certain political factors, speech-language pathologists and audiologists need a clear knowledge of their own objectives and the importance of accountability measures so that they can communicate them to their administrators. If they have not acquired these in their educational program, the readings cited would assist them in their own professional growth or would make an excellent basis for ongoing group effort at continuing education with their peers. The conditions described relative to supervision by other professionals make it imperative for educational programs to teach self-assessment and accountability procedures.

Many issues related to accountability, evaluation, termination, or dismissal are determined by organizational regulations, bargaining agents, negotiations, and other realities of the service delivery setting. These parameters vary greatly across settings and may have either negative or positive impact on the supervisor and the program.

SUPERVISOR ACCOUNTABILITY

Douglas (1983) stated that a "major consideration in clinical accountability is the effectiveness and efficiency of treatment" (p. 116). An application of this principle to supervision would assume that the effectiveness and efficiency of supervision would be the main consideration in accountability regarding the supervisory process. The meaning of effectiveness in supervision can be extrapolated from the definition of the supervisory process found in Chapter 1— ensuring optimal service to clients as well as professional growth and development in supervisees and in themselves. Efficiency is the skill with which they utilize the procedures of supervision. More specifically, effectiveness in supervision is based on whether or not what the supervisor does makes a difference in the subsequent behavior of the supervisee and ultimately in change in clients.

There has been surprisingly little concern about accountability for supervisors over the years. The ASHA Committee on Supervision report (1978a) identified the need for accountability for supervisors as one of nine major issues needing consideration by the profession, and stated: "Despite the amount of time devoted to supervision by members of the profession, the literature evidences no concern about evaluation of the activities of supervisors. Supervisors have apparently performed quite autonomously. Their decisions and methodology have been accepted and their effectiveness not questioned.... The profession must give some very serious attention to the accountability of those individuals who perform supervisory roles in academic and employment settings" (p. 484).

Early in the book, it was indicated that the Committee on Supervision had stated that there were no data to indicate that supervision makes a difference in the effectiveness of clinicians. This is a startling fact when one considers the number of hours that have been devoted to supervision in the profession since its beginning and the fact that the requirements for quantity of supervision in educational programs have steadily increased. The simple fact is that the profession has assumed that supervision is necessary and important but has done nothing until recent years to even attempt to validate its effectiveness. In that situation, speech-language pathology and audiology are not very different from other professions that utilize supervision. Even though some of them may have more theoretical and descriptive literature on supervision than speech-language pathology or audiology, statements are just beginning to appear there about the need for validation and they, too, have little data to which they can point.

Accountability for Supervision Through Research

One of the first in speech-language pathology and audiology to question the efficacy of supervision was Nelson (1974), who presented a paper at an ASHA convention entitled "Does Supervision Make a Difference?" Nelson assigned 24 inexperienced students to three different conditions—individual supervision, group supervision, and no supervision—and then rated supervisees on 24 competencies. Her data indicate that the individual and group subjects were rated higher than those who had no supervision. Thus, Nelson concluded that supervision *does* make a difference.

Other studies have since looked at the effects of different methodologies of supervision. Hall (1971) looked at behavior changes of supervisees under conditions that utilized videotape replay. Numerous variables were not controlled in this study and the conclusions are not clear-cut, but it marked the beginning of the search for answers about supervision efficacy. Goodwin (1977) looked at the results of two different lengths of conference or no conference on clinician behavior. He identified trends in his data that were interpreted as support for the conference. Engnoth (1974) investigated behavior changes under three conditions—conventional supervision, induction loop conferences (immediate feedback), and minimal supervision. Data showed both positive and negative changes under all three conditions, thus, not necessarily related to the supervision. Dowling (1977) compared conventional supervision with a form of group supervision and found that the methods did not result in different talk behaviors on the part of supervisees during conference. In a later study, Nilsen (1983) studied the results of direct and indirect verbal behaviors in the conference on subsequent behavior in the clinical session. Using a naturalistic observational methodology, she found the directive behavior of supervisors to be more influential in changing subsequent behaviors of clinicians than indirect supervision behaviors. These studies began to identify the issues, but all contained major methodological problems. The questions these researchers posed still require answers.

Another area of research related to the conference is that of perceptions of its effectiveness, that is, what people think is effective. Oratio, Sugarman, and Prass (1981) identified interpersonal factors as the most important ingredient of effective supervision.

Underwood (1973), on the basis of descriptive data gathered with the Blumberg analysis system and ratings of perceptions of conference effectiveness, made the following suggestions for guidelines for effective conferences: (1) there should be more clinician talk than supervisor talk, (2) silence and confusion should be followed by clinician talk, (3) the supervisor should spend a minimum amount of time asking for and giving information, and spend more time asking for clinician opinions, ideas, and suggestions, and (4) the supervisor should "perhaps" support the clinician's ideas. These are tentative guidelines at best, but both Underwood's findings and those of Smith (1977) to be discussed next are similar to the earlier studies of Blumberg and his colleagues, reported elsewhere in this book.

Smith (1977) studied both the content and the perceived effectiveness components of supervisory conferences. As a part of the study, she developed the *Individual Supervisory Rating Scale* (Smith & Anderson, 1982a) (see Appendix C). Using effectiveness ratings of supervisors, supervisees, and trained raters and the MOSAICS (Weller, 1971) to analyze the content of each conference, it was found that both direct and indirect supervisor behaviors were perceived to be effective and that each group of raters perceived an effective conference differently.

The basic questions that must be answered include, Does supervision make a difference? Is one methodology better than another? What variables in the conference make a difference in subsequent behavior of supervisees?

Two recent studies have addressed these issues. The effectiveness of commitments by supervisees to carry out specific activities in subsequent clinical sessions was examined by Shapiro (1985). Although the details are reported earlier in relation to planning (the commitment is, in essence, a form of contract), it is appropriate to this section since it is an effort to follow through a specific behavior from the conference to the subsequent clinical session, thus defining one effectiveness variable.

Gillam, Strike, and Anderson (1987), using a single-subject design, conducted a study to determine if supervisees would alter their clinical behaviors as a direct consequence of supervision conducted in accordance with the clinical supervision model of Cogan (1973) and Goldhammer (1969). Three behaviors—informative feedback, number of explanations per activity, and clinician responses to off-task utterances—were targeted for change after analysis of the first three clinical sessions. Efforts to adhere to the clinical supervision model included (1) observation plans that specified the observation and analysis roles of both supervisor and supervisee were jointly developed, and (2) written agreements specified the target behaviors for clinicians, procedures for attaining them, how data would be collected, and what the clinician would look for in the data. Results indicated that supervisees changed the targeted clinical behaviors as a result of the data-based discussions, jointly developed observation and data-analysis strategies, and written conference agreements. Controls applied in the study ensured that the supervisory procedures facilitated the changes. Results from these two studies are representative of the type of information needed to document the effectiveness of supervision.

Research in the supervisory process has shown a slow, steady increase since the 1970s. In addition to the published studies, numbers of research projects have been reported at ASHA and state conventions. It is obvious that many supervisors are beginning to ask their own questions and attempt to answer them. It is encouraging to note that many supervisors are teaming with colleagues who may be more knowledgeable than they in research techniques to conduct such studies. Research is certainly one way to accountability for a profession.

There are several obstacles to the accomplishment of research in the supervisory process. Skilled researchers have other interests; supervisors often do not have research skills. No vast body of research has accumulated over the years upon which to build current research, as exists for other areas of interest within the profession. The questions are just now being refined. Recent years have seen the validation of instruments and the use of various methodologies. Two research methodologies less commonly used in the past—the single-subject design and ethnographic research—may provide new procedures that will be effective in studying the supervisory process. They will be the topic of a later chapter.

There is no way to overemphasize the need for research in the supervisory process. For a profession that prides itself on its accountability to overlook the responsibility of determining the effectiveness of a task that has occupied so much of the time of so many of its members is unconscionable. There are signs that this is changing but, perhaps, not rapidly enough.

The adoption of the list of competencies for supervisors by ASHA (1985b) has provided a base for extensive research. All of these competencies must be validated if they are to provide a meaningful basis for supervisory procedures. They must not be accepted wholeheartedly until such validation is done.

Individual Supervisor Accountability

The lack of accountability for supervisors and their work in the past raises the question, "Who supervises the supervisor?" and the probable answer is "No one." It has been said that supervisors' work is accepted on faith, a fact that is probably too true.

The literature contains virtually nothing about organizational structure in relation to supervisors. Little is known about what educational programs or service delivery settings expect or require from their supervisors, whether or not they are evaluated, and if so, what criteria are used. If there are criteria, it is not known if they are related to actual change in the behavior of the supervisees with whom they have worked or to actual supervisor behavior. In the absence of criteria, evaluations of supervisors may be based on purely subjective perceptions of the global, and perhaps even irrelevant, behavior of supervisors.

Without more information, it can only be assumed that, like clinicians, supervisors are probably formally evaluated at some time. This evaluation may be done by their administrators who may be trained in another discipline or who may never have been a supervisor. These evaluations are probably based on personal characteristics of the supervisor, the ability to meet organizational needs, and perhaps on the basis of feedback from supervisees. Such feedback from supervisees is probably based on unknown, individual criteria for supervision and/or on the quality of the personal interaction they have had with the supervisor. Specific behaviors of supervisors in the interaction with their supervisees or growth in supervisees is probably not measured or taken into consideration in judgments about supervisors' effectiveness.

Evaluations generated from supervisees cannot be assumed to be sufficient data for evaluation of supervisors, although they may have some importance. The consensus has been stated previously that supervisees may not have sufficient understanding of the supervisory process to know what to expect or evaluate, thus rendering the value of their feedback somewhat questionable. Supervisees, as seen in the descriptive data, seldom challenge or confront their supervisors, even though they may disagree or complain in private. Further, unless complete anonymity is assured, the chances of honest feedback, even perceptual, may be questioned.

Sleight (1984b) found that supervisor self-evaluations and student ratings of supervisors were different on specific items. On the rating of overall effectiveness, however, supervisors who had rated themselves higher than students on most items rated themselves lower on overall effectiveness than students rated them. Ulrich and Watt (1977) looked at competence of supervisors, and in the process, developed an evaluation form for supervisors. Their study indicated that communicating expectations about clinical responsibilities to the student, evidence of knowledge of the communication disorder with which the student was working, and flexibility were the most critical of 20 items in predicting judgments of overall rating. They also found that supervisors and supervisee ratings differed, with supervisors rating themselves lower than supervisees. Perhaps supervisors, as well as supervisees, do not have a clear picture of what supervision is. Ulrich and Watt's evaluation form has been used rather widely, but is subject to all the problems of any formal evaluation.

An evaluation form based on the competencies first proposed by the Committee on Supervision (ASHA, 1982a) was developed by Hanner, Nilson, and Richard (1983). Competencies were rephrased and a computer scoring system included. Other individuals and organizations appear to be utilizing the competency list as a basis for evaluation, although nothing of this kind has been validated and published as yet.

If formal evaluation forms are developed in the future for supervisors, they should certainly be based on the ASHA list of competencies. Such evaluation forms will be more valuable if, and when, the competencies are validated. This is a very necessary area for research.

Supervisor Accountability Through Self-Assessment

Given the lack of validated guidelines for their activities and the unlikely prospect that such guidelines will be available in the perceptible future, supervisors must draw on other resources to obtain some sense of the results of their own behavior.

An example of the adoption of quality assurance techniques to the supervisory process was reported by Sbaschnig and Williams (1983, 1984), who based two reliability audits, one for supervisors in clinics and one for externship supervisors, on the Patient Care Audits, a quality assurance, peer-review mechanism utilized in health care services. In response to student concerns about inconsistencies in grading, a peer review system was developed. Goals were to attain greater uniformity in grading and more accountability to adminstrators and clinicians. A Reliability Audit committee evaluated the grading procedures using videotapes of therapy sessions. The Committee set up criteria and standards. They graded three tapes at four-week intervals during the term and did item-by-item analyses to determine reliability.

The study of supervision as a process has been covered in Chapter 11. The methods proposed there provide one approach to accountability, that is, learning what is actually happening. Another aspect of accountability for supervisors is found in the approach recommended for clinical accountability—setting objectives and measuring progress toward their attainment, self-assessment, peer review, continuing education.

In previous chapters, a great deal was said about planning, observing, and analyzing clinician behavior. The data on clinician behavior as it relates to what has been discussed during the conference is one measure, *perhaps*, of a supervisor's effectiveness. Shapiro's (1985) methodology to determine if commitments were actually carried out is an example of one form of accountability. Do the results of the conference show in the subsequent clinical sessions? The supervisor who wishes to measure his or her effectiveness in this manner can devise any number of data collection techniques that will help identify some answers to that question.

Supervisors may also utilize the competency list (ASHA, 1985b) for self-assessment. Casey (1985b) developed a *Supervisory Skills Self-Assessment*. Supervisors answer two questions about each competency—(1) How important is this competency for effectiveness in my program? (2) How satisfied am I with my ability to perform this skill?—and record their ideal and present score. Supervisees might answer similar questions about the competencies—How important is it to me? How satisfied am I with the way the supervisor performs this skill? This could be a good beginning to the discussion of the supervisory process as described in an earlier chapter. From such scorings supervisor and/or supervisee can determine competencies on which the supervisee and the supervisor will work. From this point, they can operationalize behaviors that lead to the competencies, and set objectives and procedures for reaching them.

For example, the supervisor may score himself or herself high on the importance of competency 8.3—the ability to involve the supervisee in jointly establishing a conference agenda—but low on satisfaction with the way it is performed. This lack of satisfaction may be related to the fact that the supervisor is aware from the conferences themselves or on the basis of a videotape or an audiotape that the supervisee usually has few ideas about what she or he wants to discuss in the conference and, therefore, participates very little. The supervisor may further decide that it appears that the supervisee is not analyzing the clinical session adequately; thus she or he has nothing to bring into the planning conference. The supervisor may then decide on certain procedures—to demonstrate the analysis process for the supervisee in the next two conferences with data collected by the supervisee, to make specific assignments for observing certain behaviors in certain categories, or any of many other ways to teach the analysis process. Thus, the supervisor can set an objective and determine whether or not it was accomplished in the conference. Follow-up can be done by measuring the supervisees' subsequent analysis behavior in conferences and their ability to identify issues for the conference agenda. Further appropriate follow-through for total accountability would be to determine change or lack of change in the clinical process that relate to the supervisees' ability to analyze.

Other suggestions have been made for studying the process, an activity that is the first step to accountability. There must be a continuing search for ways to validate and improve the actions of supervisors. At this time, it appears that any attempt to improve accountability for supervisors will probably have to come from supervisors themselves, since neither the profession nor their administrators have appeared to be particularly concerned about the specifics of their activities. Who takes care of the caretakers?

Although this lack of concern about accountability for supervisors from others may be perceived as a negative state of affairs, it should not be. Rather, it should be seen as an opportunity for supervisors to develop their own quality assurance mechanisms rather than having accountability measures imposed upon them by those who have little understanding of the supervisory process. Such efforts may come from individual supervisors or from the combined efforts of supervisors. That is, in fact, how the list of tasks and competencies referred to so frequently here (ASHA, 1985b) came into being—through the efforts of the group. But individuals, too, can take advantage of the opportunity to develop procedures that will document their efforts to provide high quality supervision.

SUMMARY

Supervisors are involved in accountability procedures at various levels. They are responsible for ensuring that clients receive the best possible service; they are also responsible for growth and development of supervisees. Recent attention to accountability regarding clients and clinical work is useful to supervisors. They must, however, continue to seek better methods of accountability for themselves.

Supervision Across Settings

Clinical supervision is a necessary and desirable component in any truly comprehensive clinical service program.

Kleffner (1964, p. 20)

The focus in each of the chapters in this book may *appear* to have been on the supervision of students in the educational program. It is true that the bulk of the supervision in speech-language pathology and audiology probably takes place in college or university programs. Supervision has been assumed to be the very necessary and important process by which students are inducted into the profession. As Kleffner has stated, however, it is of no less significance in service-delivery settings, albeit apparently not as pervasive.

The continuum of supervision has been designed specifically to illustrate its appropriateness and applicability to all settings. The varying nature of the styles of supervision and the assertion that supervisees and supervisors move back and forth on the continuum, unrelated to amount of experience or setting, is basic to understanding the function of the supervisor and supervisee in the process at all levels and in all settings.

DEMOGRAPHICS ON SUPERVISORS ACROSS SETTINGS

Data on supervisors in educational programs, including school practicum and the Clinical Fellowship Year, have been presented earlier. Flower (1984) listed a myriad of other service models, ranging from high-risk infant programs to senior centers, where speech-language pathologists and audiologists may work. Very little is known, however, about the demographics of these settings, including how supervisors function if they are even employed.

NEED FOR SUPERVISORS

Although the profession has defined, through ASHA requirements, the need for supervision in educational programs, including off-campus practicum and the Clinical Fellowship Year, less interest has been documented about supervision in other settings. Kleffner (1964) maintained that no one is "so adept, so experienced, and so insightful" (p. 20) that he or she could not gain from supervision or clinical consultation. That is exactly the point made here in relation to the Self-Supervision Stage of the continuum and its accompanying Consultative Style. Despite the assumption that the attainment of the CCC indicates the ability to work independently and with a degree of professional autonomy in providing clinical services, in a profession changing as rapidly as speech-language pathology and audiology it is foolhardy to assume anything other than a continuing need for professional growth and development. Organizations should recognize this need and realize that the knowledge gained in educational programs is only the beginning of learning by professionals. The facilitation of such continued learning is an important part of the role of the supervisor.

Early citings of need for more supervisors than were currently available in off-campus practica, university clinics, and schools are found as long ago as the report of the national study of services in the public schools (Black et al., 1961; Irwin et al., 1961) conducted by ASHA. Later, the ASHA (1978a) report on the status of supervision documented the lack of school program supervisors who were prepared in speech-language pathology or audiology and the high probability that the ratio of supervisor to supervisee was inappropriately high. School program supervisors in Anderson's (1972) survey, for example, reported supervising from 1 to 138 supervisees. It is hoped that ratio has changed appreciably, but the writer has personal knowledge of school programs currently employing 50 or more clinicians with no supervisor with educational background in the profession.

Speech-language pathologists have generally supported the need for supervisors. In a study of attitudes of clinicians in the schools, it was reported that 70 percent of 291 clinicians in the schools agreed or strongly agreed that where several clinicians are employed, one should serve as supervisor (Anderson, 1974). Only three percent strongly disagreed with one clinician serving in that role and they were from programs employing only one or two clinicians. The dynamics of those answers are not difficult to discern!

A more recent survey of audiologists working in the schools provides other data about supervision (Wilson-Vlotman & Blair, 1986). Of 245 audiologists surveyed, 27 percent were never supervised, 9 percent met with their supervisors at least once a month, and 38 percent met annually with their supervisor. The report does not indicate the professional background of the supervisors, although it is stated that they were from a variety of backgrounds. Thus, it can be assumed that they included school administrators—possibly directors of special education; members of other helping professions such as school psychologists; or in some instances, speech-language pathologists. It is impossible to speculate about how many were supervised by other audiologists.

Interestingly and understandably, 59 percent of the audiologists saw little or no value in being supervised. Thirty-two percent stated that they would prefer to be supervised by another audiologist, and nearly a quarter of the respondents would prefer supervision from an educational professional. The reasons for that finding also offer significant opportunities for speculation. In terms of the Consultative Style defined earlier, it is interesting to note that nearly half of the educational audiologists indicated they used a peer support system for professional advice rather than going to their supervisor, and 21 percent indicated a need to move out of their district for consultation with peers. Wilson-Vlotman and Blair stated, "Basically, educational audiologists received very little supervision and, while this pleased many professionals because they were left with much control over their own jobs, it also appeared to be disconcerting to them not to receive any direction. Those who were supervised felt it was provided by individuals who did not have the type of information needed by audiologists working in schools" (p. 38).

The advantages of having supervisors in school programs has been discussed elsewhere. Anderson (1974) stated that "programs without appointed leaders trained in speech-language pathology and audiology may be characterized by lack of coordination, continuity, cohesiveness, professional growth, or program development" (p. 7). Speech-language pathologists or audiologists working in such settings do not have the same type of peer support that classroom teachers may have. Writers in the field of education (Blumberg, 1980; Cogan, 1973; Mosher & Purpel, 1972) discussed the role of the supervisor in alleviating the "loneliness" of the teacher. This is no less important for speech-language pathologists or audiologists, especially those who work alone. The stimulation of interacting with someone within one's own profession, if it is a positive interaction, is extremely important to many professionals and lends support for the employment of supervisors in such settings. The writer has personally witnessed the difference in morale, efficiency, and organization in programs with supervisors as opposed to those without supervisors.

A bulletin distributed through the ASHA UPDATE system (ASHA, 1985d) stated that over 1,000 ASHA members indicated at that time that their primary or secondary employment was administration or supervision in speech-language-hearing programs in the schools. Although this seems a small number, considering the large number of clinicians working in the schools, the report also states that there had been an increase of 300 over the previous five years. The report attributes this growth to the fact that educational agencies "have seen the benefits of having a categorically qualified professional responsible for the program" (p. 1).

The need for supervisors of the CFY and the difficulty encountered by some professionals in obtaining a supervisor for that experience have been documented by Ambroe (1974) and Schubert and Lyngby (1977). It apparently remains a problem in sparsely populated areas.

No data are available to determine the amount or type of supervision provided in other settings. It can be assumed that a variety of arrangements would be found—no one in charge, part-time supervision, full-time supervision, and supervision by someone from another profession. It can also be assumed that the same needs for support, organization, and cohesiveness exist.

No strong action as ever been taken by ASHA to encourage the employment of supervisors in the service delivery setting other than the requirements for

Professional Services Board certification. The status report on supervision (ASHA, 1978a), the program standards and guidelines for school programs (ASHA, 1973–1974), and the report of a Task Force on Supervision in the Schools (ASHA, 1972) all discuss the *need* for supervisors. Although it is granted that ASHA has little direct authority over employing institutions, anyone who has been in the profession for very many years is aware of the indirect influence of ASHA guidelines and standards on individual service delivery programs, on state certification and licensing requirements, and on other aspects of service delivery. Thus, it is frustrating to those interested in increasing the availability of supervision in various settings to speculate on how things might have been different if ASHA, from the very beginning, had made strong recommendations about the need for supervision after the educational program is completed, that is, in the service delivery setting. Perhaps a pattern could have been established which would have resulted in a different situation than now exists where there are still leaderless programs or programs supervised inadequately.

There is hope for the future, however, in the Position Statement on Clinical Supervision in Speech-Language Pathology and Audiology (ASHA, 1985b). The position statement, in addition to listing tasks and competencies for supervisors, makes a strong statement about the ongoing importance of supervision across both educational and service delivery programs. These needs are documented by requirements of the Council on Professional Standards through the standards and guidelines of the Educational Standards Board and the Professional Services Board. Further, the statement maintains, "State laws for licensing and school certification consistently include requirements for supervision of practicum experiences and initial work performance. In addition, other regulatory and accrediting bodies (e.g., Joint Commission on Accreditation of Hospitals, Commission on Accreditation of Rehabilitation Facilities) require a mechanism for ongoing supervision throughout professional careers" (p. 57).

A further document has been issued by ASHA relative to generic versus categorical supervision (1985d). It repeats the Professional Services Board statement that administrative, business, and financial aspects of programs can be assigned to individuals who are not qualified speech-language pathologists or audiologists, but that responsibility for clinical services must be given to qualified professionals. "Therefore, if staff are being supervised and evaluated on their ability to provide clinical speech-language pathology services, this supervision should be carried out by a qualified speech-language pathologist" (p. 1).

SUPERVISION IN THE SERVICE DELIVERY SETTING

Organizational requirements for supervisors or their tasks in service delivery settings are not well documented in the literature. What is found is related mainly to administration or program management. Participants in a conference on supervision in the schools (Anderson, 1970) defined their roles more in terms of programming than the clinical teaching role described later by the Committee on Supervision (ASHA, 1978a). A survey of 211 school program supervisors (Anderson, 1972) revealed that they were "engaged in a multitude of activities, most of them for small amounts of time. Few activities occupy over half the time of the respondents" (p. 20). For some, those activities were observation of clinicians and conferring with clinicians about the observations, but most of the many other activities in which they participated would have to be classified as program management responsibilities. It is probable that these administrative responsibilities occupy even more time now because of the requirements to implement Public Law 94-142. The paperwork and administrative responsibilities related to health programs have probably had the same impact on other types of service delivery programs.

Engnoth (1987), in a discussion of administration of programs in the schools, called the supervisory aspects of the administrator's job "the most important responsibility the administrator fulfills" (p. 77), but defined its two components as program management and clinical management. The latter contains three areas—implementation of the goals and objectives of the program in each school, observation and evaluation of personnel, and case consultation. The first two, she said, are shared with school administrators. She did not address the clinical teaching role *per se* other than to list the tasks of supervision adopted by ASHA (1985b).

In an extensive chapter on supervision in the schools, Fisher (1982) also emphasized the program management aspect of the role. He did deal with styles of leadership, effective communication, objectivity, motivation, flexibility, being considerate, leadership of developing professionals, and the evaluation process. The supervisor, he said, is a catalyst in "the process of generating and expanding new ideas, planning program changes, and implementing them effectively" (p. 176). Pendergast (1983), in discussing accountability or quality assurance in school programs, came somewhat closer to the clinical teaching role when she discussed in-service programs, the supervisor as a consultant to clinicians, observations, and "ways of furthering the knowledge and skills of the practicing communication disorder specialist in the schools" (p. 144).

Supervision was discussed by Griffith (1987) as one aspect of the director's job in a hospital program. She stated that "speech-language pathologists and audiologists are competent individuals who are usually self-starters; they usually require only general supervision and they function well independently. When new or unexpected situations arise, it is helpful if the director consults with the staff concerning the nature of the problem and the possible options for its solution. . . . The staff should have clear policies and detailed procedures to guide them and supervision that is readily available to support and assist them" (p. 106).

Supervision in the complex interaction of a military-based program was discussed by Sedge (1987) as a "three-tiered rating system" (p. 139), by which he appeared to mean evaluation of technical skills. This involved medical personnel, at least in relation to audiology.

Miringoff (1980), in a book on management of human services, approached the concept of the clinical teaching role of the supervisor when he discussed staff development to improve the organization's overall pattern of service. Ultimately, Miringoff asserted, program effectiveness evolves from what occurs between client and worker, and thus, individual staff members' performances are important. Azarnoff and Seliger (1982), in a similar book, have also provided information on professional development in the service delivery setting.

Supervision or Administration?

What can be assumed from these few examples in the literature that treat program management or clinical teaching in the service delivery setting? Are persons in charge of programs so involved in administrative tasks that they have no time for any form of clinical teaching, which the Committee on Supervision perceived as taking place in any setting? Reading between the lines of the writings quoted here, one can see that the Consultative Style is no doubt in frequent operation. But is it enough to assume, as Griffith (1987) seems to, that *all* employed professionals are operating at the Self-Supervision Stage?

Everyone is aware of the immense amount of administrative detail currently required in any organization. It cannot be denied or ignored if the program is to continue. Yet, some school program supervisors have indicated to the writer that, because of their lack of preparation for the clinical teaching role, they feel more secure in completing the program management tasks than in undertaking the face-to-face interaction required of the clinical teaching role. Such interaction may be particularly difficult with personnel who are not operating at the Self-Supervision Stage. Further, some supervisors still seem to persist in the stereotypic belief that they must provide the answers. If they realize they do not have them, they may avoid encounters that reveal that fact. Additionally, some supervisors may be threatened by supervisees who possess information they do not have; this may cause them to avoid face-to-face encounters.

The Continuum in the Service Delivery Setting

Recognizing the many problems that may be present for supervisors in service delivery programs, it is obvious that the continuum of supervision is as applicable there as it is in the educational program. It seems overoptimistic to assume that all professionals will have reached the same level of clinical ability by the time they enter the work force or that their continuing professional development will proceed at the same rate. All program supervisors know that there is great unevenness in their staff. Thus, any or all of the components of supervision discussed here are appropriate to all settings. Certainly, interaction between supervisor and supervisee will stand a better chance of being satisfactory if there is mutual understanding of each individual's perceptions of the role or expectations of the other, if activities are planned, and if the interaction is analyzed objectively. Additionally, all the dynamics of human interaction in the conference apply across settings.

Professional Development in the Service Delivery Setting

There are ways other than one-to-one interaction between supervisor and supervisee to promote professional growth and development. Some large school programs divide the school system into segments and have a staff member other than the supervisor serve as consultant to the clinicians in each area. Others use a modified "buddy system" to provide assistance to inexperienced clinicians. Some tap the special skills of experienced clinicians for workshops or other forms of continuing or in-service education. Pendergast (1983) suggested observation of other clinicians who are experts in a certain area, peer interaction without the presence of the supervisor, viewing of videotape demonstrations, as well as "close observation" of new staff by the supervisor. The service delivery setting is rich in opportunities for professional growth and development, both within the department and outside. Supervisors can assist in formalizing such opportunities or can encourage clinicians to interact with other professionals. For example, the writer recalls interacting with social workers as a young clinician and learning more about working with parents than through any formal education or reading ever done.

All of these forms of professional development, however, do not negate the responsibility of the supervisor for the one-to-one interaction with the supervisee. This is the essence of accountability, and ultimately, it will be the supervisor who is accountable for the work done by the clinician. Perhaps one of the most important skills for the supervisor to develop is the diagnostic process for supervisees discussed under Planning. As Hersey and Blanchard (1982) emphasized, change must begin with the identification of a problem and all of the variables in the involved individuals and the environment. Problems cannot be solved until they are identified and analyzed. The utilization of the continuum of supervision is essential to this process.

The works of Cogan (1973), Goldhammer and colleagues (1980), and Acheson and Gall (1980) are useful reading for a program supervisor. Although written originally for the supervision of teachers, much of the information is applicable to any work setting. Certainly, the general attitude of colleagueship and objectivity that they emphasize are as important in one setting as another. An example of a method for utilizing the clinical supervision approach in a school system by Tanck (1980) is of interest and could be applied in speech-language pathology and audiology programs in any setting. The plan was implemented by supervisors and supervisees in a school district who worked as a group to develop a cooperative approach to the improvement of instruction. The group selected nine teaching techniques considered to be applicable in all teaching situations, for example, introducing a lesson, providing feedback, teaching to an objective, giving directions. Each of these techniques was operationalized by the listing of specific behaviors deemed to contribute to the effective accomplishment of the technique. Thus, criteria were established for self-evaluation by the supervisee as well as feedback from the supervisor, leading ultimately to the formal evaluation into which each provided input. Based on Cogan's cycles, the supervisory process was then divided into the preobservation conference, preparation for observation, observation, postobservation analysis, postobservation conference, and postconference analysis. The selected teaching techniques were the subject of observation, self-analysis by the teacher, and analysis by the supervisor. The nine techniques selected were observed first. Checklists for analysis were devised. Only after completion of joint analysis and the reaching of agreement on the level of competence of the supervisee, did the dyad go to other teaching techniques.

This plan has several advantages and would be easily adaptable in any setting. It is probably used informally or unknowingly in some form by supervisors who have already identified for themselves the most important techniques, and therefore, concentrate on those in their own observation. The Mawdsley (1985) system of data collection and analysis is somewhat similar to this approach. One advantage of the plan is that supervisees know what is expected of them and what will be observed, and they are involved in its analysis. There is less uncertainty and probably less anxiety about supervision under such a procedure. The most important characteristic of this system is that the focus is on the improvement of instruction through objective observation and joint analysis, not just evaluation from the supervisor.

Other chapters have included material directed toward the supervisor in the service delivery setting. The joint goal-setting procedures described in the Planning component are important in professional development in these sites as are other aspects of the continuum.

SUPERVISION OF THE OFF-CAMPUS PRACTICUM

The off-campus practicum experience varies greatly across educational programs. It may begin early in the student's preparation or be reserved for an "externship" experience late in the program. It may consist of a few hours per week or an intensive full-time affiliation over an academic term. The assignment may be geographically close to campus or at such a distance that the only contact is by letter or telephone. Some programs maintain a minimal on-campus clinic and depend primarily on off-campus clinical programs and their employees for their practicum assignments.

Only the school practicum has received much attention in the literature (Anderson, 1973a; Baldes et al., 1977; Flower, 1969; Larson & Smith, 1976; Monnin & Peters, 1977, 1981; O'Toole, 1973; Rees & Smith 1967, 1968). Many of the suggested guidelines and recommendations made for the schools are equally relevant to practica in other sites.

Issues in the Off-Campus Practicum

Particular issues exist in varying degrees in off-campus practicum assignments which require continuing communication between on-campus and off-campus personnel. University supervisors who are responsible for liaison between the two settings are key figures in this communication. They may serve one or a combination of several functions: (1) They may serve only as liaison for administrative purposes such as assignment of students or processing of paperwork required by the university or the practicum site. (2) They may serve in a consultant role to the off-campus supervisor, providing guidance, formal or informal teaching about the supervisory process, or consultation in relation to the work of the student supervisee. (3) They may monitor the off-campus supervisor's activities, in effect "supervising the supervisor." (4) They may directly supervise the student supervisee in places where the two sites are close enough to make this possible.

Whatever the type of assignment or the structure of supervisors' roles, there will be a variety of issues that both the university supervisor and the off-campus supervisor must face. Among the more common are (1) selection of appropriate sites and supervisors, (2) maintaining accountability while balancing supervisee and client needs, (3) unrealistic expectations for students' knowledge and skill level by the off-campus supervisor, (4) students who are inadequately prepared for the experiences they will have in the service delivery setting, (5) lack of communication between the university and the off-campus site, (6) lack of definition of roles of all participants, (7) lack of assumption of responsibility for supervision by the off-campus supervisor (perceiving the student as a helper or not engaging in supervisory activities), (8) grading and evaluation, (9) loss of autonomy by the off-campus supervisor because of the university supervisor's close or direct supervision. A few of these will be discussed in greater detail.

Selection of Site Supervisors

The selection of off-campus supervisors is an important and sometimes difficult process. Criteria are sometimes vague or nonexistent, and are usually subjective. Selection is often based on geographical location or client population as much as on the known qualifications of the supervisor. Some programs report that supervisors of the school practicum are identified and supervised by representatives of the education department of the university, rather than by the speech-language pathology and audiology department. Sometimes sites have a limited variety of experiences, or supervisors are unable, because of their heavy workloads or administrative inflexibility, to schedule adequate conference time with the supervisee.

It is helpful if the university program can set criteria for site selection. Certain requirements can be stated, especially for conference time. Organizations willing to accept the responsibility of sharing in the preparation of professionals must be willing to provide adequate time and experience. If they cannot, this should be made clear to the university and students should not be assigned to such sites. Formal agreements or contracts that specify content and procedures for the assignment may be necessary in some instances. Again, communication is essential.

Balancing Supervisee and Client Needs

The issue of balancing the needs of student supervisees and clients has been discussed earlier. It is, perhaps, a greater problem for the inexperienced supervisor than the experienced, but it must be considered by all involved in the practicum. It was suggested that much of the confusion that exists over this issue could be alleviated during the Planning component of the supervisory process. It is also an important part of the Understanding component, since it is often related to a lack of understanding of supervisee needs and communication about them.

Unrealistic Expectations by Site Supervisors

Unrealistic expectations by site supervisors about the knowledge and skill level of the student supervisee often creates dissatisfaction. This may be related to their inexperience in supervision of practicum students, inflexibility, lack of knowledge about the supervisee's place on the continuum or how to determine it, or lack of information from the university about the student. University supervisors may find themselves serving as mediators in such situations. Supervisors must accept the fact that the student is still completing his or her education, and not expect a "finished" professional. Here, an understanding of the continuum and the student's place on it are of utmost importance.

Students Who Lack Adequate Preparation

The dissatisfaction of supervisors with the level of the students who come to them may be justified. Universities have a responsibility to monitor carefully the ability of the students who enroll in an off-campus practicum. It is unfair to off-campus supervisors to expect them to assume responsibility for developing skills that should have been attained during the on-campus experience.

Definition of Roles of Supervisors

Some speech-language pathology and audiology departments, for reasons of budget, distance, or time, cannot provide adequate, or possibly any, supervision from the university. Others provide so much that the on-site supervisor loses a sense of autonomy. An understanding must be established of the differentiation in roles. This becomes particularly important in terms of grading and evaluation procedures.

Payment for Off-Campus Supervision

Recently, an issue has been raised which is not new, but which has not previously been so thoroughly discussed in a publication—the issue of payment to the off-campus site for the supervision of the experience. Generally viewed as a voluntary contribution to the profession, some service delivery sites now are beginning to consider the economic factors involved in the time spent in supervising students from the university and are requesting at least partial reimbursement. Thoroughly discussed in a provocative dialogue between university and off-campus supervisors (Ehrlich, Merten, Sweetman, & Arnold 1983), this issue will probably be raised more frequently in the future. Some supervisors of school practicum are now paid, usually only a token sum, from fees paid by the student for this experience. Some universities reimburse the school system, not the supervisor. Some provide benefits such as course credits or in-service training to off-campus supervisors. Plans in operation in two different states are described by Willbrand and Tibbits (1976), where the university training program offers clinical services to clients from the case load of a school clinician in return for supervision of a student from the university. This service might be in the form of assessment, treatment, or faculty consultation. Among advantages listed is the releasing of time within the school system for supervision of students and clinicians.

Supervision by the Off-Campus Supervisor

A continuing source of concern in relation to the off-campus experience is the type and amount of supervision provided by the off-campus supervisor. Often, supervisors are reluctant to turn over their clients to students they perceive as novices. Sometimes they fail to recognize that some students have advanced along the continuum and have been working fairly independently in the clinical program. Despite this, supervisors are unable or unwilling to refrain from more direct, close supervision than the students need. Ehrlich and colleagues (1983) presented both sides of this issue. The university viewpoint is that students have been closely supervised at the beginning of their training, but as they have progressed toward the point of the off-campus assignment, they "have been withdrawn from extensive observation and supervision before beginning an externship" (p. 27). Further, although students may not be familiar with procedures specific to every site, they are capable of delivering services or they would not be assigned to the externship. Nevertheless, because the site supervisor is ultimately responsible for the quality of the service to clients, they can be expected to provide close observation and supervision of the students at first, but should withdraw it as soon as possible. Unless they do, the university supervisors imply, students may still need intensive supervision at the end of the externship and will remain dependent on their supervisors.

The viewpoint of the externship supervisors is very different. They maintain that the demands for supervision in the professional clinic are greater than in the university clinic because the clients are usually paying for the service they receive. (The authors did not discuss the fact that clients also pay in many university-sponsored clinics.) "In our opinion," they said, "professional quality simply is not possible in a graduate student extern no matter how bright or well trained he or she is because experience is too limited at that stage of career development" (p. 26). Patient care must be the first priority and mistakes must be avoided. (This argument is, of course, based on the assumption that supervisors never make mistakes.)

Resolving the Issues

There is no easy resolution to these issues, but some comments are relevant. University personnel could ask themselves if they are providing enough information to the off-campus supervisors about the students' strengths and capabilities. Herein lies another problem. Some off-campus supervisors indicate they do not want to know about the supervisees before the practicum begins, for fear of biasing. Perhaps this is because the tendency is to communicate weaknesses, not strengths. University personnel must also ask themselves if their students really *are* adequately prepared for the demands of the site. University supervisors have not had experiences in all types of settings and they may not be as aware of the needs in certain settings or with certain types of cases as they should be. Further, they must ask themselves how far along the continuum the students really have progressed. Have they really reached a point where they can operate independently enough that they do not require an excessive amount of attention from the off-campus supervisor? There is great opportunity for a self-fulfilling prophecy here—supervisors want to believe that their supervisees have reached the highest level of competency. To admit that students have not achieved this is, to some supervisors, an admission of their own failure.

Educational program supervisors should not expect off-campus supervisors to do the parts of the preparation of professionals that are really the responsibility of the university. The off-campus experience should provide students with opportunities to apply their knowledge in new situations and with new populations, to explore new methodologies and materials, and to experience the administrative aspects (recordkeeping, planning, etc.) that are different from those used in the university. But, off-campus supervisors should not have to teach basic knowledge or skills. In the opinion of the writer, the off-campus experience should be the "frosting" on the educational program and students should have a solid understanding of the clinical process and its application before they enter these sites. Others will support the importance of utilizing off-campus sites throughout the educational program. Whatever the system, university supervisors must be as responsible as possible in determining the readiness of students for the off-campus experience—another facet of their role as "gate-keeper," discussed under accountability.

Nevertheless, despite the most objective and thoughtful judgments made by supervisors, students have different degrees of success in coping with new situations. Student who have been operating in the clinic quite independently may be overwhelmed by group therapy in the off-campus site or the demands made upon them by the severely handicapped adult with an unfamiliar disorder. It must then be the responsibility of both the university supervisor of the practicum and the site supervisor to help the students resolve this situation. Mosher and Purpel (1972) discussed this as part of helping the student change from a person to a professional person—making adjustments in professional attitudes that also become very personal at times.

Once again, knowledge of the place on the continuum is necessary. Students' own knowledge of their place on the continuum, their professional objectives, and their ability and willingness to communicate these objectives to the off-campus supervisor will make the assignment more advantageous to them. If students are confident and have enough self-knowledge about their needs to share them with the supervisor, a more profitable interaction can begin immediately.

Role and Responsibility of University Supervisors

Perhaps one of the most difficult supervisory roles in the profession is that of university supervisors of the off-campus practicum, who have the responsibility for on-site observation of the student. In some senses, they are invading the site supervisor's territory when they visit. Unless the site is in close proximity to the university and their visits are frequent, they will not know the needs of the clients they are observing. Unless the student and on-site supervisor are skillful in preparing the university supervisors for the observation, it may not be meaningful. Their intermittent visits may make it impossible for them to make any judgment about the student's work, if they need to make an evaluation, or to determine the student's needs or progress. They must, then, depend upon input from the site supervisor.

More sensitive than this is the situation where university supervisors and on-site supervisors hold very different clinical philosophies, either of which may be right or wrong, but they *are* different. Supervisees may be caught in the middle of this controversy, feeling forced to do clinical work in some way other than the way they were taught. Although it is often an opportunity for them to learn another valid approach, it may also be an outdated or ineffectual methodology. The university supervisors become mediators or may need to help the supervisee recognize ways to manage professional disagreements. The university supervisors do not have the authority nor the responsibility necessary to request major changes in another facility's program. Such a situation underscores the importance of selecting off-campus supervisors who are both knowledgeable and flexible.

The on-site supervisors' methods of supervision may cause some concern. When supervisees perceive, accurately or inaccurately, that supervisors wish them to do clinical work in exactly the way they do it, there is much opportunity for modeling and less for creativity. On the other hand, supervisors may be anxious for supervisees to use their own ideas while the supervisees are happier to retreat into the safety of modeling behavior. University supervisors may have to mediate in this instance, also.

A very important role for university supervisors is to assist off-campus supervisors in developing their skills in the supervisory process. In this role, they can assist the supervisors in data collection methods, analysis as opposed to evaluation, understanding of the continuum, and all other supervisory skills. These skills, if accepted and used by off-campus supervisors, can then be generalized to other students.

University supervisors sometimes contribute to problems that may exist. They may not be objective. Their methods may also be outdated or inappropriate.

They may not be skillful communicators. They may have no preparation in supervision themselves, making it difficult for them to assist the off-campus supervisors in developing supervisory skills when it seems necessary. Sometimes they do not understand the dynamics of the service delivery site. They may not be aware of the needs of on-site supervisors or students. They may be as threatening to some supervisors, especially those who are new to the experience, as they are to some students. They may be perceived as based in an "ivory tower" where they know little of the "real world."

All interactions in off-campus situations take skill, patience, insight, and time. Where they cannot be resolved, it is the students who lose.

Advantages of the Off-Campus Experience

Despite the negatives listed here, the fact is that probably most off-campus practicum experiences are positive, successful experiences. They are often perceived by students to be the most important part of their total preparation. Students have the opportunity to integrate what they have learned. They have experience with variations across sites. They gain some sense of independence from the relative safety and familiarity of the educational program. Or—some may see it as release from the confines of the educational program structure!

One great advantage for students is the opportunity to work with other professionals who may not be so readily available in the campus clinic—social workers, principals, physical therapists, teachers, doctors, and many others. Interaction with other speech-language pathologists and audiologists is also a valuable experience. Depending upon the responsibility they are given by the supervisor, students often mature perceptibly during the practicum.

Experience in more than one setting, as required by ASHA, also has value. It may help the student decide on future career goals. The student who has always planned to work in a medical setting may learn that the schools are an exciting place, and vice versa.

The "bottom line" is that university programs are undeniably dependent upon their off-campus colleagues for a portion of the training of their students. Many clinics in educational programs do not have some of the types of clients seen in hospitals, rehabilitation centers, nursing homes, or in many schools since the advent of Public Law 94-142. Constant changes in delivery systems make it imperative for students to have as many experiences as possible. Universities will never be able to, nor should they attempt to, simulate all the organizational structures in which their students will seek employment. Thus, if students are to receive adequate training, there must be continued cooperation between the universities and service programs. It is to the advantage of future employers and clients that this bridging experience between education and employment be the most productive experience possible.

Recommendations for the Off-Campus Experience

■ The basic concept of the continuum of supervision must be continued into the off-campus site.

■ Supervisors in off-campus sites should receive preparation in the supervisory process. (Some states now require that student-teaching supervisors in the schools have continuing education in supervision before being assigned a student. This includes speech-language pathologists and audiologists. Although probably not possible as a requirement in all settings, such education should be made available on a voluntary basis.)

■ University supervisors of the off-campus practicum should be chosen with care for their own clinical and supervisory ability, ability to deal with other professionals, capability to assist others in developing their supervisory skills, and ability to provide feedback to the university program about the performance of students in off-campus assignments. These supervisors serve dual roles, becoming representatives of the university to the service sites, and also communicating the concerns of practicing clinicians and of students back to the program.

■ Some method should be devised to provide recognition to off-campus supervisors for the role they play in the total educational program. It is not clear that financial reimbursement would be the best reward—it is difficult to place a monetary value on such a valuable experience. Token payment may not really be rewarding. Perhaps other benefits would mean more to some supervisors than the small amount of payment that now seems possible—course credit, in-service credit, opportunity to participate in training program activities (such as lecturing to classes), and opportunity to provide feedback that might result in appropriate modification of training. These and other activities should be considered. This not so easy, however, with the current practice of some programs of sending their students to practicum sites far from the campus. Certainly, some ways are already in place and must be continued for such recognition.

■ Every program should have a manual, or at least a set of guidelines, for off-campus assignments. Expectations of the university should be clearly defined. These should include clear communication of the philosophy, goals, evaluation procedures, and the interaction the off-campus supervisor can expect with the university.

As with every situation discussed here, adequate communication is essential. Respect for the roles of the others involved in the experience and consideration of all variables is essential.

SUPERVISION OF THE CLINICAL FELLOWSHIP YEAR

The Clinical Fellowship Year (CFY) was developed out of the desire of the profession to provide an internship year similar to that of other professions. Discussion of this issue took place as early as 1964, when a conference was held to discuss the guidelines for an internship year (Kleffner, 1964). The experience has evolved over the years and current regulations for obtaining the Certificate of Clinical Competence (ASHA, 1985c) require one year of professional experience supervised by a person who holds the CCC. Specific requirements for the CFY have changed frequently over the years since it was initiated and changes are currently being proposed (ASHA, 1987). Therefore, these details will not be discussed at this point. The main thrust of this discussion will be the supervision of the experience.

The proceedings of the 1964 conference on the internship year devoted a great deal of attention to the supervision provided to the intern. The supervisor was said to be a key figure in the experience, which was seen as the "final proving ground for clinical competence" (p. 10). The conference participants made a strong recommendation for extending knowledge and skill in supervision and stated, "There is a clear need in speech pathology and audiology for training for supervisors" (Kleffner, 1964, p. 5).

Interestingly, since this was one of the first pleas for preparation of supervisors and for better quality of supervision, it has been a continuing issue in the implementation of the CFY. One of the needs identified by the ASHA Committee on Supervision (ASHA, 1978c) was to attend to several problems related to the supervision of the CFY—standards and guidelines for evaluation, role definition and guidance for supervisors, a method of monitoring the activities of CFY supervisors, more accountability, and a need for providing information about supervisory techniques.

At about the same time that the report of the Committee on Supervision was being prepared, the Committee on the CFY was developing an extensive report that included guidelines for model CFY programs in schools, hospital/community centers, and university/college clinics (ASHA, 1977). This report included suggested experiences, responsibilities of all parties, procedures, and evaluation instruments. Later, ASHA (1978c) stated that one of the principles underlying the requirement of the CFY was that "Academic training alone is not sufficient for preparation to function as an independent, competent, professional person. Therefore...the Clinical Fellowship Year, if properly planned and monitored, constitutes a useful and necessary transition from trainee status to status as a mature, professional person" (p. 333).

Schubert and Lyngby (1977) surveyed 228 individuals who had completed the CFY and found a wide range of supervisory procedures, ranging from direct observation and conferences to telephone and mail communication, to the use of audio- or videotapes. Over 50 percent of the respondents were supervised on-site less than one hour per week and less than a total of 10 times throughout the year. There was a wide range of reaction to the quality of the experience, but 67 percent indicated that the year of professional experience would have been just as beneficial without the required supervision. In 1986, respondents to an ASHA Omnibus Survey responded to the supervision of the CFY as follows: 24 percent strongly agreed and 33 percent mildly agreed that participants in the CFY needed more supervision (Hyman, 1986). Others responding to an ASHA

Omnibus Survey (Fein, 1983) have indicated that their supervision was sufficient and that the experience was valuable.

Crichton and Oratio (1984) surveyed 340 individuals who had completed the CFY to determine what variables were perceived as effective in its supervision. Their findings supported other research that indicated the importance of interpersonal skills. They also identified a factor labeled Supervisory Commitment. Behaviors that reflected this commitment were observation and evaluation of the clinical performance and the ability to confront the supervisee for inadequacies. Thus, they said, it is the combination of interpersonal skills and commitment that predict effectiveness in the supervision of the CFY.

ASHA requirements for the CFY have changed frequently over the years. Current requirements and procedures are found in the *Membership and Certification Handbook* (1985a). A proposal was made to the ASHA legislative council in November, 1986, to abolish the CFY (ASHA, 1987). Many of the reasons given in support of the proposal were related to supervision issues— difficulty of finding supervisors, inadequacy of the supervision provided, and lack of evidence of the value of the supervision. The proposal was referred to the Executive Board, and the Professional Standards Board of ASHA will make the final decision about the continuation of the CFY.

As long as the CFY continues to be required, and regardless of regulations for its completion, the continuum should be the basis for determining the appropriate supervisory style. Presumably, the consultative style or the upper levels of the Collaborative Style will most frequently be the appropriate ones for use. Amount of supervision available will continue to be a problem where supervisor and supervisee are separated by distance. Organizations that provide a structure for the fellowship year must be willing to allow appropriate flexibility in staff time so that supervisors can be available to the fellow. Once again, all the supervisory principles and practices discussed here may be called upon in various situations.

SUPERVISION OF SUPPORTIVE PERSONNEL

Data are not available on the extent of involvement of speech-language pathologists and audiologists in the supervision of supportive personnel, also called aides or paraprofessionals. Their use has been discussed by Galloway and Blue (1975), Irwin (1967), Northern and Suter (1972), Scalero and Eskenozi (1976), Costello and Schoen (1977), and Hall and Knutson (1978). Two position statements have been issued by ASHA committees that recommend guidelines for the use and supervision of such personnel (ASHA, 1970; ASHA, 1981).

Because of the direct responsibility of the professionally qualified clinician and the supervisor for the clients' welfare, it is obvious that the speech-language pathologist or audiologist and the paraprofessional will usually be working at the Evaluation-Feedback Stage of the continuum of supervision. The qualified professional will be responsible for the training of paraprofessionals and the monitoring of their work. Depending upon the task and the paraprofessional's skill, experience, or educational background in the profession, the two might move to some point on the continuum in the Transitional Stage. At no time, however, would the paraprofessional work independently at the Self-Supervision Stage.

Again, a clear understanding of the continuum would be useful to paraprofessionals and to supervisors, especially if questions of authority and responsibility should arise. It is through the supervisory process that professionals maintain their accountability for the welfare of the client when aides are involved.

SUMMARY

Organizational structure, levels of supervisees, goals of the organization, objectives of the program, and other variables may create differences in procedures across settings, but do not negate the need for clinical teaching nor the fact that the principles remain the same. Supervisors and supervisees may have changing needs and their procedures may change as they progress along the continuum, but the basic objective of professional growth and development for both remains at the core of the supervisory process.

Toward Practical Research in Supervision

By Christine Strike and Ronald Gillam

It should not surprise the reader at this point to find a chapter devoted to researching supervision in a book that is primarily concerned with doing supervision. The point has been made repeatedly that there is great need for research in the supervisory process and that the most important questions come out of the actual performance of the process. Thus, it is the intersection of doing and researching that is the heart of practical research. Researching supervision is a relatively new task for speech-language pathologists and audiologists and one about which there is much to learn. Few articles dealing with supervision research have been published in speech-language-hearing journals. As has been pointed out in previous chapters, much of the research that has been done in supervision has been descriptive, based either on questionnaire responses or on conference observation. Many of the conference observation studies have been doctoral dissertation research projects.

Without question, descriptive research projects have contributed important information about the supervision process, which has advanced an initial understanding of supervision in speech-language pathology. Descriptive studies reveal something about the nature of "typical" conferences. However, descriptions of what a "typical" supervisor does in a "typical" conference are not necessarily informative to the supervisor working with the variety of supervisory needs of individual students. To be "practical," research results must be useful for supervisors who want to know what they can do to improve the interaction between themselves and their individual supervisees.

The most practical supervision research deals with questions about supervisory procedures. Practical questions concern such matters as the relationships between particular supervision procedures and various clinician variables such as clinical experience, effect, motivation, and personality; or strategies for solving various difficulties inherent in the supervisory process.

Questions that grow out of daily supervisory interactions have the greatest potential for being interesting and informative to supervisors. Furthermore, studies with a foundation in actual supervisory experience are necessary to answer the nagging questions of what makes a difference in supervision—What is effective supervision? What should supervisors be prepared to do? What changes do supervisees make as a result of their supervisory experiences? The most ecologically valid answers to these and many other "practical" questions will come from the analysis of data gathered within natural supervision settings, those that include actual interactions between supervisors and their supervisees. Thus, in order for supervisory research to proliferate, it will need to be carried out by supervisors studying routine supervisory situations. If such research is to be generated, supervisors will need to become more actively involved in the research process. This is not easily accomplished, due to some very basic roadblocks that seem inherent in the job situations of most clinical supervisors. Time and knowledge of research principles are the two most frequent factors that interfere with ongoing supervision research.

Supervisors may believe that research lies outside of their realm—that research can only be done by academics who have specific education in research methods and the time to devote to the endeavor. Therein lies much of the problem. It is an unfortunate fact that the people best trained to do research are not familiar with supervisory issues. Similarly, supervisors who know what the most relevant questions are and who have daily opportunities to gather data in natural supervisory settings are not usually experienced researchers. Dealing with this dilemma is critical. One possible solution is joint study between supervisors and researchers. In this case, each professional contributes his or her expertise to developing the research questions and methodology for answering the questions.

Another solution to the dilemma is to train supervisors to be researchers. There is no question that the profession of speech-language pathology and audiology needs more supervisors with extensive research training. But there are currently so few that it is impractical and unrealistic to wait for these professionals to generate all the research that is needed.

ACCOUNTABILITY

Aside from the issue of who shall/can do research, it is necessary to clarify the rationale for doing research. This is because relevant research questions will reflect the purpose of the research. A primary reason for studying supervision is accountability. Preparing competent speech-language pathologists and audiologists is important for the profession and its consumers. As a large element in that preparation, supervision of clinical practice deserves the scrutiny that clinical issues have received. For years, the profession has invested time and money in studying the nature of various speech, language, and hearing disorders, less time and money studying the treatment of people evidencing these disorders, and even less time and money studying the preparation of those who conduct that treatment. Although it has been recognized that supervision exists as an essential component in the preparation of speech-language pathologists and audiologists, the assumption has been that supervision was overseeing the student clinician and that effective clinicians could automatically fill the role of effective supervisors. This orientation has grown out of the "student apprentice" approach, which was the initial form of supervision in speech-language pathology and audiology.

As such, supervisees have largely been supervised from an intuitive position rather than a scientific one. From the scientific perspective, careful study of the supervisory process is essential for developing supervision theories. For educational or service delivery programs to be maximally effective, supervisors need to operate from supervision theories that lead to effective and efficient supervisory methods. The development of such theories and their associated practices requires that supervision has a scientific rather than an intuitive basis.

Levels of Accountability

When supervisors become researchers, they contribute both to the main body of professional literature in speech-language pathology and audiology and to their own understanding of supervision. These contributions correspond to two levels of accountability: (1) accountability for the supervision collective within the speech-language pathology and audiology community, and (2) accountability for the individual supervisor within the work setting. From this perspective, the ordinary business of daily supervision begins to be seen as having real value for the supervisee, the supervisor, and the profession at large. Since every supervisory session involves a large number of decisions about what to do with the supervisee and how to do it, effective supervision demands that the supervisor be concerned with the rationale and method of the task. In this sense, each supervisory session should be for the supervisor an inquiry, a further analysis of process, an active form of personal research. Underlying a scientific approach to supervision is the assumption that the ordinary mode of operation is significant, and therefore, worthy of experimental inquiry.

A primary goal of this chapter is to present an overview of three practical research designs that may be used to study questions generated by supervisors in ongoing supervisory situations. Some of the major problems involved in studying supervision will be discussed with examples of how to solve these problems through description of actual and hypothetical studies. (Examples to be given will be from educational settings, but the principles are the same across settings and could be utilized by any supervisor/supervisee dyad.)

RESEARCHING THE SUPERVISION PROCESS

In order to formulate and subsequently answer questions about effectiveness/efficiency issues in supervision, it is necessary to know about the supervisory process. The preceding chapters in this book described a model of supervision and provided a good information base for developing practical research questions. For example, from past research it is known that the supervisor typically talks more than the supervisee during supervisory interactions. However, it is not known whether this has any impact on the supervisee's learning and subsequent clinical performance. The Clinical Supervision model would predict that directive behavior such as telling a supervisee what to do gets more immediate, yet less long-term, results. But, a line of research is needed to determine how the nature of supervisory feedback (directness in this instance) influences the clinical performance of supervisees.

As has been noted in previous chapters, ASHA's Committee on Supervision presented a Position Statement regarding tasks and competencies of supervisors (ASHA, 1985b), which was accepted by the Legislative Council. The Legislative Council's acceptance of this document effectively mandated that the competencies be validated. In order for this to occur, these competencies must be operationalized and measured across various supervisory contexts. Operationalizing and measuring the competencies captures the essence of this chapter—practical research in supervision.

Much of the information presented in this chapter will be familiar to speech-language pathologists and audiologists, since basic research design and statistics are requirements of educational programs. However, the focus on application of research principles to the study of supervision will be less familiar.

Traditional experimental design is one method that can be used. However, assuming a research attitude toward supervision does not necessitate that the supervisor must function only within traditional experimental designs when conducting research. Rather, the research attitude is one of curiosity, of careful planning, of documentation, and of critical analysis. Two additional designs, single-subject and ethnography, are less frequent in the literature, but may better serve the research efforts of the working supervisor/researcher.

TRADITIONAL EXPERIMENTAL RESEARCH

Experimental research is best characterized as the precise analysis of the effects of a treatment on a specific behavior. This is accomplished by presenting a treatment within a specific context and then measuring how a related behavior changes. The behavior that the experimenter controls is typically referred to as the *independent variable*. The behavior that the experimenter measures is referred to as the *dependent variable*.

Brasseur and Anderson (1983), for example, wanted to know whether supervisors and supervisees rated direct, indirect, and direct/indirect conference behaviors differently. These investigators showed their subjects 20-minute videotapes of supervisory conferences. One of the videotaped conferences contained 80 percent direct supervisory behaviors, one contained 80 percent indirect supervisory behaviors, and the third contained 50 percent direct and 50 percent indirect supervisory behaviors. In this study, supervisor directness during conferences was the independent variable. The dependent variable was the ability to rate the directness/indirectness of supervisory conference behaviors. This ability was measured by having supervisors and supervisees complete an 18-item rating scale after viewing one of the taped conferences.

In experimental research, the experimenter first states a specific hypothesis (educated guess) about his or her prediction of how certain people (a population) will respond to the experimental tasks. The population of interest could be college-educated adults, learning-disabled adolescents, school-age stutterers, or, as in the example here, student clinicians and university supervisors. Since it would be unreasonable to try to test all the members of a specific population (e.g., all student clinicians or all supervisors), the researcher attempts to draw a *sample* (a small number of members who are believed to be representative of the entire group) from the population to provide the best possible estimate of how this population would respond to the experimental tasks (independent variable).

Once the sample has been selected, participants in the research (subjects) are grouped together and treated according to a preestablished design. Different groups usually receive different treatments. However, all subjects within each group receive the same treatment, which is delivered in a systematic way. For example, Shapiro (1985) was interested in measuring the follow-through behaviors of supervisees with respect to the commitments and assignments made during their supervisory conferences. He distributed the 32 beginning and 32 experienced student clinicians in his study into two groups. The first group received supervision under each of two conditions: (1) three weeks of supervision under one condition in which only the supervisor kept track of the commitments and assignments made during supervisory sessions, and (2) three weeks of supervision under another condition in which the supervisor and supervisee together documented, in writing, the commitments and assignments they had made during each supervisory session. Shapiro then reversed the order in which the conditions were presented for the second group.

In experimental research, the measured behavior (the dependent variable) is observed before and after the treatment and a statistical test is used to determine if there are significant (probability that is greater than chance) differences between the performance of the groups. Based upon the results, the researcher is able to support or refute the original hypothesis. The design of the Shapiro (1985) study allowed him to analyze the cause and effect relationships between the completion of the commitments that were made and the treatment condition, the order in which the treatments were presented, the experience level of the supervisee, and the type of commitment. Among many other significant results, Shapiro found that experienced clinicians completed more commitments in the not-written agreement condition, whereas beginning clinicians completed more commitments when written agreement was required. He interpreted this finding as suggesting that experienced clinicians had more confidence in their own ability and were more flexible in changing their clinical behaviors, whereas beginning clinicians, with less background knowledge and experience, needed greater structure in their supervisory conferences.

The quality of an experiment is concerned with its validity, reliability, and generality. *Validity* concerns the difference that the treatment made on the dependent variable. For an experiment to be valid, the researcher must demonstrate that observed changes in the dependent variable were caused by the treatment and not from lack of control of other interfering variables (Campbell & Stanley, 1963; Ventry & Schiavetti, 1980). *Reliability* concerns the stability, consistency, and reproducibility of the research (Huck, Cormier, & Bounds, 1974; Thorndike, 1982). Reliability means that the reported research results would be the same if the experiment was repeated. *Generality* (most often referred to as external validity) refers to the extent that the experimental results apply to nontested populations, settings, or treatments. Generality means that research findings will be applicable for conditions and participants that are not identical to those in the experiment.

Lack of validity, reliability, and generality pose serious threats to the value of a research project. Results that cannot be replicated, or results that cannot be applied to anyone other than the subjects in a particular experiment, are of questionable value to practicing supervisors. Researchers address such threats by careful attention to experimental control.

Control

Traditional experimental research requires that the researcher manipulate and observe an individual subject's behavior in a precise and reliable fashion. Experimental control concerns the extent to which the researcher is able to eliminate all explanations other than the independent (treatment) variable as causing change in the dependent (measured) variable. For example, a supervisor/researcher might be interested in the effect that clinician data-keeping has on the number of neutral/social comments made by the clinician during a clinical session. An experiment may be designed to demonstrate that having the clinician keep data on the types of utterances produced within the sessions (the independent variable) causes a decrease in the number of neutral/social comments that are made in each session (the dependent variable). But how can the researcher be certain that it was the data-keeping that caused the reduction in neutral/social utterances and not something else? Ensuring such experimental control is primarily achieved through the design of the research.

True experimental designs have built-in controls for threats to the validity of an experiment (Campbell & Stanley, 1963; Huck et al., 1974). The simplest "true" experimental design is the two-group pretest-posttest design. This design usually employs a control group that does not receive treatment. However, it would be a violation of ASHA standards, as well as unethical, for a supervisor/researcher to withhold supervision from a group of student clinicians. Therefore, a variation of this design which employs two treatment groups is more suited to supervision research.

Returning to the question about the effects of clinician data-keeping on neutral/social comments posed earlier, a hypothetical example will illustrate the principles of this design. Ten clinicians might randomly be assigned to a data-keeping supervision group and 10 other clinicians to a traditional (control) supervision group. The subjects in the data-keeping group would be asked to analyze audiotapes of each of their clinical sessions for the number of neutral/social comments they made. The clinical supervisors working with clinicians in the control group would be told to help students decrease neutral-social comments as they supervise in their usual manner. The experimenter would need to be sure that the supervisors in this group were not asking supervisees to collect data. The subjects and supervisors in both groups would be blind to the specific objectives of the study. That is, they would know that they were participating in a research project but would not know the precise nature of the research. Both groups would be measured on the number of neutral/social comments they used per session at the beginning of the semester, and again after 10 weeks of supervision. If, at the end of the 10 weeks of treatment, the average number of neutral/social comments per session of the data-keeping group was significantly lower than that of the traditional supervision group, it could be reasonably claimed that the clinician data-keeping treatment was responsible for the decreases in neutral/social comments observed for the experimental group.

Remember, however, in order to interpret the results with confidence, it is necessary to control several variables. For instance, in the hypothetical example, the subjects were randomly assigned to groups and were blind to the research objectives. Since research in supervision is young, variables that may influence results are not well known. Still, it is important to examine the literature and try to account for as many variables as possible.

As has been shown, experimental research essentially involves comparisons of groups or individuals. Subjects are independently treated and individual scores are assembled together to form like groups, which are compared with each other to demonstrate controlled effects. Experimental research is, at best, difficult to apply to supervision issues. One of the primary reasons for this is theoretical. The clinical supervision model advocated in this book is *nonlineal*, since it proposes that the supervisory relationship is triadic. That is, supervision involves the supervisor-supervisee relationship, the clinician-client relationship, and the supervisor-client relationship. These relationships are held in synergistic balance as transacting entities within networks of interpersonal exchanges. Keeney (1983) referred to such interrelationships as "recursive" connections. The assumption is that the client's actions have implications for the supervisor-supervisee relationship, the supervisor's actions both result from and create changes in the clinician-client relationship, and the clinician's actions have cause-and-effect relationships with both client and supervisor actions. It is the goal of practical research to determine the specifics of these interactions and the impact on behaviors. Even multivariate (use of more than one dependent variable) designs are linear since they operate on the assumption of independence. That is, it is assumed that the multiple dependent variables that are compared are not interrelated. However, it is not known that the variables of interest in supervisory interactions are not related, and in fact, there is reason to believe that many variables are intimately related. The researcher interested in examining the multiple relationships that exist within the supervisory context is simply not able to do so within the rigorous experimental research paradigm.

Other difficulties supervisors might have with using traditional experimental design for supervision research are primarily pragmatic. First, experimental designs demand larger numbers of subjects. A rule of thumb for experimental research is that to be representative, a group should not be composed of less than 10 members. Since all experimental designs employ at least two groups, the supervisor must be able to assemble at least 20 supervisee participants. Additionally, the researcher organizing a two-group study may need to coordinate these subjects' supervisory experiences across multiple supervisors. This is an extremely important consideration for the full-time supervisor interested in conducting research. Unless the experiment is to be a collaborative effort among a number of supervisors, the task of assembling 20 or more clinicians and coordinating their supervision can be monumental.

Even if the research project is a collaborative effort between two or more supervisors, there are additional problems inherent in experimental research in supervision. The supervisor/researcher must ensure that supervisory procedures are identical across supervisors within each treatment condition. In the two-group pretest-posttest design discussed previously, the researcher would have to demonstrate that all supervisors in the data-keeping treatment condition were following the same supervisory procedures. The same difficulty applies to the supervisors in the traditional treatment condition. If four separate supervisors were assigned to clinician-subjects in the traditional treatment condition, and all were using somewhat different supervisory procedures, an important element of experimental control would be lost.

Another difficulty with control in experimental treatment studies involves the number of clients and supervisors the subjects may have. Ideally, each clinician/subject should have one client and one supervisor. If the subjects have more than one client at the time they are participating in a study, they should be supervised by only one supervisor and should conference with that supervisor about all of their clients at the same time. In the event that two supervisors are supervising a given subject at the same time, the researcher must ensure that (1) both supervisors are using the same supervisory procedures, and (2) that every other subject in the study is being supervised by more than one supervisor as well. Why is this important? Consider the case in which clinician/subjects are being supervised by one supervisor who is participating in the study and another supervisor who is not. If significant results obtain under these conditions, the researcher cannot be certain that the change in the supervisees' behavior was caused by the experimental treatment, by the supervision received from the supervisor not involved in the study, or by a combination of both.

There are numerous other variables that could interfere with validity, reliability, and generality and that should be controlled in experimental studies in supervision. These variables include supervisor experience, the supervisee's clinical and supervisory experience, the type of client the participants are working with, the length of the conferences and the topics discussed, and the number of conferences. At this point in the development of research in supervision in speech-language pathology and audiology, little is known about the influence of these variables on clinician and client behavior. As such, they must be controlled.

Additionally, supervisor/researchers working within experimental paradigms are going to have to deal with such potential problems as semester time-lines, canceled clinical and supervisory sessions, client progress, and supervisee commitment. The point is not that these problems are limited to experimental research; they are not. But, the inflexibility of experimental design together with the large number of subjects that experimental research requires make traditional experimental research extremely difficult (if not impossible) for the working supervisor/researcher to manage.

This is not to say that experimental research is unnecessary, for it most certainly is necessary. The point is that the multitude of problems posed by the prospect of using traditional experimental designs for supervisory research are disadvantageous to the supervisor who is thinking about beginning a research project. There are other research models that are less problematic but just as useful for answering the kinds of practical research questions that are being advocated in this chapter. Attention is now turned to the first of two of these models.

SINGLE-SUBJECT RESEARCH

A less rigid, and therefore more manageable, approach to research is the use of single-subject experimental research designs. These are also called time-series designs, within-subject designs, and single-case designs (Connell & Thompson, 1986; Kearns, 1986; McReynolds & Thompson, 1986; McReynolds & Kearns, 1983). Single-subject designs have appeared occasionally in the speech-language pathology and audiology literature, more frequently during the past few years.

McReynolds and Kearns (1983) pointed out that single-subject designs are well suited to the needs of the interventionist, since they are useful for exploring the effectiveness of treatments. In single-subject designs, the researcher specifies the problem and the intervention plan, measures the behavior(s) of interest repeatedly before intervention is begun, and continues repeated measurements during treatment. Experimental control is demonstrated when untreated behaviors are unvarying at the same time that treated behaviors are changing. The data are charted and visually inspected for evidence of meaningful change.

The major differences between single-subject and aggregate (group) experimental research are related to the collection and interpretation of data and the mechanisms for demonstration of experimental control. In group experimental research, data are collected only a few times, usually once before and once after intervention. The experimentalist assumes that the behavior patterns being studied are static enough so that if a sufficient number of subjects are included in the research, the range of behaviors common to the population of interest will be sampled. In single-subject research, data are collected frequently in regular intervals before, during, and sometimes after the intervention. The single-subject researcher does not assume behavior to be static, but rather considers behavior to be variable beyond that which can be experimentally controlled (Bloom & Fischer, 1982).

Ventry and Schiavetti (1980) characterized the experimental researcher as an active rather than passive investigator who controls and manipulates variables and who observes the effects of the manipulation on variables. As noted previously, the variable that the investigator manipulates is the independent variable. In supervision research, this might be contracting with the supervisee, training the supervisor, or meeting individually versus in a group. The variable that is observed and measured for change is the dependent variable. Examples in supervision research are supervisee implementation of a goal behavior in the clinical session, supervisor talk-time, and use of questions by the supervisor.

Dependent Measures

Choosing the Dependent Measure

Data from single-subject studies are typically evaluated through visual inspection of charted (graphed) data points. Direct measurements are taken of the target behavior (dependent variable). For example, assume that after listening to an audiotape of a clinical session, a supervisor and supervisee agree that the supervisee was giving far too many explanations of the therapy activity to the client. They might decide to collect data on this behavior and could do so in a number of different ways. The method and metric chosen for the dependent measure is very important and must be selected carefully. The dependent measure should reflect the research question and must be a valid and reliable account of the dependent variable.

The reliability of the dependent measures are extremely critical in single-subject research, since the credibility of the study rests, to a great extent, on the accuracy and reproducibility of the observer's measurements. Space constraints do not allow for adequate presentation of reliability considerations in this chapter, but issues pertinent to inter- and intrajudge reliability in single-subject research were discussed by McReynolds and Kearns (1983) and Bloom and Fischer (1982).

McReynolds and Kearns (1983) presented four types of measurement typically found in single-subject studies: frequency, rate of occurrence, duration of occurrence, and percentage.

FREQUENCY. In the previous example, simply counting the number of explanatory utterances given by the clinician during the session yields frequency data. This appears to be an acceptable measure of the dependent variable; however, several factors may affect the validity of frequency data. For example, if the clinical sessions varied in length, the frequency of explanations would be expected to vary also. Thus, an increase/decrease of number of explanations may reflect the length of the session rather than clinician variability. This would be true for most behaviors.

Also consider factors that relate to this specific dependent variable. Explanations usually occur at the beginning of an activity, and to a lesser extent, intermittently as clarification. The number of explanations during two 30-minute sessions might differ significantly if one session contained four activities and the other contained only two or three. Also, fewer explanatory remarks would be expected for activities that were familiar to the client. Thus, if the supervisor/researcher wanted to monitor the clinician's ability to give a greater number of explanations that were both more concise and appropriate for the client's linguistic level, it would be necessary to control for the length of the session, the number of activities, and the familiarity of the activities. This could be accomplished by requesting that the clinician maintain a consistent length of session and also regulating the number of new and familiar activities in each session.

RATE. If the frequency measurement total is divided by the number of minutes of the clinical session, rate of occurrence data are obtained. Rate of occurrence can also be computed by dividing the frequency data by the number of activities. The denominator in the rate computation is chosen based on what the researcher knows about the subject and about the research question being asked.

DURATION. Getting back to the example—perhaps a clinician tended to start each activity with long explanations that were composed of several sentences, but rarely gave explanatory comments for clarification. The amount of time during the session used to introduce therapy activities might be measured. The clinician's introductions could be timed with a stopwatch to get an estimate of the number of minutes during a session that were spent introducing an activity. This could also be converted to a "minutes per activity" rate by dividing the total duration by the number of activities.

If the clinician used many explanatory remarks in the introduction as well as throughout the session, the unit of interest might again be the duration of occurrence. This time duration might be determined by timing all the clinician's explanatory turns. This could be expressed as rate of duration by dividing the total explanation time by the length of the session or the number of activities.

PERCENTAGE. If, on the other hand, the clinician tended to give single-sentence explanations about the various procedures of an activity following every client utterance, a percentage-of-response measurement would be more practical and informative than a duration or frequency metric. This measurement could be obtained by dividing the number of explanatory utterances by the total number of utterances spoken by the clinician during the session. Charting this clinician's percentage of response data over the span of 10 clinical sessions would reveal something similar to Figure 15–1.

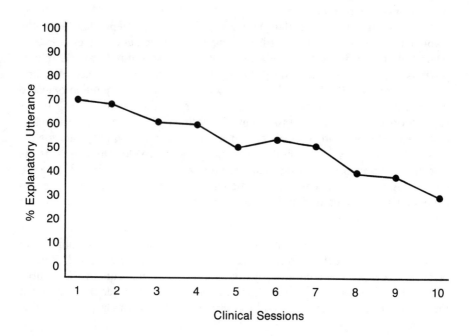

FIGURE 15-1. *RESULTS OF A HYPOTHETICAL STUDY DEMONSTRATING THE GENTLE DOWNWARD SLOPE OF A CLINICIAN'S EXPLANATORY UTTERANCES OVER 10 CLINICAL SESSIONS.*

Graphing the Dependent Measures

McReynolds and Kearns (1983) suggested three parameters of visual interpretation of charts or graphs. The term *trend* is used to refer to the direction of change as revealed by the graph. The hypothetical data in Figure 15–1 show a decreasing trend as the clinician/supervisee lowered the percentage of explanatory utterances across the 10 sessions. *Slope* refers to the degree of change and indicates how strong the trend is. Figure 15–1 presents a gentle slope, suggesting that the clinician gradually decreased the percentage of explanations. Finally, it is apparent that the clinician/supervisee began at a relatively high level and reached a relatively low level of percentage.

It was mentioned in the experimental design section that nuisance variables are controlled in experimental research mainly through the use of a control group that does not receive the independent variable. Control groups are not necessary in single-subject designs because each subject participates in no-treatment and treatment periods. Effectively, they act as their own controls during no-treatment periods.

Not all single-subject designs can be interpreted in terms of cause-effect relationships. Experimental control is best demonstrated through designated *experimental* single-subject designs (A-A-B, A-B-A-B) and multiple-baseline designs. Bloom & Fischer (1982) provided criteria for inferring causality in single-subject designs. Causal inferences may be made when the independent and dependent variables change together (covary) and other factors are equal. The seven criteria are that the (1) change in dependent variable occurs after the independent variable has been manipulated; (2) the observed change occurs in such a way that the two variables may be considered co-present; (3) absence of change is noted in the absence of this intervention; (4) there is repeated co-presence of intervention and subsequent change; (5) attempts are made to determine whether alternate explanations for the change exist; (6) the desired change is consistent over time; and (7) the relationship is theoretically and practically plausible.

Single-Subject Experimental Designs

A-B-A Design

In standard single-subject design, notation "A" refers to the no-treatment or baseline phase, and "B" refers to the treatment phase (Bloom & Fischer, 1982; Herson & Barlow, 1976; McReynolds & Kearns, 1983; Tawney & Gast, 1984). Using the previous hypothetical example, assume that the clinician/supervisee began collecting data after the topic of explanations was discussed in the first supervisory session. Subsequently, percentage data for explanations were charted for the first 10 weeks of the semester. In this instance, there would be B-only data, since no data were collected before the treatment was administered (i.e., before the supervisory session). Thus, there was no baseline period. A downward sloping (decreasing) line graph of the data would signify improvement, but there would be no way of knowing if this improvement was due in any way to the supervision. It is quite possible that the clinician would have lessened the percentage of explanations during the sessions independently of meeting with the supervisor. There also would be no knowledge of the consistency of explanatory comments before that first supervisory session.

A second hypothetical case will be used to explain the difference between the nonexperimental B-only design and the experimental A-B-A design. In this instance, assume that the supervisor met with the clinician before the semester began to discuss general supervisory procedures and client-related issues. As is the case in most college and university programs, this client had received services during the previous semester and end-of-the-semester data and recommendations were detailed in the client's chart. With this in mind, the clinician was advised to spend the majority of the time in the first three clinical sessions providing intervention based on the previous recommendations. The supervisor and supervisee agreed that they would not meet again until after the third session with the client. The three clinical sessions were audiotaped and the supervisor directly observed all or part of each one. This continued to be true for clinical sessions throughout the semester.

During the second supervisory conference (held after the third clinical session), the supervisor and clinician discussed the first three sessions and reached consensus on possible client and clinician objectives. Like the clinician in the previous example, this clinician also spent a great deal of session time giving explanations to the client about how to play the games provided as intervention contexts. Following the clinical supervisory model, the supervisor and supervisee did the following. First, they decided what an explanation was while listening to the tape together. Second, they decided what data to take and how to analyze those data. Third, they decided on a strategy for the supervisee to use in trying to reduce her abundant use of explanations. In this hypothetical instance, the supervisor and supervisee decided that any sentence that had as its topic the performance of the activity rather than the performance of the goal would be counted as an explanation. It was also decided that the supervisee would listen again to the first three tapes and would calculate the total number of explanations given in each session. A line graph of this frequency data might look like Figure 15–2.

The data in Figure 15–2 represent the A-phase (baseline data), since it was collected before supervisory intervention began. It is shown that the trend in the data was basically stable with a slight upward slope. One could argue that the clinician's use of between 72 and 78 explanations dealing with the procedures of the therapy activities during a 30-minute session represented a rather high level of occurrence. This clinician presents a stable baseline of the behavior of concern.

Knowing what the clinician routinely does and the frequency with which the behavior occurs does not in itself address the problem of how to bring about change. The supervisor and supervisee dyad developed a three-part strategy to try to decrease the number of explanations the clinician used in the session. First,

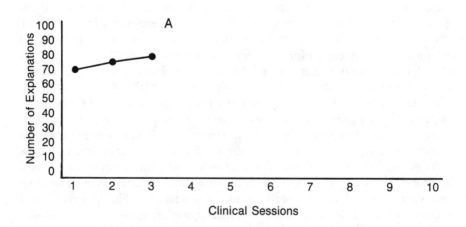

FIGURE 15–2. BASELINE (A-PHASE) POINTS REPRESENTING THE FREQUENCY OF A CLINICIAN'S EXPLANATORY UTTERANCES DURING THREE CLINICAL SESSIONS BEFORE INTERVENTION (I.E., BEFORE SUPERVISORY CONFERENCES).

it was decided that the clinician's goal would be to make her explanations as brief and informative as possible. To help her do this, before each session she would write out the explanations she would give for each of the three different activities she did in each session. Second, during the session the clinician would keep track of each explanatory utterance she gave. This would serve to focus attention on this aspect of the clinical behavior as the session was in progress. Finally, the clinician would review the audiotape of each session, continuing to collect frequency data on the number of explanations and transcribing the explanations that were used. This latter activity would demonstrate to the clinician how closely she could follow the preplanning that she had done. Over the next three sessions, the frequency data might look like Figure 15–3.

Figure 15–3 now demonstrates the outlines of an A-B single-subject design. It is readily apparent that the intervention plan instituted by this supervisor and supervisee to deal with the supervisee's frequent use of explanations was effective. The line graph of the B-phase shows a marked downward trend, a gradual slope, and a significantly smaller number of explanations per session.

Once it had been established that the clinician had made significant progress on the target behavior (i.e., reached a predetermined criterion), the supervisor and supervisee decided to focus their attention on another aspect of the clinical process. The supervisor could, during the next three or four sessions, continue to tally the number of explanations used by the clinician. Data collected after explanations are no longer being discussed during the supervisory conferences is termed withdrawal phase data, since the treatment has, in a sense, been withdrawn. If these data are added to the chart, the A-B-A outline would look like that in Figure 15–4.

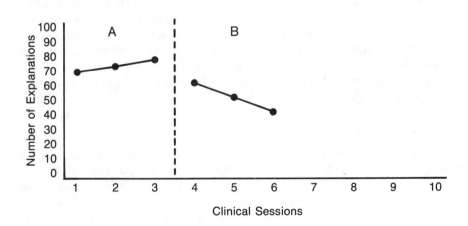

FIGURE 15-3. RESULTS OF A HYPOTHETICAL STUDY REPRESENTING THE BASELINE (A) AND TREATMENT (B) PHASES OF THE A-B DESIGN.

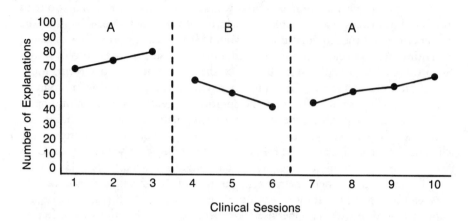

FIGURE 15-4. *RESULTS OF A HYPOTHETICAL STUDY REPRESENTING THE BASELINE (A), TREATMENT (B), AND WITHDRAWAL (A) PHASES OF THE A-B-A WITHDRAWAL DESIGN.*

Bloom and Fischer (1982) referred to this A-B-A design as an "experimental removal of intervention design" (p. 309). As noted by Bloom and Fischer, the important question in the A-B-A design is the maintenance of the intervention effect. For control to be demonstrated in the A-B-A design, the experimental behavior must be changed when treatment is initiated (B-phase) and changed again when treatment is discontinued. In the hypothetical example, when the clinician began to attend to other aspects of the clinical process, the number of explanations she used began to rise again. This is informative for two reasons. First, there is reasonably strong evidence that the intervention strategies (independent variable) developed were responsible for the change noted during the treatment phase and not some other unknown variable. Second, this clinician needed a longer period of intervention on this particular behavior in order to stabilize the explanatory behavior at acceptable levels. When the behavior approaches baseline or near-baseline levels during the second A-phase, it may be trained again to further demonstrate the effectiveness of the training program. This would result in an A-B-A-B design.

Multiple-Baseline Designs

The A-B-A design is the most basic of the experimental single-subject designs, because it deals with only one behavior of one subject. The A-B-A model may be built into more complex designs that involve multiple elements. For example, once the first target behavior has been trained to an acceptable level, an alternative way to demonstrate experimental control is by introducing training of a second target behavior—regardless of whether the first behavior level is maintained or drops off. Thus, the multiple-baseline designs do not require return to the baseline level of performance in order to demonstrate control. These designs replicate A-B-A phases across subjects, behaviors, or settings.

Now, returning to the hypothetical example, assume that this clinician was prone to engaging with the client in off-task conversations. Directive responses to the client's off-task utterances might be chosen as a second experimental behavior. In this case, both behaviors would be analyzed and charted throughout the semesters. The decision to use a multiple-baseline design is preferably made at the initiation of the study. However, an A-B-A design can be converted to a multiple-baseline design in retrospect. The audiotapes of the previous sessions could be reanalyzed and used to collect the A-phase (baseline) data.

Figure 15–5 illustrates line graphs of the data collected through the end of the B-phase of the first behavior for the clinician in the hypothetical example. The bottom line graph represents the long baseline (A-phase) of the second behavior, which is typical of the multiple-baseline design.

When the first behavior has reached the criterion level during the B-phase, the focus of the supervisory sessions would shift from decreasing explanatory remarks to increasing directive responses. The "training" procedures used for modifying directive responses must be the same as those used for training explanatory comments so that the *nature* of the training for the two behaviors is not a factor. Other single-subject designs are appropriate for comparing different treatment programs.

When the directive-response data from the example are graphed, it is apparent that the clinician responded well to the training, as revealed by the upward slope of the B-phase after a relatively stable baseline period. These data are shown in Figure 15–6.

The multiple baseline across behaviors design provides experimental control within the subject by the sequential training of two behaviors. That is, control comes from a replication of treatment effects on the second behavior which remained at a baseline level while the initial behavior was being trained. Two assumptions are specific to the multiple-baseline design. The first is that each target behavior is predicted to be functionally independent, so that the dependent measure remains stable until training occurs. According to the second assumption, the behaviors need to be functionally similar in order to compare them for replication purposes and they must respond to the same intervention.

One factor that cannot be ruled out in the one-subject, multiple-baseline design is the cumulative effect of training the first behavior on the training of the second behavior. This can be controlled by adding a second subject who is trained on the same two behaviors using the same training procedures. However, the order in which the two behaviors are trained is reversed. This procedure is referred to as *counterbalancing*, and in this example, it is the order of the behaviors that is counterbalanced.

The hypothetical example implemented a multiple-baseline design across two behaviors. More than two behaviors may be used for added control. In supervision research, time constraints limit the number of behaviors that can reasonably be trained. It is desirable to complete supervisory studies within the time frame of an academic (or clinical) semester/quarter, since many factors change from semester to semester.

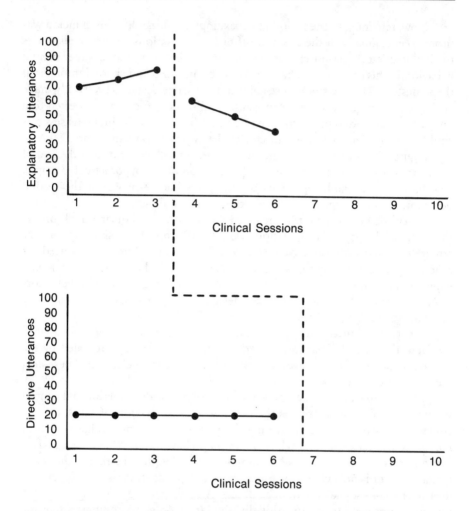

FIGURE 15-5. *INCOMPLETE RESULTS OF A HYPOTHETICAL STUDY ILLUSTRATING THE LONG BASELINE PERIOD FOR BEHAVIOR 2 IN THE MULTIPLE BASELINE ACROSS BEHAVIORS DESIGN. IN THIS EXAMPLE BEHAVIOR 1 IS THE NUMBER OF EXPLANATORY UTTERANCES AND BEHAVIOR 2 IS THE NUMBER OF DIRECTIVE UTTERANCES.*

There are several variations of the multiple-baseline design—some are more complex versions of the across-behaviors design, others implement control by means other than training subsequent behaviors in the same subject. For example, the multiple-baseline-across-subjects design compares sequential phases of the same behavior (similar behavior) in two subjects; multiple-baseline-across-settings design compares the same behavior of the same subject, but in two or more different contexts. McReynolds and Kearns (1983) and Bloom and Fischer (1982) provided more comprehensive treatment of these and other more complex designs.

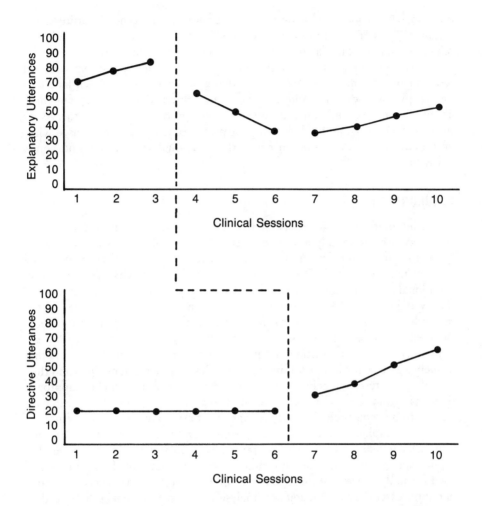

FIGURE 15-6. *RESULTS OF A HYPOTHETICAL STUDY ILLUSTRATING THE SEQUENTIAL TREATMENT PHASES OF TWO BEHAVIORS IN A COMPLETED MULTIPLE BASELINE ACROSS BEHAVIORS DESIGN.*

Generality of Findings in Single-Subject Research

The single-subject designs allow for experimental study of individual subjects and reveal information that is important for supervisors in their work settings. But what do the results reveal about the general population of supervisors and supervisees within the speech-language pathology and audiology community? The solution to the question of generality of research results is found in replication of the results using additional subjects (Bloom & Fischer, 1982; McReynolds & Kearns, 1983; Ventry & Schiavetti, 1980). Similar findings with more than one subject provide convincing evidence supporting the general nature of the findings. The inability to replicate across subjects may relate to any number of reliability and validity factors, or to individual differences in the subjects.

It is now apparent that both single-subject and aggregate experimental research designs may be useful in studying supervision in speech-language pathology and audiology. Additionally, single-subject designs reveal something about the nature of individual differences of the participants in the supervisory process. The third, and final, design to be presented in this chapter is used when even more detailed information about the individual subject and situation is desired.

ETHNOGRAPHY

Ethnography has its roots in the social sciences of anthropology and sociology. It is essentially a research method that involves the study of human behavior through the description or reconstruction of events that are observed as they naturally occur. Ethnographic research is somewhat different from traditional experimental research or single-subject experimental research in both theory and method. Experimental research is conducted on the premise that the research results are applicable for nontested members of the population being sampled and to settings that may be somewhat different than those within the experiment. The experimenter attempts to demonstrate the precise factors that influence a behavior by controlling the variables and their interactions and then recording the resulting behavioral changes. Experimental researchers approach their task from the assumption that there are universal principles of behavior and learning that appear across settings and participants in those settings.

Ethnographers, on the other hand, work from the assumption that learning and behavior are socially and situationally constituted. They believe that knowledge is advanced when information from the analysis of one situation is used for analyzing yet another situation. For example, what a supervisor learned about the careful reconstruction and analysis of supervisee behavior from reading an ethnographic study could be used as a guide for analyzing the behavior of her or his own supervisees. The premise of an ethnography is not that the results are directly generalizable, but that knowledge gained from close situational analysis is useful for analyzing other events in other situations.

The Nature of Ethnographic Research

The ethnographer collects naturalistic data which is then arranged to render complete descriptions of activities and interactions. This logically leads to the generation of *categories* of analysis and the explanation of relationships between the categories. The interpretation of the data becomes the ethnographer's explanation of the categories and their relationships. Pickering (1979, 1984) used ethnographic techniques to describe aspects of interpersonal communication in clinical sessions and supervisory conferences. She transcribed 10-minute samples from videotaped therapy sessions and audiotaped supervisory sessions and analyzed individual statements within the conferences. Four "sensitizing concepts" (loosely defined categories for analyzing the conference verbalizations) served as a heuristic for beginning to analyze the data. After multiple passes through the data, the loose sensitizing categories began to be defined according to the shape of the data set. Through this process, Pickering was able to systematically describe the interpersonal phenomena at work in the sessions; to generate and refine the conceptual categories she began with to fit the data; to discover and validate associations among the interpersonal phenomena observed; and to compare constructs and postulates generated from phenomena specific to the supervisees working with one supervisor with those phenomena specific to supervisees working with two other supervisors.

In considering the data, the ethnographer attempts to go beyond the analysis of individual behaviors (Cicourel, 1974; Corsaro, 1985). The purpose of doing an ethnography is to uncover meaning—the meanings the participants give to a situation as well as the meanings that grow out of the situation as a whole. *Triangulation* is a research technique used by ethnographers to discover and reconstruct the multiple meanings at work in the situations they study. The ethnographer's use of triangulation has been compared to the surveyor's attempt to locate specific points on a map (Glaser & Strauss, 1967). The ethnographer uses several sources of data to converge on a meaningful conclusion in the same way that the surveyor "triangulates" on several sights to determine his or her location on a chart. The triangulation process involves the collection of a variety of data as well as the collection of multiple interpretations of the data. For example, in the study mentioned previously, Pickering (1979, 1984) went beyond the analysis of individual conference speech acts to determine how the participants themselves interpreted their interactions. The supervisors who participated in the research kept journals in which they reflected on their interpretation of the interaction that occurred within each conference. This information provided Pickering with participant perspectives on the meaning of the supervisor-supervisee interactions that took place. For Pickering, the triangulation process extended the scope and clarity of the constructs developed during the course of the investigation. She was able to negotiate the meanings and interpretations given to the phenomena under study between herself and the sources from which the data were drawn (Lincoln & Guba, 1985).

Subject Selection

Another difference between ethnographic and experimental research involves subject selection. Ethnographers often use "theoretical" (Glaser & Strauss, 1967) or "purposive" (Lincoln & Guba, 1985) sampling in which researchers choose those subjects that will help generate categories. The number of subjects and their characteristics do not have to be preplanned. The researchers may add to or modify the characteristics of the groups observed as the theory evolves. For example, supervisor/researchers might be interested in the development of collaborative relationships between supervisors and supervisees. In particular, they may want to analyze this development while working with two supervisors who are interested in learning to supervise according to the clinical supervision model. As they begin meeting with these supervisors to explain the model, the researchers may watch some of the participants' supervisory sessions from behind a one-way mirror and may videotape others. They may also want to audiotape all of their own meetings with the two supervisors in which they discuss the clinical supervision model and the supervisors' attempts to apply the model to their own supervision. If, after three weeks of the semester, another supervisor wants to join the group, the additional supervisor may be incorporated into the study without difficulty.

Data Collection

Ethnographers primarily use three means of data collection: participant observation, interview, and nonparticipant observation. Participant observation is the primary data elicitation technique used. The collection of anecdotes, stories, and interpretations of events is considered to be as important to the ethnographic process as the rote transcription of detail. Lincoln and Guba (1985) suggested that the ethnographer augment observational data with information from structured interviews. The interview questions the ethnographer asks are usually open-ended and variable, depending upon information that is being explored. Nonparticipant observation exists where data are gathered from video- or audiotaped sources or through one-way mirrors. Observers may label themselves as nonparticipants when direct contact with the participants is avoided.

What kinds of data might supervisor/researchers gather in the hypothetical ethnographic research project discussed previously? A decision might be made to have the participating supervisors and supervisees keep daily journals in which they reflected on their understanding of the relationships they were developing, their roles in that development, and their interpretations of what they gained from the experience. Participant observations could come from the meetings the researchers had with the supervisor. The videotaped conferences and the observation of conferences from behind a one-way mirror could serve as nonparticipant observations.

Ethnographers tend to work with data that is not enumerative or standardized. The classic conceptionalization of ethnographic data is the field note. Field notes usually consist of narrative accounts of events, the ethnographers' interpretations of the meaningfulness of events, and discussions of participant interpretations. The ethnographers in the hypothetical study could take field notes during meetings with the supervisors, during the conferences they observed, and while they watched the videotapes. Later, as they attempted to reconstruct the situation and develop a theory to account for the data, the researchers could make liberal use of field notes as a reminder of how they originally interpreted the events being studied.

Data Analysis

There are numerous differences between the analytic processes involved in ethnography and those used in experimental research. Rather than analyze the data as a whole after compilation, ethnographers analyze data throughout the study and again after the data collection process has been completed (Goetz & LeCompte, 1984). The ongoing analysis informs decisions about possible changes in selection strategies and data collection. The ethnographers are free to modify or change methodology at any time throughout the data collection phase of the research. If, after collecting data for a month or so, the hypothetical supervisor/researchers decided that they needed to observe some of the supervisee's clinical sessions in order to better understand what was happening in the supervisory sessions, they could begin doing so without fear of invalidating the study.

Once the data are obtained, ethnographers attempt to interpret and present the significance of the events from multiple perspectives. Geertz (1973) characterized an ethnographic account of something as a "thick description." Through thick description, ethnographers attempt to clarify and understand the conceptions and formulae which the participants in a situation use to define what happens to them (Schieffelin, 1979). Leech (1976) described thick description as a decoding process in which ethnographers view the details of an event as elements of a complex. Single details are not thought to have meaning in isolation; rather, they come to have meaning by virtue of their relationship with other details. Ethnographers look for structural patterns that are contained in the multiple relationships that are being examined by separating and recombining the details in the data. Rather than converting complex data into numbers, which are then tested according to assumptions about the similarity or variability of data points across all possible situations (the central limit theorem), ethnographic methodology treats detail "holistically," as it relates to the whole context. Each detail is used to raise questions about, provide justification for, and contribute to the interpretation of all others. The significance of an observed event is determined by describing the relationship that the event has with all other events. This is quite different from comparing a calculated number with a numerical position represented on a hypothetical curve (i.e., statistical significance).

Supervisor/researchers could begin data analysis by making a decision about what information they want to work with. Given the high assortment of data contained in the videotapes, audiotapes, journal entries, and field notes that would have been collected, they could not possibly analyze everything. While reviewing the data, they could begin to develop codes or categories for various incidents. For example, incidents might be grouped into such broad categories as changing beliefs, collaborative interactions, discoveries, and instances of support. During the coding process, the supervisor/researchers could compare the coding of each incident with previously coded incidents in the same category.

Glaser and Strauss (1967) believe that such constant comparison begins to generate the specific properties of the categories that have been chosen. The categories themselves could change several times throughout the process.

After the ethnographers categorized their data, they could move from comparing incidents within each category to comparing the different categories with each other. This procedure would force them to make related sense of each comparison, enabling them to begin to see patterns that exist in the data. When they felt they had been able to categorize all the significant data and were able to explain the patterns of relationship that exist between the categories, the analysis would be complete.

Returning to an example from an actual ethnography, Pickering (1979, 1984) identified, described, illustrated, and coded the phenomena on the tapes of clinical and supervisory sessions she collected. She viewed each clinical session tape sample in its entirety and her first impressions were written down. A handwritten transcript of the continuous interactions that were relevant for data analysis was then generated. Using the sensitizing concepts discussed earlier, Pickering analyzed the transcripts and noted her interpretations and comments about the analysis. She then listed the major incidents, patterns, and issues by taped sample. Logs from the clients' files that corresponded to the dates of the 40 therapy sessions were selected and the log information was compared to the content of the corresponding analyses. Pickering followed the same procedure for the analysis of the audiotapes of the supervisory conferences with one variation: she transcribed the audiotapes almost verbatim, omitting only those interactions that clearly and redundantly focused on irrelevant issues.

The final analysis revealed that the predominant communicative focus in clinical sessions was directly or indirectly task-related. Student clinicians interacted within therapeutic, social, or disciplinary situations in objective, cognitive and nonaffective ways. As expected, the communication in the supervisory conferences typically followed these same lines. Even though reinforcing types of utterances appeared frequently in the clinical sessions, it often sounded stylized and ritualized. In the supervisory conferences, supervisors usually expressed their support in verbalizations such as "mmmm," "Right," "Uh huh," or "Good." Pickering found that supervisors rarely provided their supervisees with help or support in developing, expanding, or extending their feelings during supervisory sessions, and clinical sessions focused on preplanned instruction or on a client's specific action rather than on feelings or on the existential significance of a behavior. Pickering used these and other findings to demonstrate the congruences between supervisor behavior with supervisees' and clinicians' behavior with their clients and to develop a theory about the interdependent nature of supervision and therapy.

Qualitative research involves inductive, generative, constructive, and subjective processes of data gathering and analysis. As such, it is very different from the deductive, verificative, enumerative, and objective processes involved in experimental research (Goetze & LeCompte, 1984). Supervisor researchers, whether engaging in experimental research, single-subject research, or ethnographic research, can develop research questions from their own understanding of the supervisory process and their experiences as supervisors; can choose data sources that will provide evidence about the problem; can develop methods for obtaining the data they need; and can analyze the data they have collected for its relevance to their focus or problem.

SUMMARY

Kuhn (1970), in agreement with the earlier views of Boring (1950), described the continuing evolution of science as a paradigm structure. For Kuhn, progress in science is limited by ignorance and community. Ignorance, because one discovery opens the way for others to follow; community, because the thought style and scientific habits of a community of scientists delimit the discovery and acceptance of alternative ideas. Writing in this same genre, Fleck (1979) suggested that "facts" are grounded in the thought styles of particular thought *collectives*, the collective being a group of persons whose intellectual constitution is "thought stylized."

Speech-language pathologists and audiologists who are interested in supervision represent a collective within the larger speech-language pathology and audiology community. As such, the development of the science of supervision will both parallel and intersect with that of the larger community of which supervisors are but one part. Because of the indefinite nature of supervisors' membership in the larger community and the tendency of the esoteric core of the larger community to consider supervision inquiry as extraneous, it is vital that the supervision collective achieve consensus about its past and present accomplishments, the worth of its endeavors, and the course of its future exploration.

The supervisor's goal is to help facilitate clinicians' learning about the clinical process, the diagnostic process, the nature of communication disorders, and, most of all, about their own developing abilities to offer effective intervention to their clients. To be effective at their job, supervisors must also be concerned with their own learning and development. Reading and conducting research are the two primary means by which supervisors can increase their own knowledge about supervision. Given the parallels between learning, supervision, and research, it seems appropriate that a book that attempts to clarify what has been learned about the supervision process end with a discussion of ways that supervisors can become active participants in their own and others' learning processes. This is perhaps best accomplished when supervisors become active researchers.

The term *practical research* has been used to point a direction for future supervision research. The most informative supervision research concerns supervisory practices and their effects. Supervision is an activity; research finds are discoveries; practical research is a process by which discovery is brought into balance with daily supervisory activities. The supervisor/researcher essentially enters the business of learning by experiment.

Basic research in supervision has much in common with basic research in speech-language intervention and education. The agenda ahead for supervisors is to develop research methodologies that jointly meet their needs as practitioners and researchers. The suggestion is not for lack of rigor in modes of inquiry, but rather, for methodologies which can be both individually and collectively useful. Single-subject and ethnographic design are well suited for the purposes delineated here, since these designs are flexible enough to allow the supervisor/researcher to approach research within the confines of the daily supervision routine. When the clinical supervision process proceeds as inquiry, personal discoveries have the potential for becoming collective discoveries. From this perspective, research does not need to be an esoteric experience. When research becomes practical, the intersection between deliberate research projects and day-to-day supervisory experiences is revealed.

The ordinary business of daily supervision should indeed be taken seriously. Supervision and research can exist as interrelated modes of inquiry, in the same order that learning and doing can be interrelated. If the full potential of the training enterprise is to be realized, the interactive roles of supervisor and researcher must be assumed to reveal the supervisor as "practical researcher."

References and Suggested Readings

Acheson, K., & Gall, M. (1980). *Techniques in the clinical supervision of teachers.* New York: Longman, Inc.

Adair, M. (1983). Accountability in hospitals. *Seminars in Speech and Language, 4,* 159–169.

Alfonso, R., Firth, G., & Neville, R. (1975). *Instructional supervision.* Boston: Allyn & Bacon, Inc.

Ambroe, M. (1974). Locating supervisors for the CFY experience: A report from Minnesota. *Asha, 16,* 738.

American Speech and Hearing Association. (1942). Amendments to By-Laws. *Journal of Speech and Hearing Disorders, 7,* 61–63.

American Speech and Hearing Association. (1946). Membership Requirements, *Journal of Speech and Hearing Disorders, 11,* 54–55.

American Speech and Hearing Association. (1961). F. Darley (Ed.), Public school speech and hearing services. *Journal of Speech and Hearing Disorders.* (Monograph Suppl. 8).

American Speech and Hearing Association. (1970). Report of Committee on Supportive Personnel. Guidelines on the role, training, and supervision of the communication aide. *Asha, 12,* 78–80.

American Speech and Hearing Association. (1972). Supervision in the schools. Report of task force on supervision. *Language, Speech and Hearing Services in Schools, 3,* 4–10.

American Speech-Language-Hearing Association. (1973). *Essentials of program planning, development, management, and evaluation.* W. Healey, Project Director, Washington, DC.

American Speech and Hearing Association. (1973–1974). *Program Supervision Guidelines for Comprehensive Language, Speech and Hearing Services in the Schools.* Rockville, MD: American Speech and Hearing Association.

American Speech-Language-Hearing Association. (1977). Report of the Committee on the Clinical Fellowship Year. Models for Clinical Fellowship Year experiences. *Asha, 19,* 624–642.

American Speech and Hearing Association. (1978a). Committee on Supervision in Speech-Language-Pathology and Audiology. Current status of supervision of speech-language pathology and audiology [Special report]. *Asha, 20,* 478–486.

American Speech and Hearing Association. (1978b). *Patient care audit manual.* Rockville, MD: American Speech and Hearing Association.

American Speech and Hearing Association (1978c). Principles underlying the requirements for the Certificate of Clinical Competence adopted. *Asha, 20,* 331–333.

American Speech-Language-Hearing Association (1981). Employment and utilization of supportive personnel in audiology and speech-language pathology. *Asha, 23,* 165–169.

American Speech-Language-Hearing Association. (1982a). Committee on Supervision in Speech-Language-Pathology and Audiology. Minimum qualifications for supervisors and suggested competencies for effective clinical supervision. *Asha, 24,* 339–342.

American Speech-Language-Hearing Association. (1982b). Suggested competencies for effective supervision. *Asha, 24,* 1021–1023.

American Speech-Language-Hearing Association. (1982c). *Child services review manual.*

Rockville, MD: American Speech-Language-Hearing Association.

American Speech-Language-Hearing Association. (1984). Committee on Supervision in Speech-Language-Pathology and Audiology. Clinical supervision in speech-language pathology and audiology [Draft form]. *Asha, 5,* 45–48.

American Speech-Language-Hearing Association. (1985a). ASHA demographic update. *Asha, 27,* 55.

American Speech-Language-Hearing Association. (1985b). Committee on Supervision in Speech-Language-Pathology and Audiology. Clinical supervision in speech-language pathology and audiology. A position statement. *Asha, 27,* 57–60.

American Speech-Language-Hearing Association. (1985c). *ASHA membership and certification handbook.* Rockville, MD: American Speech-Language-Hearing Association.

American Speech-Language-Hearing Association. (1985d). Generic vs. categorical supervisors. *ASHA UPDATE.* Rockville, MD: American Speech-Language-Hearing Association.

American Speech-Language-Hearing Association. (1986). *Planning and development of quality services in the schools.* Rockville, MD: American Speech-Language-Hearing Association.

American Speech-Language-Hearing Association. (1987). Legislative council report. *Asha, 29,* 38.

Amidon, E., & Flanders, N. (1967). *The role of the teacher in the classroom.* Minneapolis: Association for Productive Teaching, Inc.

Amidon, E., & Hough, J. (1967). *Interaction analysis: Theory, research, and application.* Reading, MA: Addison-Wesley Publishing Co.

Amidon, P. (1971). *Nonverbal interaction analysis.* Minneapolis, MN: Paul S. Amidon and Associates, Inc.

Andersen, C. (1980a). Oratio Transactional System. In J. Anderson (Ed.), *Proceedings—Conference on Training in the Supervisory Process in Speech-Language Pathology and Audiology.* Bloomington, IN: Indiana University.

Andersen, C. (1980b). The analysis stage. In J. Anderson (Ed.), *Clinical supervision: What does it mean?* Mini-seminar presented at Annual Convention of the American Speech-Language-Hearing Association, Detroit.

Andersen, C. (1981). The effect of supervisor bias on the evaluation of student clinicians in speech/language pathology and audiology. (Doctoral dissertation, Indiana University, 1981). *Dissertation Abstracts International, 41,* 4479B. (University Microfilms No. 81-12, 499)

Anderson, J. (Ed.). (1970). *Proceedings of Conference on Supervision of Speech and Hearing Programs in the Schools.* Bloomington, IN: Indiana University.

Anderson, J. (1972). Status of supervision in speech, hearing and language programs in the schools. *Language, Speech and Hearing Services in Schools, 3,* 12–23.

Anderson, J. (1973a). Status of college and university programs of practicum in the schools. *Asha, 15,* 60–68.

Anderson, J. (1973b). Supervision: The neglected component of the profession. In L. Turton (Ed.), *Proceedings of a Workshop on Supervision in Speech Pathology.* Ann Arbor, MI: University of Michigan.

Anderson, J. (1974). Supervision of school speech, hearing and language programs—an emerging role. *Asha, 16,* 7–10.

Anderson, J. (Ed.). (1980). *Proceedings—Conference on Training in the Supervisory Process in Speech-Language Pathology and Audiology.* Bloomington, IN: Indiana University.

Anderson, J. (1981). Training of supervisors in speech-language pathology and audiology. *Asha, 23,* 77–82.

Anderson, J. (1982). *Report of survey of speech-language pathologists and audiologists in public schools of Indiana.* Unpublished manuscript.

Anderson, J. (1985). Doctoral level emphasis. In K. Smith (Moderator), *Preparation and training models for the supervisory process.* Short course presented at Annual Convention of American Speech-Language-Hearing Association, Washington, DC.

Anderson, J., Brasseur, J., Casey, P., Roberts, J., & Smith, K. (1979, November). *Studying the supervisory process.* Short course presented at the annual convention of the American

Speech and Hearing Association, Atlanta.

Anderson, J., Dowling, S., Goodwin, W., Ingrisano, D., McCrea, E., & Smith, K. (1978). *The supervisory process in speech-language pathology and audiology: Research.* Miniseminar presented at the annual convention of the American Speech and Hearing Association, San Francisco.

Anderson, J., & Kirtley, D. (Eds.). (1966). *Institute on Supervision of Speech and Hearing Programs in the Public Schools.* Indianapolis, IN: Department of Public Instruction.

Anderson, J. & Milisen, R. (1965). *Report on Pilot Project in Student Teaching in Speech and Hearing.* Bloomington, IN: Indiana University.

Andrews, J. (1971). Operationally written therapy goals in supervised clinical practicum. *Asha, 13,* 385–387.

Aptekar, H. (1965). *Supervision and the development of professional responsibility: An application of systems thought.* Paper presented at the Institute for Field Instructors, Yeshiva University.

Argyris, C. (1962). *Interpersonal competence and organizational effectiveness.* Homewood, IL: Richard D. Irwin.

Avert, J., & Michel, L. (1979, November). *Supervision and the consistency of beginning clinician behavior.* Paper presented at the annual convention of the American Speech and Hearing Association, Atlanta.

Azarnoff, R., & Seliger, J. (1982). *Delivering Human Services.* Englewood Cliffs, NJ: Prentice Hall.

Backus, O. (1953). Letters to the editor. *Journal of Speech and Hearing Disorders, 18,* 193–203.

Baer, D., Wolf, M., & Risley, T. R. (1968). Some current dimensions of applied behavior analysis. *Journal of Applied Behavior Analysis, 1,* 91–97.

Baker, E., & Popham, W.J. (1973). *Expanding dimensions of instructional objectives.* Englewood Cliffs, NJ: Prentice-Hall, Inc.

Baker, R., & Ryan, B. (1971). *Programmed conditioning for articulation.* Monterey, CA: Monterey Learning Systems.

Baldes, R., Goings, R., Herbold, D., Jeffrey, R., Wheeler, G., & Freilinger, J. (1977). Supervision of student speech clinicians. *Language, Speech and Hearing Services in Schools, 8,* 76–84.

Bales, R. (1951). *Interaction process analysis.* Reading, MA: Addison-Wesley Publishing Co.

Bales, R. (1950). *Interaction process analysis: A method for the study of small groups.* Reading, MA: Addison-Wesley Publishing Co.

Barlow, D., & Hersen, M. (1973). Single-case experimental designs: Uses in applied clinical research. *Archives of General Psychiatry, 29,* 319–325.

Battin, R. (1983). Clinical accountability: Private practice. *Seminars in Speech and Hearing, 4,* 147–159.

Beegle, C., & Brandt, R. (1973). *Observational Methods in the Classroom.* Washington, DC: Association for Supervision and Curriculum Development.

Bellack, A., Kliebard, H., Hyman, R., & Smith, F. (1966). *The Language of the Classroom.* New York: Teachers College Press, Columbia University.

Benjamin, A. (1969). *The helping interview.* Boston: Houghton Mifflin Co.

Berliner, D., & Tikunoff, W. (1976). The California beginning teacher evaluation study: Overview of the ethnographic study. *Journal of Teacher Education, 27,* 24–30.

Berne, E. (1966). *Principles of group treatment.* New York: Oxford University Press.

Bernthal, J. (Ed.). (1985). *Conference Proceedings-Sixth Annual Conference on Graduate Education.* Lincoln, NE: Department of Special Education and Communication Disorders.

Bernthal, J., & Bankson, N. (1981). *Articulation Disorders.* Englewood Cliffs, NJ: Prentice-Hall.

Bernthal, J., & Beukelman, D. (1975). Self-evaluation by the student clinician. *National Student Speech and Hearing Association Journal,* 39–44.

Bess, F. (1987). Community-based speech-language-hearing clinic administration. In H. Oyer (Ed.), *Administration of programs in speech-language pathology and audiology.* Englewood Cliffs, NJ: Prentice-Hall, Inc.

Biddle, B., & Thomas, E. (1966). *Role theory: Concepts and research.* New York: John Wiley and Sons.

Birdwhistell, R. (1952). *Introduction to kinesics.* Louisville: University of Louisville Press.

Birdwhistell, R. (1970). *Kinesics and context.* Philadelphia: University of Pennsylvania.

Black, M., Miller, A., Anderson, J., & Coates, N. (1961). Supervision of speech and hearing programs. In F. Darley (Ed.), Public school speech and hearing services. *Journal of Speech and Hearing Disorders.* (Monograph Suppl. 8).

Blanton, S. (1936). Helping the handicapped school student. *Journal of Speech Disorders, 1,* 97–100.

Block, F. (1982). The preconference observation system: Supervisor's point of view. *SUPERvision, 6,* 1–6.

Blodgett, E., Schmitt, J., & Scudder, R. (1987). Clinical session evaluation: The effect of familiarity with the supervisee. *The Clinical Supervisor, 5,* 33–43.

Bloom, B.E. (Ed.). (1956). *Taxonomy of educational objectives, Handbook I: Cognitive domain.* NY: David McKay Co., Inc.

Bloom, M., & Fischer, J. (1982). *Evaluating practice: Guidelines for the accountable professional.* Englewood Cliffs, NJ: Prentice-Hall.

Blumberg, A. (1968, Spring). Supervisory behavior and interpersonal relations. *Educational Administration,* 34–35.

Blumberg, A. (1974). *Supervisors and teachers: A private cold war.* Berkeley, CA: McCutchan Publishing Corp.

Blumberg, A. (1980). *Supervisors and teachers: A private cold war* (2nd ed.). Berkeley, CA: McCutchan Publishing Corp.

Blumberg, A., & Amidon, E. (1965). Teacher perceptions of supervisor-teacher interaction. *Administrator's Notebook, 14,* 1–4.

Blumberg, A., Amidon, E., & Weber, W. (1967). *Supervisor-teacher interaction as seen by supervisors.* Unpublished manuscript, Temple University.

Blumberg, A., & Cusick, P. (1970). Supervisor-teacher interaction: An analysis of verbal behavior. *Education, 91,* 126–134.

Blumberg, A., & Weber, W. (1968). Teacher morale as a function of perceived supervisor behavior style. *Journal of Educational Research, 62,* 109–113.

Boone, D. (1970). A close look at the clinical process. In J. Anderson (Ed.), *Proceedings of Conference on Supervision of Speech and Hearing Programs in the Schools.* Bloomington, IN: Indiana University.

Boone, D., & Goldberg, A. (1969). An experimental study of the clinical acquisition of behavioral principles by videotape self-confrontation. *Final Report.* (Project No. 4071—Grant No. OEG-8-071319-2814). Washington, DC: U.S. Department of Health, Education, and Welfare.

Boone, D., & Prescott, T. (1972). Content and sequence analysis of speech and hearing therapy. *Asha, 14,* 58–62.

Boone, D., & Stech, E. (1970). The development of clinical skills in speech pathology by audiotape and videotape self-confrontation. *Final Report.* (Project No. 1381—Grant No. OEG-9-071318-2814). Washington, DC: U.S. Department of Health, Education, and Welfare.

Borg, W., & Gall, M. (1983). *Educational research.* NY: Longman, Inc.

Boring, E. (1950). *A history of experimental psychology.* NY: Appleton-Century-Crofts, Inc.

Bowers, N.D., & Scofield, A.C. (1959). Evaluating the supervision of student teachers. *Journal of Teacher Education, 10,* 461–467.

Boyd, J. (1978). *Counselor supervision.* Muncie, IN: Accelerated Development, Inc.

Boylston, W., & Tuma, J. (1972). Training of mental health professionals through the use of the "bug-in-the-ear." *American Journal of Psychiatry, 129,* 92–95.

Brammer, L. (1985). *The helping relationship.* Englewood Cliffs, NJ: Prentice-Hall, Inc.

Brammer, L., & Wassmer, A. (1977). Supervision in counseling and psychotherapy. In D. Kurpius, R. Baker, & I. Thomas (Eds.), *Supervision of applied training.* Westport, CT: Greenwood Press.

Brandt, R. (1975). An historical overview of systematic approaches to observation in school settings. In R. Weinberg, & F. Wood (Eds.), *Observation of pupils and teachers in mainstream and special education settings: Alternative strategies.* Minneapolis, MN: Leadership Training Institute/Special Education.

Brasseur, J. (1978). *Personal model of consultation.* Unpublished manuscript.

Brasseur, J. (1980a). System for analyzing supervisor-teacher interaction—Arthur Blumberg. In J. Anderson (Ed.), *Proceedings Conference on Training in the Supervisory Process in Speech-Language Pathology and Audiology,* (pp. 71–73). Bloomington, IN: Indiana University.

Brasseur, J. (1980b). The observed differences between direct, indirect, and direct/indirect videotaped supervisory conferences by speech-language pathology supervisors, graduate students, and undergraduate students. (Doctoral dissertation. Indiana University, 1980). *Dissertation Abstracts International, 41,* 2131B. (University Microfilms No. 80–29, 212)

Brasseur, J. (1980c). Underwood Category System for analyzing supervisor-clinician behavior. In J. Anderson (Ed.), *Proceedings Conference on Training in the Supervisory Process in Speech-Language Pathology and Audiology,* (pp. 73–74). Bloomington, IN: Indiana University.

Brasseur, J. (1985). External-internal practicum. In K. Smith (Moderator), *Preparation and training models for the supervisory conference.* Short course presented at the Annual Convention of the American Speech-Language-Hearing Association, Washington, DC.

Brasseur, J., & Anderson, J. (1983). Observed differences between direct, indirect, and direct/indirect videotaped supervisory conferences. *Journal of Speech and Hearing Research, 26,* 349–355.

Brooks, R., & Hannah, E. (1966). A tool for clinical supervision. *Journal of Speech and Hearing Disorders, 31,* 383–387.

Brookshire, R. (1967). Speech pathology and the experimental analysis of behavior. *Journal of Speech and Hearing Disorders, 32,* 215–227.

Brookshire, R., Nicholas, L., & Krueger, K. (1978). Sampling of speech pathology treatment activities: An evaluation of momentary and interval sampling procedures. *Journal of Speech and Hearing Research, 21,* 652–666.

Brookshire, R., Nicholas, L., Krueger, K., & Redmond, K. (1978). The Clinical Interaction Analysis System: A system for observational recording of aphasia treatment. *Journal of Speech and Hearing Disorders, 43,* 437–447.

Brown, S. (1952). Letters to the editor. *Journal of Speech and Hearing Disorders, 17,* 260–262.

Buckberry, E. *Videotape teams: A tape scheduling approach to student peer evaluation and supervision.* Athens, OH: School of Speech and Hearing Sciences, Ohio University.

Burke, P.B. (1985). *Vica.* Oxford: Oxford University Press.

Butler, K. (1974). Videotaped self-confrontation. *Language, Speech and Hearing Services in Schools, 3,* 162–170.

Butler, K. (1976). *The supervision of clinicians: The three C's. . .competition, complaints and competencies.* Paper presented at the annual convention of the American Speech and Hearing Association, Houston.

Butler, K. (1980). Supervision issues in speech-language-pathology and audiology: A personal and professional perspective. In J. Anderson (Ed.), *Proceedings—Conference on Training in the Supervisory Process in Speech-Language Pathology and Audiology.* Bloomington, IN: Indiana University.

Byng-Hall, J. (1982). The use of the earphone in supervision. In R. Whiffen & J. Byng-Hall (Eds.), *Family therapy supervision.* NY: Grune and Stratton.

Byng-Hall, J., & Whiffen, R. (1982). Evolution of supervision: An overview. In R. Whiffen, & J. Byng-Hall (Eds.), *Family Therapy Supervision.* NY: Grune and Stratton.

Campbell, D., & Stanley, J. (1963). *Experimental and quasi-experimental designs for research.* Chicago: Rand McNally and Co.

Campbell, J. (1975). Macroanalysis: A new development for interaction analysis. *Journal of Educational Research, 68,* 261–269.

Campbell, J., & Barnes, C. (1969). Interaction analysis—A breakthrough? *Phi Delta Kappan, 50,* 587–590.

Campbell, R. J., Kagan, N., & Krathwohl, D. (1971). The development and validation of a scale to measure affective sensitivity (empathy). *Journal of Counseling Psychology, 18*, 407–412.

Caracciolo, G. (1977). Perceptions by speech pathology student-clinicians and supervisors of interpersonal conditions and professional growth during the supervisory conferences. (Doctoral dissertation, Columbia University Teachers College, 1976). *Dissertation Abstracts International, 37*, 4411B. (University Microfilms No. 77–04, 183).

Caracciolo, G., Rigrodsky, S., & Morrison, E. (1978a). A Rogerian orientation to the speech-language pathology supervisory relationship. *Asha, 20*, 286–290.

Caracciolo, G., Rigrodsky, S., & Morrison, E. (1978b). Perceived interpersonal conditions and professional growth of master's level speech-language pathology students during the supervisory process. *Asha, 20*, 467–477.

Carin, A., & Sund, R. (1971). *Developing questioning techniques*. Columbus, OH: Charles E. Merrill Publishing Co.

Carkhuff, R. (1967). Toward a comprehensive model of facilitative processes. *Journal of Counseling Psychology, 14*, 67–72.

Carkhuff, R. (1969a). *Helping and human relations: A primer for lay and professional helpers—I*. NY: Holt, Rinehart and Winston.

Carkhuff, R. (1969b). *Helping and human relations—II*. NY: Holt, Rinehart and Winston.

Carkhuff, R., & Berensen, B. (1967). *Beyond counseling and therapy*. NY: Holt, Rinehart and Winston.

Carkhuff, R., & Truax, C. (1964). Concreteness: A neglected variable in research in psychotherapy. *Journal of Clinical Psychology, 20*, 264–267.

Cartwright, C., & Cartwright, G. (1984). *Developing observation skills*. NY: McGraw-Hill Book Co.

Cartwright, D., & Zander, A. (1960). *Group dynamics* (2nd ed.). New York: Harper and Row.

Carrell, J. (1946). State certification of speech correctionists. *Journal of Speech Disorders, 11*, 91–95.

Casey, P. (1980). The validity of using small segments for analyzing supervisory conferences with McCrea's Adapted System. (Doctoral dissertation, Indiana University, 1980). *Dissertation Abstracts International, 41*, 1729B. (University Microfilms No. 80–24, 566).

Casey, P. (1985a). Course and practicum in supervision at graduate level. In K. Smith (Moderator), *Preparation and training models for the supervisory process*. Short course presented at Annual Convention of American Speech-Language-Hearing Association, Washington, D.C.

Casey, P. (1985b). *Supervisory skills self-assessment*. Wisconsin: University of Wisconsin-Whitewater.

Champagne, D., & Morgan, J. (1978). *Supervision-A study guide for educational administrators*. Ft. Lauderdale, FL: Nova University.

Chapman, M. (1942). The speech clinicians and the classroom teachers cooperate in a speech correction program. *Journal of Speech Disorders, 7*, 57–61.

Cicourel, A. (1974). *Cognitive sociology*. NY: Free Press.

Cimorell-Strong, J., & Ensley, K. (1982). Effects of student clinician feedback on the supervisory conference. *Asha, 24*, 23–29.

Cogan, M. (1973). *Clinical supervision*. Boston, MA: Houghton Mifflin Co.

Collins, P., & Cunningham, G. (1976a). *Writing individualized programs: A workbook for speech pathologists*. Tigard, OR: C.C. Publications, Inc.

Collins, P., & Cunningham, G. (1976b). *Writing individualized programs: A workbook for learning disabilities specialists*. Gladstone, OR: C.C. Publications.

Condon, J. (1977). *Interpersonal communication*. New York: Macmillan Publishing Co.

Connell, P., Spradlin, J., & McReynolds, L. (1977). Some suggested criteria for evaluation of language programs. *Journal of Speech and Hearing Disorders, 42*, 563–567.

Connell, P., & Thompson, C. (1986). Flexibility of single-subject experimental design. Part III: Using flexibility to design or modify experiments. *Journal of Speech and Hearing Disorders, 51*, 214–215.

Conover, H. (1979). *Conover Analysis System*. Unpublished manuscript. Athens, OH: Ohio University.

Conture, E. (1973). *Special study institute: Management and supervision of programs for speech and hearing handicapped.* Syracuse, NY: Syracuse University.

Cooper, H., & Good, T. (1983). *Pygmalion grows up: Studies in the expectation communication process.* New York: Longman, Inc.

Copeland, W. (1980). Affective dispositions of teachers in training toward examples of supervisory behavior. *Journal of Educational Research, 74,* 37–42.

Copeland, W., & Atkinson, D. (1978). Student teachers' perceptions of directive and nondirective supervisory behavior. *Journal of Educational Research, 71,* 123–226.

Corsaro, W.A. (1985). *Friendship and peer culture in the early years.* Norwood, NJ: Ablex Publishing.

Costello, J. (1977). Programmed instruction. *Journal of Speech and Hearing Disorders, 42,* 3–28.

Costello, J., & Onstine, J. (1976). The modification of multiple articulation errors based on distinctive feature theory. *Journal of Speech and Hearing Disorders, 41,* 199–215.

Costello, J., & Schoen, J. (1977). The effectiveness of paraprofessionals and a speech clinician as agents of articulation intervention using programmed instruction. *Language, Speech and Hearing Services in the Schools, 9,* 118–128.

Crago, M. (1987). Supervision and self-exploration. In M. Crago & M. Pickering (Eds.), *Supervision in human communication disorders: Perspectives on a process.* San Diego: Little Brown-College Hill Press.

Crago, M., & M. Pickering (Eds.). (1987). *Supervision in human communication disorders: Perspectives on a process.* San Diego: Little Brown-College Hill Press.

Crichton, L., & Oratio, A. (1984). Retrospective study: Speech-language pathologists' clinical fellowship training. *Asha, 26,* 39–43.

Cronbach, L., & Snow, R. (1981). *Aptitudes and instructional methods: A handbook for research on interactions.* New York: Irvington Publishers.

Cruise, R., & Cruise, P. (1979). Research for practicing nurses. *Supervisor Nurse, 10,* 54–55.

Culatta, R., Colucci, S., & Wiggins, E. (1975). Clinical supervisors and trainees: Two views of a process. *Asha, 17,* 152–157.

Culatta, R., & Helmick, J. (1980). Clinical Supervision: The state of the art—Part I. *Asha, 22,* 985–993.

Culatta, R., & Helmick, J. (1981). Clinical Supervision: The state of the art—Part II. *Asha, 23,* 21–31.

Culatta, R., & Seltzer, H. (1976). Content and sequence analyses of the supervisory session. *Asha, 18,* 8–12.

Culatta, R., & Seltzer, H. (1977). Content and sequence analysis of the supervisory session: A report of clinical use. *Asha, 19,* 523–526.

Cunningham, R. (1971). Developing question-asking skills. In J. Weigand (Ed.), *Developing teacher competencies.* Englewood Cliffs, NJ: Prentice-Hall, Inc.

Danish, S.J., & Kagan, N. (1971). Measurement of affective sensitivity: Toward a valid measurement of interpersonal perception. *Journal of Counseling Psychology, 18,* 51–54.

Darley, F. (1964). *Diagnosis and appraisal of communication disorders.* Englewood Cliffs, NJ: Prentice-Hall.

Darley, F., & Hanley, T. (1961). Summary: New horizons. In F. Darley (Ed.), Public school speech and hearing services. *Journal of Speech and Hearing Disorders.* (Monograph Suppl. 8).

Darley, F., & Spriestersbach, D.C. (1978). *Diagnostic methods in speech pathology* (2nd ed.). NY: Harper and Row, Publishers.

Darley, J., Glucksberg, S., & Kinchla, R. (1986). *Psychology.* Englewood Cliffs, NJ: Prentice Hall, Inc.

Davies, I. (1981). *Instructional techniques.* New York: McGraw-Hill Co.

Deetz, S., & Stevenson, S. (1986). *Managing interpersonal communication.* New York: Harper and Row.

Delaney, D., & Moore, J. (1966). Student expectations of the role of supervisor. *Counselor Education and Supervision, 6(1),* 11–17.

Denzin, N. (1970). *The research act.* Chicago: Aldine Publishing.

Diedrich, W. (1969). Assessment of the clinical process. *Journal of Kansas Speech and Hearing Association.*

Diedrich, W. (1971a). Functional description of therapy and revised multidimensional scoring system. In T. Johnson (Ed.), *Clinical interaction and its measurement.* Logan, UT: Utah State University.

Diedrich, W. (1971b). Procedures for counting and charting a target phoneme. *Language, Speech and Hearing Services in Schools, 2,* 18–32.

Diggs, C. (1983). Professional accountability: Present and future directions. *Seminars in Speech and Language. 4,* 169–184.

Dopheide, W., Thornton, B., & McCready, V. (1984). *A preliminary validation of a practicum performance assessment scale.* Paper presented at the American Speech-Language-Hearing Association Annual Convention.

Douglas, R. (1983). Defining and describing clinical accountability. *Seminars in Speech and Language. 4,* 107–119.

Dowling, S. (1977). A comparison to determine the effects of two supervisory styles, conventional and teaching clinics, in the training of speech pathologists. (Doctoral dissertation, Indiana University, 1977). *Dissertation Abstracts International, 37,* 889B. (University Microfilms No. 77-01, 883.)

Dowling, S. (1979a). The teaching clinic: A supervisory alternative. *Asha, 21,* 646–649.

Dowling, S. (1979b). Developing student self-supervisory skills in clinical training. *Journal of National Student Speech and Hearing Association, 7,* 37–41.

Dowling S. (1981). Observation analysis: Procedures for training coders and data collection. *Journal of National Student Speech and Hearing Association, 9,* 82–88.

Dowling, S. (1982). Supervisor and supervisee responsibilities in the supervisory process. *Tejas Journal of Audiology and Speech Pathology, 7,* 26–29.

Dowling, S. (1983a). An analysis of conventional and teaching clinic supervision. *The Clinical Supervisor, 1,* 15–29.

Dowling, S. (1983b). Teaching clinic conference participant interactions. *Journal of Communication Disorders, 16,* 385–397.

Dowling, S. (1984). Clinical evaluation: A comparison of self, self with videotape, peers, and supervisors. *The Clinical Supervisor, 2,* 71–79.

Dowling, S. (1985). Clinical performance characteristics failing, average and outstanding clinicians. *The Clinical Supervisor, 3,* 49–55.

Dowling, S. (1986). Supervisory training: Impetus for clinical supervision. *The Clinical Supervisor, 4,* 27–35.

Dowling, S., & Bliss, L. (1984). Cognitive complexity, rhetorical sensitivity: Contributing factors in clinical skill? *Journal of Communication Disorders, 7,* 9–17.

Dowling, S., Sbaschnig, K., Williams, C. (1982). Culatta & Seltzer. Content and Analysis of the Supervisory Session: Question of reliability and validity. *Journal of Communication Disorders, 15,* 353–362.

Dowling, S., & Shank, K. (1981). A comparison of the effects of two supervisory styles, conventional and teaching clinic, in the training of speech and language pathologists. *Journal of Communication Disorders, 14,* 51–58.

Dowling, S., & Wittkopp, M. (1982). Students' perceived supervisory needs. *Journal of Communication Disorders, 15,* 319–328.

Dublinske, S. (1970). Program-planning-evaluation. In J. Anderson (Ed.), *Conference on supervision of speech and hearing programs in the schools.* Bloomington, IN: Indiana University.

Dublinske, S. (1978). Special reports: P.L. 94-142: Developing the Individualized Education Program (IEP). *Asha, 20*(5), 393–397.

Dublinske, S., & Grimes, J. (1979). Program planning evaluation. In *Health management institute syllabus.* Rockville, MD: American Speech-Language-Hearing Association.

Dublinske, S., & Healey, W. (1978, March). P.L. 94-142: Questions and answers for the speech-language pathologists and audiologists. *Asha, 20,* 188–205.

Dussault, G. (1970). *Theory of supervision in teacher education.* NY: Teachers College, Columbia University.

Ehrlich, C., Merten, K., Sweetman, R., & Arnold, C. (1983). Training issues—graduate student externship. *Asha, 25,* 25–28.

Elbert, M., & Geirut, J. (1986). *Handbook of clinical phonology.* San Diego: College-Hill Press, Inc.

Elbert, M., Shelton, R., & Arndt, W. (1967). A task for evaluation of articulation change. I. Development of methodology. *Journal of Speech and Hearing Research, 10,* 281–288.

Emerich, L., & Hatten, J. (1979). *Diagnosis and evaluation in speech pathology.* Englewood Cliffs, NJ: Prentice-Hall.

Engnoth, G. (1974). A comparison of three approaches to supervision of speech clinicians in training. (Doctoral dissertation, University of Kansas, 1973). *Dissertation Abstracts International, 34,* 6261B. (University Microfilms No. 74–12, 552).

Engnoth, G. (1987). Public school speech-language-hearing administration. In H. Oyer (Ed.), *Administration of programs in speech-language pathhology and audiology.* Englewood Cliffs, NJ: Prentice Hall, Inc.

Erickson, R., & Van Riper, C. (1967). Demonstration therapy in a university training center. *Asha, 9,* 33–35.

Ervin-Tripp, S. (1970). Discourse agreement: How children answer questions. In J. Hayes (Ed.), *Cognitions and the development of language.* New York: John Wiley and Sons.

Evertson, C., & Green, J. (1986). Observation as inquiry and method. In M. Wittrock (Ed.), *Handbook of research on teaching.* New York: Macmillan Publishing Co.

Farmer, J., & Farmer, S. (1986). *Unilateral and bilateral styles of dyadic and group clinical education/supervision.* Short course presented at convention of American Speech-Language-Hearing Association, Detroit.

Farmer, S. (1980). *Interview Analysis System.* Paper presented at the annual convention of the American Speech-Language-Hearing Association, Detroit.

Farmer, S. (1984). Supervisory conferences in communicative disorders: Verbal and non-verbal interpersonal communication pacing. (Doctoral dissertation, University of Colorado, 1983). *Dissertation Abstracts International, 44,* 2715B. (University Microfilms No. 84–00, 891).

Farmer, S. (1985–1986). Relationship development in supervisory conferences: A tripartite view of the process. *The Clinical Supervisor, 4,* 5–22.

Farmer, S. (1987). Visual literacy and the clinical supervisor. *The Clinical Supervisor, 5,* 45–73.

Farmer, S. (Ed.). (1987). *Clinical supervision: A coming of age.* Proceedings of a conference held at Jekyll Island, GA: Las Cruces, NM, New Mexico State University.

Farris, G.F. (1974). Leadership and supervision in formal organizations. In J.G. Hunt & L.L. Larson (Eds.), *Contingency approaches to leadership.* Carbondale, IL: Southern Illinois University Press.

Fein, D. (1983). Survey report: 1982 ASHA Omnibus. *Asha, 25,* 53–57.

Fein, D. (1984). Findings from the 1983 ASHA Omnibus survey. *Asha, 26,* 45–48.

Fey, M. (1986). *Language intervention with young children.* San Diego: College-Hill Press.

Fiedler, F.E. (1967). *A theory of leadership effectiveness.* New York: McGraw Hill.

Fisher, L. (1982). Supervision. In R. Van Hattum (Ed.), *Speech-language programming in the schools.* Springfield, IL: Charles C. Thomas.

Flanders, N. (1967). Teacher influence in the classroom. In E. Amidon & J. Hough (Eds.), *Interaction analysis: Theory, research, and application.* Reading, MA: Addison-Wesley Publishing Co.

Flanders, N. (1969). Classroom interaction patterns, pupil attitudes, and achievement in the second, fourth and sixth grades. (Cooperative Research Project No. 5–1055 [OE 4–10–243]). Ann Arbor, MI: The University of Michigan.

Flanders, N. (1970). *Analyzing teacher behavior.* Reading, MA: Addison-Wesley Publishing Co.

Fleck, L. (1979). *Genesis and development of a scientific fact.* Chicago: University of Chicago Press.

Fleishman, E. A. (1953). The description of supervisor behavior. *Journal of Applied Psychology, 37,* 1–6.

Fleming, R. (1973). The supervisor as observer. In C. Beegle (Ed.), *Observational methods in the classroom.* Washington, DC: Association for Supervision and Curriculum Development.

Flower, R. (Ed.). (1969). *Conference on standards for supervised experience for speech and hearing specialists in public schools.* Los Angeles, CA: Department of Education.

Flower, R. (1983). Professional standards and accountability. *Seminars in Speech and Language, 4,* 119–131.

Flower, R. (1984). *Delivery of speech-language pathology and audiology services.* Baltimore, MD: Williams and Wilkins.

Fox, R. (1983). Contracting in supervision: A goal oriented process. *The Clinical Supervisor, 1,* 37–49.

Frassinelli, L., Superior, K., & Myers, J. (1983). A consultation model for speech and language intervention. *Asha, 25,* 25–30.

Freeman, G. (1982). Consultation. In R. Van Hattum, *Speech-language programming in the schools.* Springfield, IL: Charles C. Thomas.

Frick, T., & Semmel, M. (1978). Observer agreement and reliabilities of classrooms observation measures. *Review of Educational Research, 48,* 157–184.

Fristoe, M. (Ed.). (1975). *Language intervention systems for the retarded: A catalogue of original structured language programs in use in the U.S.* Montgomery: State of Alabama Department of Education.

Froehle, T., & Kurpius, D. (1980). The interpersonal aspects of the supervising process. In J. Anderson (Ed.), *Conference on training in the supervisory process in speech-language pathology and audiology.* Bloomington, IN: Indiana University.

Gage, N. (Ed.). (1963). *Handbook of research on teaching.* Chicago, IL: Rand McNally and Co.

Gallagher, T., & Prutting, C. (1983). *Pragmatic assessment and intervention issues in language.* San Diego: College Hill Press, Inc.

Galloway, H., & Blue, C. (1975). Paraprofessional personnel in articulation therapy. *Language, Speech, and Hearing Services in the Schools, 6,* 125–130.

Ganz, C., & Hunt-Thompson, J. (1985). Speech-language intern supervisor training program. In K. Smith (Moderator), *Preparation and training models for the supervisory process.* Short course presented at ASHA convention. Washington, DC.

Garbee, F. (1982). The speech-language pathologist as a member of the educational team. In R. Van Hattum (Ed.), *Speech-language programming in the schools.* Springfield, IL: Charles C. Thomas.

Garrett, E.R. (1963). An automated speech correction: A pilot study. *Asha, 5,* 796.

Gavett, E. (1987). Career development: An issue for the Master's degree supervisor. In M. Crago & M. Pickering (Eds.), *Supervision in human communication disorders*: perspectives on a process. San Diego, CA: College Hill Press.

Gazda, G. (1974). *Human relations development—A manual for educators.* Boston: Allyn and Bacon.

Gazda, G., Asbury, F., Balzer, F., Childers, W., & Walters, R. (1977). *Human relations development—A manual for educators* (2nd ed.). Boston, MA: Allyn and Bacon, Inc.

Geertz, C. (1973). *The interpretation of cultures.* New York: Basic Books.

Geoffrey, V. (1973). *Report on supervisory practices in speech and hearing.* Unpublished report, College Park, MD: University of Maryland, Department of Hearing and Speech Sciences.

George, R., & Cristiani, T. (1981). *Theory, methods, and processes of counseling and psychotherapy.* Englewood Cliffs, NJ: Prentice-Hall.

Gerstman, H. (1977). Supervisory relationships: Experiences in dynamic communication. *Asha, 19,* 527–529.

Getzel, J., & Guba, E. (1954). Role, role conflict and affectiveness: An empirical study. *American Sociological Review, 19,* 164–175.

Gibb, J. (1969). Defensive communication. *Journal of Communication, 11,* 141–148.

Gillam, R., Strike, C., & Anderson, J. (1987). *Facilitating change in clinical behaviors: An investigation of supervisory effectiveness.* Unpublished manuscript, Indiana University, Bloomington.

Glaser, B., & Strauss, A. (1967). *The discovery of grounded theory: Strategies for qualitative research.* Hawthorne, NY: Adline Publishing.

Goetz, J., & LeCompte, M. (1984). *Ethnography and qualitative design in educational research.* Orlando, FL: Academic Press.

Goldhammer, R. (1969). *Clinical supervision.* New York: Holt, Rinehart and Winston.

Goldhammer, R., Anderson, R., & Krajewski, R. (1980). *Clinical supervision* (2nd ed.). New York: Holt, Rinehart and Winston.

Golper, L., McMahon, J., & Gordon, M. (1976). *The use of interaction analysis for training in observation.* Paper presented at ASHA convention.

Goodman, R. (1985). The live supervision model in clinical training. *The Clinical Supervisor, 3,* 43–59.

Goodwin, W. (1977). The frequency of occurrence of specified therapy behaviors of student speech clinicians following three conditions of supervisory conferences. (Doctoral dissertation, Indiana University, 1976). *Dissertation Abstracts International, 37,* 3889B. (University Microfilms No. 77–01, 892).

Gouran, D. (1980). Leadership skills for supervisors. In J. Anderson (Ed.), *Conference on training in the supervisory process in speech-language pathology and audiology.*

Gray, B., & Ryan, B. (1973). *A language program for the nonlanguage child.* Champaign, IL: Research.

Griffith, T. (1987). Administration of community hospital speech-language-hearing programs. In H. Oyer (Ed.), *Administration of programs in speech-language pathology and audiology.* Englewood Cliffs, NJ: Prentice-Hall, Inc.

Gross, N., & Herriot, R. E. (1965). *Staff leadership in public schools.* New York: John Wiley and Sons.

Guinty, C., & Scudder, R. (1980, November). *Effects of training on observer's ability to count nonverbal behaviors.* Paper presented at the annual convention of the American Speech-Language-Hearing Association, Detroit.

Gunter, C. (1985). Clinical reports in speech-language pathology: Nature of supervisory feedback. *Australian Journal of Human Communication Disorders. 13,* 37–51.

Gyshers, N., & Johnson, J. (1965). Expectations of a practicum supervisor's role. *Counselor Education and Supervision, 4*(1), 68–74.

Hackney, H., & Nye, S. (1973). *Counseling strategies and objectives.* Englewood Cliffs, NJ: Prentice-Hall, Inc.

Hagler, P. (1986). *Effects of verbal directives, data, and contingent social praise on amount of supervisor talk during speech-language pathology supervision conferencing.* Unpublished dissertation, Indiana University, Bloomington, IN.

Hagler, P., & Fahey, R. (1987). The validity of using short segments for analyzing supervisory conferences in speech pathology. *Human Communication Canada.*

Halfond, M. (1964). Clinical supervision—stepchild in training. *Asha, 6,* 441–444.

Halfond, M., & Russell, L. (1986). *An expanded view of the evaluative component of clinical instruction: Written commentaries.* Paper presented at ASHA convention, Detroit.

Hall, A. (1971). The effectiveness of videotape recordings as an adjunct to supervision of clinical practicum by speech pathologists. (Doctoral dissertation, Ohio State University, 1970). *Dissertation Abstracts International, 32,* 612B. (University Microfilms No. 71–18, 014).

Hall, E. (1959). *The silent language.* Garden City, NY: Doubleday.

Hall, E. (1966). *The hidden dimension.* Garden City, NY: Doubleday.

Hall, P., & Knutson, C. (1978). The use of preprofessional students as communication aides in the schools. *Language, Speech and Hearing Services in Schools, 9,* 162–168.

Hampton, D.R., Summer, C.E., & Webber, R.A. (1982). *Organizational behavior and the practice of management.* Glenview, IL: Scott, Foresman and Co.

Hanner, M., Nilson, J., & Richard, G. (1983). *A supervisory evaluation form based on ASHA's suggested competencies.* Paper presented at ASHA convention, Washington, DC.

Hansen, J.C. (1965). Trainees' expectations of supervision in the counseling practicum. *Counselor Education and Supervision, 2,* 75–80.

Hardick, E., & Oyer, H. (1987). Administration of speech-language-hearing programs within the university setting. In H. Oyer (Ed.), *Administration of programs in speech-language pathology and audiology.* Englewood Cliffs, NJ: Prentice-Hall, Inc.

Harris, B. (1975). *Supervisory behavior in education.* Englewood Cliffs, NJ: Prentice-Hall.

Hart, G. (1982). *The process of clinical supervision.* Baltimore, MA: University Park Press.

Hartman, D. (Ed.). (1982). *Using observers to study behavior.* San Francisco: Jossey-Bass Inc.

Hatfield, M., Caven, C., Bartlett, C., & Ueberle, J. (1973). *Supervision: The supervisee speaks.* Papers presented at the annual convention of the American Speech and Hearing Association, Detroit.

Hatten, J. (1966). A descriptive and analytical investigation of speech therapy supervisors-therapist conferences. (Doctoral dissertation, University of Wisconsin, 1965). *Dissertation Abstracts International, 26,* 5595–5596. (University Microfilms No. 71–18, 014).

Hatten, J., Bell, J., & Strand, J. (1983). *A comparative study of supervisor evaluation of a clinical session.* Paper presented at ASHA convention, Washington, DC.

Haverkamp, K. (1983). The orientation experience for the adult learner. In R. Smith. (Ed.), *Helping adults learn how to learn.* San Francisco: Jossey-Bass Inc., Publishers.

Hawk, S. (1936). Speech defects in handicapped children. *Journal of Speech Disorders, 1,* 101–106.

Hawkins, R. (1982). Developing a behavior code. In D. Hartman (Ed.), *Using observers to study behavior.* San Francisco: Jossey-Bass, Inc.

Hawthorne, L. (1975). Games supervisors play. *Social Work, 20,* 179–183.

Hayek, F.A. (1979). *The counter-revolution of science.* Indianapolis: Liberty Press.

Hays, W. (1981). *Statistics.* (3rd ed.). New York: CBS College Publishing.

Healey, W. (1982). Systems for program planning, management, and evaluation. In R. Van Hattum (Ed.), *Speech-language programming in the schools.* Springfield, IL: Charles C. Thomas.

Hegde, M. (1985). *Treatment procedures in communicative disorders.* San Diego, CA: College-Hill Press, Inc.

Heidelbach, R. (1967). The development of a tentative model for analyzing and describing the verbal behavior of cooperating teachers engaged in individualized teaching with student teachers (Doctoral dissertation, Columbia University, 1967). *Dissertation Abstracts, 28,* 1326-A. (University Microfilms No. 67–12, 689)

Herbert, J., & Attridge, C. (1975). A guide for developers and users of observation systems and manuals. *American Educational Research Journal, 12,* 1–20.

Hersey, P., & Blanchard, K. (1982). *Management of organizational behavior* (4th ed.). Englewood Cliffs, NJ: Prentice-Hall, Inc.

Herson, M., & Barlow, D. (1976). *Single case experimental design: Strategies for studying behavioral change.* NY: Pergamon.

Hess, A. (1986). Growth in supervision: Stages of supervisee and supervisor development. *The Clinical Supervisor, 4,* 51–67.

Hess, A., & Hess, K. (1983). Psychotherapy supervision: A survey of internship training practices. *Professional Psychology, 14,* 504–513.

Heward, Wm., Heron, T., Hill, D., & Trap-Porter, J. (1984). *Focus on behavior analysis in education.* Columbus: Merril Publishing Co.

Hicks, C. (1964). *Fundamental concepts in the design of experiments.* New York: Holt, Rinehart, and Winston.

Ho, M.K. (1976, January). Evaluation: A means of treatment. *Social Work*, 20, p.

Holland, A. (1970). Case studies in aphasia rehabilitation using programmed instruction. *Journal of Speech and Hearing Disorders, 35*, 377–390.

Holland, A., & Matthews, J. (1963). Application of teaching machine concepts to speech pathology and audiology. *Asha, 5*, 474–482.

House, R.J., Filley, A.C., & Gujarati, D.N. (1971). Leadership style, hierarchical influence and the satisfaction of subordinate role expectations: A test of Likert's influence propositions. *Journal of Applied Psychology, 55*, 422.

Huck, S., Cormier, W., & Bounds, W. (1974). *Reading statistics and research.* New York: Harper and Row Publishers.

Hunt, J., & Kauzlarich, M. (1979). *Enhancing the effectiveness of the supervisory process.* Paper presented at the Annual Convention of the American Speech-Language-Hearing Association, Atlanta, GA.

Hunt, J.G., & Larson, K.L. (Eds.). (1974). *Contingency approaches to leadership.* Carbondale, IL: Southern Illinois University Press.

Hyman, C. (1986). The 1986 Omnibus Survey—Implications for strategic planning. *Asha, 28*, 19–24.

Hymes, D. (1974). *Foundations in sociolinguistics: An ethnographic approach.* Philadelphia: University of Philadelphia Press.

Ingrisano, D. (1979). An experiment in clinical process reactivity. (Doctoral dissertation, Indiana University, 1978). *Dissertation Abstracts International, 40*, 3231B. (University Microfilms No. 79-00, 395)

Ingrisano, D. (1980, November). *Solving clinical and supervisory process problems through time series designs.* Paper presented at the annual convention of the American Speech-Language-Hearing Association, Detroit.

Ingrisano, D., & Boyle, K. (1973). *A study of effectiveness and efficiency variables in a supervisory interaction.* Unpublished manuscript, University of Wisconsin, Madison.

Ingrisano, D., Guinty, C., Chambers, D., McDonald, J., Clem, R., & Cory, M. (1979). *The relationship between supervisory conference performance and supervisor experience.* Paper presented at the ASHA convention, Atlanta.

Irwin, J. (1967). Supportive personnel in speech pathology and audiology. *Asha, 9*, 348–354.

Irwin, R. (1948). Ohio looks ahead in speech and hearing therapy. *Journal of Speech and Hearing Disorders, 13*, 55–60.

Irwin, R. (1949). Speech and hearing therapy in the public schools of Ohio. *Journal of Speech and Hearing Disorders, 14*, 63–68.

Irwin, R. (1953). State program in speech and hearing therapy: II. Certification. *The Speech Teacher, 4*, 254–258.

Irwin, R. (1972). *Microsupervision—A study of the behaviors of supervisors of speech clinicians.* Unpublished manuscript, Ohio State University, Columbus.

Irwin, R. (1975). Microcounseling interview skills of supervisors of speech clinicians. *Human Communication, 4*(spring), 5–9.

Irwin, R. (1976). Verbal behavior of supervisors and speech clinicians during microcounseling. *Central States Speech Journal, 26*, 45–51.

Irwin, R. (1981a). Training speech pathologists through microtherapy. *Journal of Communication Disorders, 14*, 93–103.

Irwin, R. (1981b). Video self-confrontation on speech pathology. *Journal of Communication Disorders, 14*, 235–243.

Irwin, R., & Hall, A. (1973). Microtherapy—A study of the behaviors of speech clinicians. *Central States Speech Journal, 24*, 297–303.

Irwin, R., & Nickles, A. (1970). Use of audiovisual films in supervised observation. *Asha, 12*, 363–367.

Irwin, R., Van Riper, C., Breakey, M., & Fitzsimmons, R. (1961). Professional standards in training. In F. Darley (Ed.), Public school speech and hearing services. *Journal of Speech and Hearing Disorders.* (Monograph Suppl. 8).

Ivey, A.E. (1971). *Microcounseling*. Springfield, IL: Charles C. Thomas.

James, H. *Life of Nathaniel Hawthorne*. In Oxford Dictionary of Quotations (p. 271). Oxford: Oxford University Press.

James, S. & Seebach, M. (1982). The pragmatic function of children's questions. *Journal of Speech and Hearing Research, 25*, 2–11.

Johnson, C., & Fey, S. (1983). Comparative effects of teaching clinic versus traditional supervision methods. *SUPERvision, 7*, 2–4.

Johnson, T. (1970). The development of a multidimensional scoring system for observing the clinical process in speech pathology. (Doctoral dissertation, University of Kansas, 1970). *Dissertation Abstracts International, 30*, 5735B–5736B. (University Microfilms No. 70–11, 036)

Johnson, T. (Ed.). (1971). *Clinical interaction and its measurement*. UT: Utah State University, Department of Communicative Disorders, Logan.

Johnson, W., Darley, F., & Spriestersbach, D. (1963). *Diagnostic methods in speech pathology*. NY: Harper and Row.

Johnston, M., & Harris, F. (1968). Observation and recording of verbal behavior in remedial speech work. In H.N. Sloane & B.D. MacAulay (Eds.), *Operant procedures in remedial speech and language training*. NY: Houghton Mifflin.

Kadushin, A. (1968). Games people play in supervision. *Social Work, 13*, 23–32.

Kadushin, A. (1976). *Supervision in social work*. New York: Columbia University Press.

Kagan, N. (1970). Human relationships in supervision. In J. Anderson (Ed.), *Conference on supervision of speech and hearing programs in the schools*. Bloomington, IN: Indiana University.

Kagan, N., & Werner, A. (1977). Supervision in psychiatric education. In D. Kurpius, R. Baker, & I. Thomas (Eds.), *Supervision of applied training*. Westport, CT: Greenwood Press.

Kaplan, N., & Dreyer, D. (1974). The effect of self-awareness training on student speech pathologist client relationships. *Journal of Communication Disorders, 7*, 329–342.

Karr, J., & Geist, G. (1977). Facilitation on supervision as related to facilitation on therapy. *Counselor Education and Supervision, 16*, 263–268.

Kaslow, F. (1977). Training of marital and family therapists. In F. Kaslow & Associates (Ed.), *Supervision, consultation, and staff training in the helping professions*. San Francisco, CA: Jossey-Bass Publishers.

Katz, D., Macoby, E., & Morse, N. (1950). *Productivity, supervision and morale in an office situation*. Ann Arbor: Institute for Social Research Center, University of Michigan.

Kavanagh, M. (1975). Expected supervisory behavior, interpersonal trust and environmental preferences. *Organizational Behavior and Human Performance, 13*, 17–30.

Kazdin, Alan. (1982). Observer effects: Reactivity of direct observation. In D. Hartman (Ed.), *Using observers to study behavior*. San Francisco: Jossey-Bass Publishers.

Keeney, B. (1983). *Aesthetics of change*. New York: The Guilford Press.

Kelly, J. (1980). *Organizational behavior*. Homewood, IL: Richard D. Irwin, Inc.

Kennedy, K. (1981). The effect of two methods of supervisor preconference written feedback on the verbal behaviors of participants in individual speech pathology supervisory conferences. (Doctoral dissertation, University of Oregon, 1981). *Dissertation Abstracts International, 42*, 2071A. (University Microfilms No. 81–23, 492)

Kennedy, K. (1985). Clinical supervision in a university setting—Hidden dynamics related to the supervisory role. In J. Bernthal (Ed.), *Proceedings: Sixth Annual Conference on Graduate Education*. Lincoln, NE: Department of Special Education and Communication Disorders.

Kent, L.P. (1977). *Problem-oriented record for clinical service and supervision in speech pathology and audiology*. Paper presented at the annual convention of the American Speech and Hearing Association, Chicago.

Kent, L.P., & Chabon, S. (1980). Problem-oriented record in a university speech and hearing clinic. *Asha, 22*, 151–155.

Kent, R. (1985). Science and the clinician: The practice of science and the science of practice. *Seminars in Speech and Language, 6*, 1–13.

Kearns, K. (1986). Flexibility of single-subject experimental design. Part II: Design selection and arrangement of experimental phases. *Journal of Speech and Hearing Disorders, 51,* 204–214.

Kirk, R. (1982). *Experimental design: Procedures for the behavioral sciences* (2nd ed.). Monterey, CA: Brooks/Cole Publishing.

Kirtley, D. (Ed.). (1967). *Supervision of student teaching in speech and hearing therapy.* Indianapolis, IN: Department of Public Instruction.

Kleffner, F. (Ed.). (1964). *Seminar on guidelines for the internship year.* Washington, DC: American Speech and Hearing Association.

Klevans, D., & Semel, B. *Nonverbal behavior system.* Unpublished manuscript, State College, PA.

Klevans, D., & Volz, H. (1974). Development of a clinical evaluation tool. *Asha, 16,* 489–491.

Klevans, D., & Volz, H. (1976, November). *The nonverbal behavior system: A procedure for evaluating clinical interactions.* Paper presented at the American Speech and Hearing Association, Houston.

Klevans, D., Volz, H., & Friedman, R. (1981). A comparison of experimental and observational approaches for enhancing the interpersonal communication skills of speech-language pathology students. *Journal of Speech and Hearing Disorders, 46,* 208–213.

Knapp, M. (1972). *Nonverbal communication in human interaction.* New York: Holt, Rinehart and Winston, Inc.

Knight, H., Hahn, E., Ervin, J., & McIsaac, G. (1961). The public school clinician: professional definition and relationships. In F. Darley (Ed.), Public school speech and hearing services. *Journal of Speech and Hearing Disorders.* (Monograph Suppl. 8).

Knowles, M. (1984). *The adult learner: A neglected species.* Houston: Gulf Publishing Co.

Korner, I., & Brown, W. (1952). The mechanical third ear. *Journal of Consulting Psychology, 16,* 81–84.

Kounin, J. (1970). Observing and delineating techniques of managing behaviors in classrooms. In Systematic Observation. *Journal of Research and Development in Education, 4,* 62–72.

Krajewski, R. (Ed.). (1976). Clinical supervision. *Journal of Research and Development in Education, 9,* 1–99.

Kuhn, T. (1970). *The structure of scientific revolutions* (2nd ed.). Chicago: University of Chicago Press.

Kunze, L. (1967). Program for training in behavioral observation. In A. Miner, A symposium: improving supervision of clinical practicum. *Asha, 9,* 473–497.

Kurpius, D., Baker, R., & Thomas, I. (1977). *Supervision of applied training.* Westport, CT: Greenwood Press.

Kurpius, D., & Robinson, S. (1978). An overview of consultation. *Personal and Guidance Journal, 3,* 231–323.

Kutzik, A. (1977a). The medical field. In F. Kaslow (Ed.), *Supervision, consultation, and staff training in the helping professions.* San Francisco: Jossey-Bass Publishers.

Kutzik, A. (1977b). The social work field. In F. Kaslow (Ed.), *Supervision, consultation, and staff training in the helping professions.* San Francisco: Jossey-Bass Publishers.

Laccinole, M. (1985). Supervisory course at graduate level. In K. Smith (Moderator), *Preparation and training models for the supervisory process.* Short course presented at the Annual Convention of the American Speech-Language-Hearing Association, Washington, DC.

Laney, M. (1982). Research and evaluation in the public schools. *Language, Speech and Hearing Services in Schools, 13,* 53–60.

Lao-tse. (1962). *The way of life according to Laotzu* (W. Bynner, Trans.). New York: Capricorn Books.

Larkins, P. (1987). Determining quality of speech-language-hearing services—Program Evaluation System. *Asha, 29,* 21–24.

Larson, L. (1982). Perceived supervisory needs and expectations of experienced vs. inexperienced student clinicians. (Doctoral dissertation, Indiana University, 1981). *Dissertation Abstracts Interternational, 42,* 4758B. (University Microfilms No. 82–11, 183)

Larson, L., & Smith, K. (1976, November). *Development of minimum clinical competencies for speech pathology school practicum form during student teaching experience.* Paper presented at the annual convention of the American Speech and Hearing Association, Houston.

Leach, E. (1972). Interrogation: A model and some implications. *Journal of Speech and Hearing Disorders, 37,* 33–46.

Leddick, G., & Barnard, J. (1980). The history of supervision—A critical review. *Counselor Education and Supervision. 19,* 186–196.

Leech, E. (1976). *Culture and communication.* Cambridge: Cambridge University Press.

Lemme, M. (1986). Clinical supervision of language intervention in adult aphasia. In R. Chapey (Ed.), *Language intervention strategies in adult aphasia.* Baltimore: Williams and Wilkins.

Lemmer, E., & Drake, M. (1983). Client management and professional development. *Asha, 25,* 33–39.

Lewin, K., Lippett, R., & White, R. (1939). Patterns of aggressive behavior in experimentally created "social climates." *Journal of Social Psychology, 10,* 271–299.

Likert, R. (1961). *New patterns of management.* NY: McGraw-Hill.

Likert, R. (1967). *The human organization: Its management value.* NY: McGraw-Hill.

Lincoln, Y., & Guba, E. (1985). *Naturalistic inquiry.* Beverly Hills: Sage Publications.

Lindsey, M. (1969). *Inquiry into teaching behavior of supervisors in teaching education laboratories.* New York: Teachers College Press, Columbia University.

Lindsley, O.R. (1964). Direct measurement and prosthesis of retarded behavior. *Journal of Education, 147,* 62–81.

Link, C. (1971). Teacher-supervisor conference interaction: A study of perceptions and their relation in selected variables. (Doctoral dissertation, Western Michigan University, 1970). *Dissertation Abstracts International, 31,* 3824A. (University Microfilms No. 71–4376).

Loewenstein, S., & Reder, P. (1982). The consumers' response: Trainees' discussion of the experience of live supervision. In R. Whiffen & J. Byng-Hall (Eds.), *Family therapy supervision.* New York: Grune and Stratton.

Loganbill, G., & Hardy, E. (1983). Developing training programs for clinical supervisors. *The Clinical Supervisor, 1,* 15–21.

Lovell, J., & Wiles, K. (1983). *Supervision for better schools* (5th ed.). Englewood Cliffs, NJ: Prentice-Hall, Inc.

Lowery, L. (1970). *Learning about instruction: Questioning strategies: A personal workshop.* (ERIC Research Document #ED 113 297).

Luft, J. (1969). *Of human interaction.* Palo Alto, CA: National Press Books.

Lund, N., & Duchan, J. (1983). *Assessing children's language in naturalistic contexts.* Englewood Cliffs, NJ: Prentice-Hall, Inc.

Luterman, D. (1979). *Counseling parents of hearing–impaired children.* Boston: Little, Brown and Co.

Luterman, D. (1984). *Counseling the communicatively disordered and their families.* Boston: Little, Brown and Co.

MacLearie, E. (1947). Suggestions for supervised teaching in speech correction. *Journal of Speech Disorders, 12,* 369–372.

MacLearie, E. (1958). Appraisal form for speech and hearing therapists. *Journal of Speech and Hearing Disorders, 23,* 612–614.

Mager, R. (1962). *Preparing instructional objectives.* Palo Alto, CA: Fearon Publishers, Inc.

Mager, R. (1972). *Goal analysis.* Belmont, CA: Fearon Publishers/Lear Siegler, Inc.

Mager, R., & Pipe, P. (1970). *Analyzing performance problems.* Belmont, CA: Fearon Publishers/Lear Siegler, Inc.

Mandell, T. (1952). Letters to the editor. *Journal of Speech and Hearing Disorders, 17,* 433–435.

Maslow, A.H. (1954). *Motivation and personality.* New York: Harper and Bros.

Mawdsley, B. (1985a). *The integrative task-maturity model of supervision.* Presentation at Annual Meeting of the American Speech-Language-Hearing Association, Washington, DC.

Mawdsley, B. (1985b). *Kansas inventory of self-supervision.* Paper presented at convention of the American Speech-Language-Hearing Association, Washington, DC.

Mawdsley, B. (1987). Kansas inventory of self-supervision. In S. Farmer (Ed.), *Clinical supervision: A coming of age*. Proceedings of a conference held at Jekyll Island, GA: Las Cruces, NM, New Mexico State University.

Mayo, E. (1933). *The human problems of an industrial civilization*. New York: The MacMillan Co.

McAvoy, R. (1970). Measurable outcome with systematic observation. In Systematic Observation. *Journal of Research and Development in Education, 4*, 10–13.

McCrea, E. (1980). Supervisee ability to self-explore and four facilitative dimensions of supervisor behavior in individual conferences in speech-language pathology (Doctoral dissertation, Indiana University, 1980). *Dissertation Abstracts International, 41*, 2134B. (University Microfilms No. 80–29, 239)

McCrea, E. (1985). Supervision component in undergraduate clinical management class. In K. Smith (Moderator), *Preparation and training models for the supervisory process*. Short course presented at ASHA Convention, Washington, DC.

McCready, V., Shapiro, D., & Kennedy, K. (1987). Identifying hidden dynamics in supervision: Four scenarios. In M. Crago & M. Pickering (Eds.), *Supervision in human communication disorders: Perspectives on a process*. San Diego, CA: College Hill Press.

McGregor, D.M. (1960). *The human side of enterprise*. New York: McGraw-Hill Book Co.

McReynolds, L. (1974). Introduction to developing systematic procedures. In L. McReynolds (Ed.), *Developing systematic procedures for training children's language*. (ASHA Monograph 18). Washington, DC: American Speech and Hearing Association.

McReynolds, L., & Kearns, K. (1983). *Single-subject experimental designs in communicative disorders*. Baltimore: University Park Press.

McReynolds, L., & Thompson, C. (1986). Flexibility of single-subject experimental designs. Part I: Review of the basics of single-subject designs. *Journal of Speech and Hearing Disorders, 51*, 194–203.

Medley, D. (1975). Systematic observation schedules as measuring instruments. In R. Weinberg & F. Word (Eds.), *Observation of pupils and teachers in mainstream and special education settings: Alternative strategies*. Minneapolis: University of Minnesota, Leadership Training Institute.

Medley, D., & Mitzel, H. (1963). Measuring classroom behavior by systematic observation. In N. Gage (Ed.), *Handbook of research on teaching*. Chicago: Rand, McNally.

Mehrabian, A. (1969). *Methods and designs: Some referents and measures of nonverbal behavior*. Behavioral Research Methods and Instrumentation I.

Mehrabian, A. (1971). *Silent messages*. Belmont, CA: Wadsworth.

Michalak, D. (1969). Supervisory conferences improve teaching. *Florida Educational Research and Development Council Research Bulletin. 5.*

Milisen, R. (1939). Speech correction in the schools. *Journal of Speech Disorders, 4*, 241–245.

Miller, E. (1948). A public school program for hard of hearing children. *Journal of Speech Disorders, 13*, 256–259.

Miller, J. (1981). *Assessing language production in children*. Baltimore: University Park Press.

Miner, A. (1967). A symposium: Improving supervision of clinical practicum. *Asha, 9*, 471–482.

Miringoff, M. (1980). *Management in human service organizations*. NY: Macmillan Publishing Co., Inc.

Molyneaux, D., & Lane, V. (1982). *Effective interviewing: Techniques and analysis*. Boston: Allyn and Bacon, Inc.

Monnin, L., & Peters, K. (1977). Problem solving supervised experience in the schools. *Language, Speech and Hearing Services in Schools, 8*, 99–106.

Monnin, L., & Peters, K. (1981). *Clinical practice for speech-pathologists in the schools*. Springfield, IL: Charles C. Thomas.

Montalvo, B. (1973). Aspects of live supervision. *Family Process, 12*, 343–359.

Mosher, R., & Purpel, D. (1972). *Supervision: The reluctant profession*. Boston, MA: Houghton Mifflin Co.

Monly, G. (1960). *Psychology for effective teaching*. New York: Holt, Rinehart and Winston, Inc.

Mowrer, D. (1969). Evaluating speech therapy through precision recording. *Journal of Speech and Hearing Disorders, 34,* 239–245.

Mowrer, D. (1972). Accountability and speech therapy. *Asha, 14,* 111–115.

Mowrer, D. (1977). *Methods of modifying speech behaviors.* Columbus, OH: Charles E. Merrill Publishing Co.

Mullendore, J., Koller, D., & Payne, P. (1976). *The use of live closed circuit television for direct supervision.* Paper presented at the American Speech-Language-Hearing Association Annual Convention, Houston, TX.

Munson, C. (1983). *An introduction to clinical social work supervision.* New York: The Haworth Press.

Murray, K. (Ed.). (1970a). Systematic observation. *Journal of Research and Development in Education, 4*(1).

Murray, K. (1970b). The systematic observation movement. In Systematic Observation. *Journal of Research and Development in Education, 4*(1).

Myers, F. (1980). Clinician needs in the practicum setting. *SUPERvision. 4.*

Myers, R. (1971). Research on educational and vocational counseling. In A. Bergin & S. Garfield (Eds.), *Handbook of psychology and behavior analysis.* New York: John Wiley and Sons.

Naisbitt, J. (1984). *Megatrends.* NY: Warner Books, Inc.

Neale, J., & Liebert, R. (1973). *Science and behavior: An introduction to methods of research.* Englewood Cliffs, NJ: Prentice-Hall, Inc.

Neidecker, E. (1980). *School programs in speech-language.* Englewood Cliffs, NJ: Prentice-Hall, Inc.

Nelson, G. (1974). *Does supervision make a difference?* Paper presented at the annual convention of the American Speech and Hearing Association, Las Vegas, Nevada.

Nilsen, J. (1983). Supervisor's use of direct/indirect verbal conference style and alteration of clinical behavior. (Doctoral dissertation, University of Illinois, 1983). *Dissertation Abstracts International, 43,* 3935B. (University Microfilms No. 83–09, 991).

Northern, J., & Suter, A. (1972). Supportive personnel in audiology. *Asha, 14,* 354–357.

Oas, D., & Sparks, S. (1983, August). *Supervisor and self ratings of student clinical performance.* Unpublished manuscript, Western Michigan University, Kalamazoo.

Olsen, B.D. (1972). Comparisons of sequential interaction patterns in therapy of experienced, inexperienced clinicians in the parameters of articulation, delayed language, prosody and voice disorders (Doctoral dissertation, University of Denver, 1972). (University Microfilms, 72–33, 052)

O'Neil, J. (1985). The clinical supervisor—proctor or accountant? *Asha, 27,* 23–24.

O'Neil, J., & Peterson, M. (1964). The use of closed circuit television in a clinical speech training program. *Asha, 6,* 445–447.

Oratio, A. (1976). A factor-analytic study of criteria for evaluating student clinicians in speech pathology. *Journal of Communication Disorders, 9,* 199–210.

Oratio, A. (1977). *Supervision in speech pathology: A handbook for supervisors and clinicians.* Baltimore, MD: University Park Press.

Oratio, A. (1978). Comparative perceptions of therapeutic effectiveness by student clinicians and clinical supervisors. *Asha, 20,* 959–962.

Oratio, A. (1979). Computer-assisted interaction analysis in speech-language pathology and audiology. *Asha, 21,* 179–184.

Oratio, A., Sugarman, M., & Prass, M. (1981). A multivariate analysis of clinicians' perceptions of supervisory effectiveness. *Journal of Communication Disorders, 14,* 31–42.

O'Toole, T. (1973). Supervision of the clinical trainee. *Language, Speech and Hearing Services in Schools, 4,* 132–139.

Owens, R. (1970). *Organizational behavior in schools.* Englewood Cliffs, NJ: Prentice Hall, Inc.

Oyer, H. (Ed.). (1987). *Administration of programs in speech language pathology and audiology.* Englewood Cliffs, NJ: Prentice-Hall, Inc.

Paden, E. (1970). *A history of the American Speech and Hearing Association.* Washington, DC: American Speech and Hearing Association.

Palin, M., & Cohen, C. (1986). Technology in the schools. *Asha, 35.*

Pappas, F. (1983). *Managing the clinically marginal student in university training programs.* Paper presented at conference of American Speech-Language-Hearing Association.

Pascale, R.T., & Athos, A.G. (1981). *The art of Japanese management.* NY: Warner Books, Inc.

Peaper, R. (1984). An analysis of student perceptions of the supervisory conference and student developed agendas for that conference. *The Clinical Supervisor, 2,* 55–64.

Peaper, R., & Mercaitis, P. (1987). The nature of narrative written feedback provided to student clinicians: A descriptive study. In S. Farmer (Ed.), *Clinical supervision: A coming of age.* Proceedings of a conference held at Jekyll Island, GA: Las Cruces, NM, New Mexico State University.

Peaper, R., & Wener, D. (1984). A comparison of perceptions of written clinical plans and reports. *Asha, 26,* 37–41.

Pendergast, K. (1983). Accountability in a public school setting. *Seminars in Speech and Language, 4,* 131–147.

Perkins, W. (1962). Our profession—what is it? *Asha, 4,* 339–344.

Peters, T.J., & Waterman, R.H. (1982). *In search of excellence: Lessons from America's best-run companies.* New York: Harper and Row Publishers.

Pickering, M. (1977). An examination of concepts operative in the supervisory process and relationship. *Asha, 19,* 607–610.

Pickering, M. (1979). Interpersonal communication in speech-language pathology clinical practicum: A descriptive humanistic perspective. (Doctoral dissertation, Boston University School of Education, 1979). *Dissertation Abstracts International, 40,* 2140B. (University Microfilms No. 79–23, 892)

Pickering, M. (1980). *Introduction to qualitative research methodology: purpose, characteristics, procedures, examples.* Paper presented at the annual convention of the American Speech-Language-Hearing Association, Detroit.

Pickering, M. (1981). *Supervisory interaction: The subjective side.* Paper presented at the CUSPSPA meeting during the annual convention of the American Speech-Language-Hearing Association, Los Angeles.

Pickering, M. (1982). *Interpersonal communication in student-conducted therapy sessions.* Paper presented at the annual convention of the American Speech-Language-Hearing Association, Los Angeles.

Pickering, M. (1984). Interpersonal communication in speech-language pathology supervisory conferences: A qualitative study. *Journal of Speech and Hearing Disorders, 49,* 189–195.

Pickering, M. (1985). Clinical supervision in a university setting. In J. Bernthal (Ed.), *Proceedings: Sixth Annual Conference on Graduate Education.* Lincoln, NE: Department of Special Education and Communication Disorders.

Pickering, M. (1986). Communication. *Explorations—A journal of research at the University of Maine.* Orono, ME: University of Maine.

Pickering, M. (1987a). Interpersonal communication and the supervisory process: A search for Ariadne's thread. In M. Crago, and J. Pickering, (Eds.), *Supervision in human communication disorders: Perspectives on a process.* San Diego: College-Hill Press.

Pickering, M. (1987b). Supervision: A person-focused process. In J. Crago, & M. Pickering (Eds.), *Supervision in human communication disorders: Perspectives on a process.* San Diego: College-Hill Press.

Pickering, M., & McCready, V. (1983). *Supervisory journals: An 'inside' look at supervision.* SUPERvision, 7, 5–7.

Pittinger, A. (1972). An analysis of the patterns of verbal interaction and their relationship to self-reported satisfaction ratings and a measure of empathic accuracy in selecting secondary student teaching supervisory conferences. (Doctoral dissertation, University of Maryland, 1971). *Dissertation Abstracts International, 32,* 5658A. (University Microfilms No. 72–12, 847)

Popham, W.J., & Baker, E. (1970). *Establishing instructional goals.* Englewood Cliffs, NJ: Prentice-Hall, Inc.

Porch, B. (1967). *Porch index of communicative ability: Theory and development.* Palo Alto, CA: Consulting Psychologists Press.

Powell, T. (1987). A rating scale for measurement of attitudes toward clinical supervision. *SUPERvision 11,* 31–34.

Prather, E. (1967). An approach to clinical supervision. In A. Miner, A symposium: Improving supervision of clinical practicum. *Asha, 9,* 471–482.

Prescott, T. (1971). The development of a methodology for describing speech therapy. In T. Johnson (Ed.), *Clinical interaction and its measurement.* Logan: Utah State University.

Prescott, T., & Tesauro, P. (1974). A method for quantification and description of clinical interactions with aurally handicapped children. *Journal of Speech and Hearing Disorders, 39,* 235–243.

Prutting, C., Bagshaw, N., Goldstein, H., Juskowitz, S., & Umen, I. (1978). Clinician-child discourse: Some preliminary questions. *Journal of Speech and Hearing Disorders, 43,* 123–139.

Prutting, C., & Kirchner, D. (1983). Applied pragmatics. In T. Gallagher & C. Prutting (Eds.), *Pragmatic assessment and intervention issues in language.* San Diego: College-Hill Press.

Prutting, C., & Kirchner, D. (1987). A clinical appraisal of the pragmatic aspects of language. *Journal of Speech and Hearing Disorders, 52,* 105–119.

Rassi, J. (1978). *Supervision in audiology.* Baltimore, MD: University Park Press.

Rassi, J. (1985). Supervision in audiology. In K. Smith (Moderator), *Preparation and training models for the supervisory process.* Short course presented at the Annual Convention of American Speech-Language-Hearing Association, Washington, DC.

Rassi, J. (1987). The uniqueness of audiology supervision. In M. Crago & M. Pickering (Eds.), *Supervision in human communication disorders: Perspectives on a process.* San Diego: Little Brown-College Hill Press.

Rathnel, B. (1959, November). *The effect of operationalizing low-rated competencies from the Wisconsin Procedure for Appraisal of Clinical Competencies.* Paper presented at the annual convention of the American Speech and Hearing Association, Detroit.

Rees, M., & Smith, J. (1967). Supervised school experience for student clinicians. *Asha, 9,* 251–257.

Rees, M., & Smith, J. (1968). Some recommendations for supervised school experience for student clinicians. *Asha, 10,* 93–103.

Reid, J. (1982). Observer training in naturalistic research. In D. Hartman (Ed.), *Using observers to study behavior.* San Francisco: Jossey-Bass.

Reitz, J. (1970). The role of leadership. In J. Anderson (Ed.). *Conference on Supervision of Speech and Hearing Programs in the Schools.* Bloomington, IN: Indiana University.

Reitz, J. (1981). *Behavior in organizations.* Homewood, IL: Richard D. Irwin, Inc.

Robbins, S. (1937). Federal aid for speech defectives near. *Journal of Speech Disorders, 2,* 30–34.

Robbins, S. (1939). Changes in election of new members. *Journal of Speech Disorders, 4,* 78.

Roberts, J. (1980). Content and sequence analysis system. In J. Anderson, *Proceedings—Conference on Training in the Supervisory Process in Speech-Language Pathology and Audiology.* Bloomington, IN: Indiana University.

Roberts, J. (1982). An attributional model of supervisors' decision-making behavior in speech-language pathology. (Doctoral dissertation, Indiana University, 1981). *Dissertation Abstracts International, 42,* 2794B. (University Microfilms No. 81–28, 040)

Roberts, J., & Naremore, R. (1983). An attributional model of supervisors' decision-making behavior in speech-language pathology. *Journal of Speech and Hearing Research, 26,* 537–549.

Roberts, J., & Smith, K. (1982). Supervisor-supervisee role differences and consistency of behavior in supervisory conferences. *Journal of Speech and Hearing Research, 25,* 428–434.

Rockman, B. (1977). *Supervisor as clinician: A point of view.* Paper presented at the annual convention of the American Speech and Hearing Association, Chicago.

Rogers, C. (1951). *Client-centered therapy.* Boston: Houghton-Mifflin Company.

Rogers, C. (1957). The necessary and sufficient conditions of therapeutic personality change. *Journal of Consulting Psychology, 21,* 95–103.

Rogers, C. (1961). *On becoming a person: A therapist's view of psychotherapy.* Boston: Houghton Mifflin.

Rogers, C. (1962). The interpersonal relationship: The core of guidance. *Harvard Educational Review. 32,* 116–129.

Rogers, C. (1980). *A way of being.* Boston: Houghton Mifflin Co.

Rosaldo, M.Z. (1980). *Knowledge and passion: Mongol nations of self and social life.* Cambridge: Cambridge University Press.

Rosenshine, B. (1970). Evaluation of classroom instruction. *Review of Educational Research, 40,* 282.

Rosenshine, B. (1971). Research on teacher performance criteria. In B. Smith (Ed.), *Research in teacher education.* Englewood Cliffs, NJ: Prentice-Hall.

Rosenshine, B., & Furst, N. (1973). The use of direct observation to study teaching. In R. Travers (Ed.), *Second handbook of research on teaching.* Chicago, IL: Rand McNally College Publishing Company.

Runyan, S., & Seal, B. (1985). A comparison of supervisors' ratings while observing a language remediation session. *The Clinical Supervisor. 3,* 61–75.

Russell, L. (1976). *Aspects of supervision.* Unpublished manuscript, Temple University.

Russell, L., & Engle, B. (1977). *A study of the supervisory process.* Paper presented at the New Jersey Speech and Hearing Association Convention.

Russell, L., & Halfond, M. (1985). *An expanded view of the evaluative component of clinical supervision.* Paper presented at ASHA convention, Washington, DC.

Sales, S. (1966). Supervisory style and productivity: Review and theory. *Personnel Psychology, 19,* 575–586. Reading, MA: Addison-Wesley Publishing Co.

Sanders, N. (1966). *Classroom questions: What kinds?* New York: Harper and Row.

Sbaschnig, K., & Williams, C. (1983). *A reliability audit for supervisors.* Paper presented at the Annual Meeting of the American Speech-Language-Hearing Association. Cincinnati, OH.

Sbaschnig, K., & Williams, C. (1984). *A reliability audit for externship supervisors.* Paper presented at Annual Convention of the American Speech-Language-Hearing Association, San Francisco.

Scalero, A., & Eskenozi, C. (1976). The use of supportive personnel in a public school speech and language program. *Language, Speech and Hearing Services in Schools. 7,* 150–158.

Schieffelin, B. (1979). Getting it together: An ethnographic approach to the study of the development of communicative competence. In E. Ochs & B. Schieffelin (Eds.), *Developmental pragmatics.* New York: Academic Press.

Schneider, D., Hastorf, A., & Ellsworth, P. (1979). *Person perception.* Reading, MA: Addison-Wesley Publishing Co.

Schubert, G. (1974). Suggested minimal requirements for clinical supervisors. *Asha, 16,* 305.

Schubert, G. (1978). *Introduction to clinical supervision.* St. Louis, MO: W.H. Green.

Schubert, G., & Aitchison, C. (1975). A profile of clinical supervisors in college and university speech and hearing training programs. *Asha, 17,* 440–447.

Schubert, G., & Glick, A. (1974). A comparison of two methods of recording and analyzing student clinician-client interaction: ABC system and the "Boone" system. *Acta Symbolica, 5,* 39–56.

Schubert, G., & Gudmundson, P. (1976, November). *Effects of videotape feedback and interaction upon nonverbal behavior of student clinicians.* Paper presented at the ASHA convention, Houston.

Schubert, G., & Laird, B. (1975, December). The length of time necessary to obtain a representative sample of clinician-client interaction. *Journal of National Student Speech and Hearing Association,* 26–32.

Schubert, G., & Lyngby, A. (1977). The clinical fellowship year (CFY). *Journal of National Student Speech and Hearing Association, 5,* 22–29.

Schubert, G., & Mercer, A. (1975). Nonverbal behavior used by two different groups of clinicians during therapy. *Acta Symbolica, 6,* 41–58.

Schubert, G., Miner, A., & Till, J. (1973). *The analysis of behavior of clinicians (ABC) system.* Unpublished manuscript, University of North Dakota, Grand Forks.

Schubert, G., & Nelson, J. (1976). *Verbal behaviors occurring in speech pathology supervisory conferences.* Paper presented at ASHA convention, Houston.

Schwartz, P., & Ogilvy, J. (1980). *The emergent paradigm: Toward an aesthetics of life.* Paper presented at ESOM AR, Barcelona, Spain.

Sedge, R. (1987). Administration of a military-based program of speech-language pathology and audiology. In H. Oyer (Ed.), *Administration of programs in speech-language pathology and audiology.* Englewood Cliffs, NJ: Prentice-Hall, Inc.

Shanks, S. (1984). Expanding the clinic cubicle through the use of media. In H. Winitz (Ed.), *Treating articulation disorders.* Baltimore: University Park Press.

Shapiro, B.J., & Shapiro, P.P. (1971). *The relationship between satisfaction and performance in student teaching.* U.S. Department of Health, Education and Welfare. (ERIC Document Reproduction Service No. ED 056 997).

Shapiro, D. (1985). An experimental and descriptive analysis of supervisees' commitments and follow-through behaviors as one measure of supervisory effectiveness in speech-language pathology and audiology. (Doctoral Dissertation, Indiana University, 1984). *Dissertation Abstracts International, 45,* 2889B. (University Microfilms No. 84–26, 682)

Shapiro, D. (1985). Clinical supervision: A process in progress. *National Student Speech-Language-Hearing Association Journal*

Shefte, L. (1959). *An evaluation of certain aspects of student teaching programs for public school speech and hearing therapists.* Unpublished dissertation, University of Wisconsin.

Shelton, R., Elbert, M., & Arndt, W. (1967). A task for evaluation of articulation change: II. Comparison of task scores during baseline and lesson series testing. *Journal of Speech and Hearing Research, 10,* 578–586.

Shipley, K. (1977). *Analysis of interview behavior by categories.* Paper presented at the American Speech-Language-Hearing Association Annual Convention.

Shriberg, L., Filley, F., Hayes, D., Kwiatkowski, J., Shatz, J., Simmons, K., & Smith, M. (1974). *The Wisconsin procedure for appraisal of clinical competence (W-PACC).* Madison, WI: Department of Communicative Disorders, University of Wisconsin-Madison.

Shriberg, L., Filley, F., Hayes, D., Kwiatkowski, J., Shatz, J., Simmons, K., & Smith, M. (1975). *The Wisconsin procedure for appraisal of clinical competence (W-PACC): Model and data. Asha, 17,* 158–165.

Sidman, M. (1960). *Tactics of scientific research: Evaluating experimental data in psychology.* New York: Basic Books.

Siegel, G. (1975). The high cost of accountability. *Asha, 17,* 796–797.

Silverman, F. (1977a). Tutorial: Criteria for assessing therapy outcome on speech pathology and audiology. *Journal of Speech and Hearing Research, 20,* 5–20.

Silverman, F. (1977b). *Research design in speech pathology and audiology* (2nd ed.). Englewood Cliffs, NJ: Prentice-Hall, Inc.

Simon, A., & Boyer, E. (Eds.). (1970a). *Mirrors for behavior: An anthology of classroom observation instruments.* (Vol. A). Philadelphia: Research for Better Schools.

Simon, A., & Boyer, E. (Eds.). (1970b). *Mirrors for behavior: An anthology of classroom observation instruments.* (Vol. B). Philadelphia: Research for Better Schools.

Simon, A., & Boyer, E. (1974). *Mirrors for Behavior III.* Wyncote, PA: Communications Materials Center.

Skinner, B.F. (1954). The science of learning and the art of teaching. *Harvard Educational Review, 24,* 86–97.

Sleight, C. (1984a). Games people play in clinical supervision. *Asha, 26,* 27–29.

Sleight, C. (1984b). Supervisor self-evaluation in communication disorders. *The clinical supervisor, 2,* 31–42.

Sleight, C. (1985). Confidence and anxiety in student clinicians. *The Clinical Supervisor, 3,* 25–48.

Sloane, H., & MacAulay, B. (Eds.). (1968). *Operant procedures in remediating speech and language training.* Boston: Houghton Mifflin.

Smith, D., & Wiliamson, L. (1985). *Interpersonal communication: Roles, rules, strategies, and games.* (3rd ed.). Dubuque, IA: Wm. C. Brown Publishers.

Smith, G. (1977). Supervisory thought and practice in teacher education. In D. Kurpius, R. Baker, & I. Thomas (Eds.), *Supervision of applied training.* Westport, CT: Greenwood Press.

Smith, K. (1978). Identification of perceived effectiveness components in the individual supervisory conference in speech pathology and an evaluation of the relationship between ratings and content in the conference. (Doctoral dissertation, Indiana University, 1977). *Dissertation Abstracts International, 39,* 680B. (University Microfilms No. 78–13, 175)

Smith, K. (1979). *Supervisory conferences questions: Who asks them and who answers them.* Paper presented at Annual Convention of the American Speech and Hearing Association, Atlanta, Georgia.

Smith, K. (1980). Multidimensional Observational System for the Analysis of Interactions in Clinical Supervision (MOSAICS). In J. Anderson (Ed.), *Proceedings—Conference on Training in the Supervisory Process in Speech-Language Pathology and Audiology.* Bloomington, IN: Indiana University.

Smith, K. (Moderator). (1985). *Preparation and training models for the supervisory process.* Short course presented at ASHA convention, Washington, DC.

Smith, K., & Anderson, J. (1982a). Development and validation of an individual supervisory conference rating scale for use in speech-language pathology. *Journal of Speech and Hearing Research, 25,* 252–261.

Smith, K., & Anderson, J. (1982b). Relationship of perceived effectiveness to content in supervisory conferences in speech-language pathology. *Journal of Speech and Hearing Research, 25,* 243–251.

Smith, K., & Larson, L. (1975, November). *Minimum clinical competencies for speech pathology school practicum.* Paper presented at the ASHA convention, Washington, DC.

Snow, C., Midkiff-Borunda, S., Small, A., & Proctor, A. (1984). Therapy as social interaction: Analyzing the context for language remediation. *Topics in Language Disorders. 4,* 72–85.

Stace, A., & Drexler, A. (1969). Special training for supervisors of student clinicians: What private speech and hearing centers do and think about training their supervisors. *Asha, 11,* 318–320.

Starkweather, C.W. (1974). Behavior modification in training speech clinicians: Procedures and implications. *Asha, 16,* 607–611.

Stevens, S.S. (1968). Measurement, statistics, and the schemapiric view. *Science, 161,* 849–856.

Stewart, J., & D'Angelo, G. (1975). *Together: Communicating interpersonally.* Reading, MA: Addison-Wesley Publishing Company.

Stogdill, R., & Coons, A. (1957). (Eds.). *Leader behavior: Its description and measurement.* Columbus, OH: Bureau of Business Research, Ohio State University.

Strike, C., & Anderson, J. (in progress). *Training verbal behaviors of supervisors during the supervisory conference in speech-language pathology.* Bloomington, IN: Indiana University.

Stuntebeck, S.U. (1975). Perceived need satisfaction and teaching effectiveness: A study of university faculty. (Doctoral dissertation, University of Notre Dame, 1974). *Dissertation Abstracts International, 35.* (Microfilms No. 74–13, 451)

Sullivan, C. (1980). Clinical supervision: *A state of the art review.* Alexandria, VA: Association for Supervision and Curriculum Development.

Tanck, M. (1980). *A cooperative approach to improving instruction through supervision.* Presentation at Conference on Administration of Special Education. Bloomington: Indiana University.

Tannenbaum, A. (1966). *Social psychology of the work organization.* Belmont, CA: Wadsworth Publishing Co., Inc.

Tawney, J.W., & Gast, D.L. (1984). *Single-subject research in special education*. Columbus: Charles E. Merrill Publishing Company.

Taylor, F. (1911). *The principles of scientific management*. New York: Harper and Bros.

Thorndike, R. (1982). *Data collection and analysis*. NY: Gardener Press Co.

Tihen, L. (1984). Expectations of student speech/language clinicians during their clinical practicum. (Doctoral dissertation, Indiana University, 1983) *Dissertation Abstracts International, 44*, 3048B. (University Microfilms No. 84–01, 620)

Till, J. (1976, December). The use and misuse of evaluation forms. *Journal of National Student Speech and Hearing Association*, 48–53.

Travers, R. (Ed.). (1973). *Second handbook of research on teaching*. Chicago: Rand McNally College Publishing Company.

Trow, R. (1960). Role functions of the teacher in the instructional group. In *Dynamics of instructional groups*. National Society for the Study of Education Yearbook.

Tufts, L. (1984). A content analysis of supervisory conferences in communicative disorders and the relationship of the content analysis system to the clinical experience of supervisees. (Doctoral dissertation, Indiana University, 1983). *Dissertation Abstracts International, 44*, 3048B. (University Microfilms No. 84–01, 588)

Turton, L. (Ed.). (1973). *Proceedings of a Workshop on Supervision in Speech Pathology*. Ann Arbor: University of Michigan, Institute for the Study of Mental Retardation and Related Disabilities.

Turton, L. (1973). Diagnostic implications of articulation testing. In W.D. Wolfe & D.J. Goulding (Eds.), *Articulation and learning*. Springfield, IL: Charles Thomas.

Tyack, D., & Ingram, D. (1977). Children's production and comprehension of questions. *Journal of Child Language. 4*, 211–224.

Ulrich, S. (1985). Continuing education model of training. In K. Smith (Moderator), *Preparation and training models for the supervisory process*. Short course presented at Annual Convention of American Speech-Language-Hearing Association, Washington, DC.

Ulrich, S. (1987). Supervision: A developing speciality. In M. Crago & M. Pickering (Eds.), *Supervision in human communication disorders: perspectives on a process*. San Diego, CA: College-Hill Press.

Ulrich, S., & Giolas, T. (1977, November). *Status of clinical supervisors: A model for reappointment and promotion*. Paper presented at ASHA convention, Chicago.

Ulrich, S., & Watt, J. (1977, November). *Competence of clinical supervisors: A statistical analysis*. Paper presented at ASHA convention, Chicago.

Underwood, J. (1973). Interaction analysis between the supervisor and the speech and hearing clinician. (Doctoral dissertation, University of Denver, 1973). *Dissertation Abstracts International, 34*, 2995B. (University Microfilms No. 73–29, 608).

Underwood, J. (1979). *Underwood category system*. Unpublished manuscript, University of Northern Colorado, Greeley.

Van Dersal, C. (1974, September). The relationship of personality, values, and race to anticipation of the supervisory relationship. *Rehabilitation Counseling Bulletin*, 41–46.

Van Hattum, R., Page, J., Baskerville, R., Duguay, M., Conway, L., & Davis, T. (1974). The speech improvement system (SIS) taped program for remediation of articulation problems in the schools. *Language, Speech and Hearing in the Schools. 5*, 91–97.

Van Riper, C. (1965). Supervision of clinical practice. *Asha, 3*, 75–77.

Vander Kolk, C. (1974, September). The relationship of personality, values, and race to anticipation of the supervisory relationship. *Rehabilitation Counseling Bulletin*, 41–46.

Vargus, I. (1977). Supervision in social work. In D. Kurpius, R. Baker, & I. Thomas, I. (Eds.), *Supervision of applied training*. Westport, CT: Greenwood Press.

Ventry, I. M., & Schiavetti, N. (1980). *Evaluating research in speech pathology and audiology*. Reading, MA: Addison-Wesley Publishing Company.

Vetter, D. (1985). Evaluation of clinical intervention: Accountability. *Seminars in Speech and Language, 6*, 55–67.

Villareal, J. (Ed.). (1964). *Seminar on guidelines for supervision of clinical practicum.* Washington, DC: American Speech and Hearing Association.

Volz, H. (1976). The effects on clinician performance, client progress, and client satisfaction of two programs to enhance the helping skills of undergraduate students in speech pathology. (Doctoral dissertation, University of Pennsylvania, 1976). *Dissertation Abstracts International, 37,* 716B. (University Microfilms No. 76–17, 239.)

Volz, H., Klevans, D., Norton, S., & Putens, D. (1978). Interpersonal communication skills of speech-language pathology undergraduates: The effects of training. *Journal of Speech and Hearing Disorders, 43,* 524–541.

Ward, C. H. (1960). An electronic aide for teaching interviewing techniques. *Archives of General Psychiatry, 3,* 357–358.

Ward, L., & Webster, E. (1965a). The training of clinical personnel: I. Issues in conceptualization. *Asha, 7,* 38–41.

Ward, L., & Webster, E. (1965b). The training of clinical personnel: II. A concept of clinical preparation. *Asha, 7,* 103–106.

Webster's II New Riverside University Dictionary. (1984). Boston: The Riverside Publishing Co.

Weinberg, R., & Wood, F. (1975). *Observation of pupils and teachers in mainstream and special education settings: Alternative strategies.* Minneapolis: College of Education, University of Minnesota.

Weller, R. (1969). An observational system for analyzing clinical supervision of teachers. (Doctoral dissertation, Harvard University, 1969). *Dissertation Abstracts 29,* 1904A. (University Microfilms No. 69–18, 245).

Weller, R. (1971). *Verbal Communication in Instructional Supervision.* NY: Teachers College Press, Columbia University.

Wernimont, P.F. (1966). Intrinsic and extrinsic factors in job satisfaction. *Journal of Applied Psychology, 50*(1), 41–50.

Whiffen, R., & Byng-Hall, J. (1982). *Family therapy supervision.* NY: Grune & Stratton.

White, R., & Lippett, R. (1960). Leader behavior and member reaction in three "social climates." In D. Cartwright and A. Zander (Eds.), *Group dynamics: Research and theory* (2nd ed.). Evanston, IL: Row, Peterson and Co.

Whiteside, J. (1981). *Analysis of question type in supervisory conferences and classroom in speech-language pathology.* Unpublished manuscript, Indiana University, Bloomington.

Wiles, K. (1950). *Supervision for better schools.* Englewood Cliffs, NJ: Prentice Hall, Inc.

Willbrand, M., & Tibbitts, D. (1976). Compensation for supervisors of clinical practicum in public school settings. *Language, Speech and Hearing Services in the Schools, 7,* 128–131.

Wilson-Vlotman, A., & Blair, J. (1986). A survey of audiologists working full-time in school systems. *Asha, 28,* 33–38.

Wisconsin Speech-Language-Hearing Association, Inc. (1980). *Quality assurance program manual.* Milwaukee, WI: Wisconsin Speech-Language-Hearing Association.

Wittmer, J., & Myrick, R. (1974). *Facilitative teaching.* Pacific Palisades, CT: Goodyear Publishing Co.

Wollman, I.L., & Conover, H.B. (1979). The student clinician's reception of the supervisory process. *Ohio Journal of Speech and Hearing, 14,* 192–201.

Worchel, S., & Cooper, J. (1983). *Understanding social psychology.* Homewood, IL: The Dorsey Press.

Worthington, E., Jr., & Roehlke, H. J. (1979). Effective supervision as perceived by beginning counselors-in-training. *Journal of Consulting Psychology, 26,* 64–73.

A · P · P · E · N · D · I · C · E · S

Appendix A:
Supervisory Expectations Rating Scale
Lillian Larson

Please give your assessment of what you expect will happen during your future individual supervisory conferences. Circle the number that best represents the expected <u>level of occurrence</u> of the behaviors suggested by each item. The numbers correspond to the following categories:

1 — To a very little extent
2 — To a little extent
3 — To some extent
4 — To a great extent
5 — To a very great extent

1. Do you expect your supervisors will help you set goals for your client?   1   2   3   4   5

2. Do you expect your supervisors will use conference time to discuss ways to improve materials?   1   2   3   4   5

3. Do you expect your supervisors will motivate you to perform at your highest potential?   1   2   3   4   5

4. Do you expect you will state the objectives of your conferences?   1   2   3   4   5

5. Do you expect your supervisors will pay attention to what you are saying whenever you talk with them?   1   2   3   4   5

6. Do you expect you will ask many questions during your conferences?   1   2   3   4   5

7. Do you expect your supervisors will use your ideas in discussion during conferences?   1   2   3   4   5

8. Do you expect your supervisors will function as teachers who are instructing you?   1   2   3   4   5

9. Do you expect you will inform your supervisors of your needs?   1   2   3   4   5

10. Do you expect your supervisors will tell you the weaknesses in your clinical behavior?   1   2   3   4   5

11. Do you expect you will use conference time to provide information about the clinical session to your supervisors?   1   2   3   4   5

12. Do you expect your supervisors will be willing to listen to your professional problems?   1   2   3   4   5

13. Do you expect your supervisors will be available to talk to you immediately following clinical sessions?   1   2   3   4   5

14. Do you expect your supervisors will be the superiors and you the subordinate in the relationship?   1   2   3   4   5

15. Do you expect you will give value judgments about your clinical behavior?   1   2   3   4   5

16. Do you expect your supervisors will give suggestions on therapy techniques to be used in subsequent clinical sessions?   1   2   3   4   5

17. Do you expect your supervisors will be supportive of you?   1   2   3   4   5

From Larson, L. (1982). Perceived supervisory needs and expectations of experienced vs. inexperienced student clinicians. (Doctoral dissertation, Indiana University, 1981). *Dissertation Abstracts International, 42,* 4758B. (University Microfilms No. 82–11, 183)

18. Do you expect discussions with your supervisors will be focused
    on clients' behaviors rather than on your behavior?   1   2   3   4   5

19. Do you expect your supervisors will give a rationale for their
    statements or suggestions?   1   2   3   4   5

20. Do you expect your supervisors will demonstrate how to improve
    your performance?   1   2   3   4   5

21. Do you expect your supervisors will give you the opportunity
    to express your opinions?   1   2   3   4   5

22. Do you expect your supervisors will ask you to think about
    strategies that might have been done differently or that may
    be done in the future?   1   2   3   4   5

23. Do you expect your supervisors will be willing to listen to your
    personal problems?   1   2   3   4   5

24. How often do you expect your supervisors will meet with you
    for an individual conference?

    Please check each applicable time and then rate only those   **1** — most expected
    times checked according to your level of *expectation*.   **5** — least expected

    _____ weekly throughout practicum   1   2   3   4   5
    _____ weekly at beginning and end of practicum   1   2   3   4   5
    _____ at your request   1   2   3   4   5
    _____ at supervisor's request   1   2   3   4   5

25. What information sources have influenced your responses to
    the previous questions?

    Please check all applicable sources and then rate only those   **1** — most influential
    sources checked according to level of *influence*.   **5** — least influential

    _____ peer group (students at same training level)   1   2   3   4   5
    _____ graduate student clinicians (at more advanced level
            than you)   1   2   3   4   5
    _____ clinical supervisors   1   2   3   4   5
    _____ academic courses   1   2   3   4   5
    _____ training program policies (i.e. practicum manual) 1   2   3   4   5
    _____ other (please specify)

    _____   1   2   3   4   5

26. Do you have any expectations about supervision which have
    not been covered in the previous questions? If so, please specify
    in the space below.

Supervisory Needs Rating Scale
Lillian Larson

Regardless of what you indicated about your expectations, now indicate to what extent you need the same behaviors to occur during your future individual supervisory conferences. Circle the number that best represents the level of occurrence at which the behaviors suggested by each item are needed. The numbers correspond to the following categories:

1 — To a very little extent
2 — To a little extent
3 — To some extent
4 — To a great extent
5 — To a very great extent

1. To what extent do you need your supervisors to give suggestions on therapy techniques to be used in subsequent clinical sessions?　　1　2　3　4　5

2. To what extent do you need your supervisors to pay attention to what you are saying whenever you talk with them?　　1　2　3　4　5

3. To what extent do you need to inform your supervisors of your needs?　　1　2　3　4　5

4. To what extent do you need your supervisors to use your ideas in discussion during conferences?　　1　2　3　4　5

5. To what extent do you need your supervisors to be available to talk to you immediately following clinical sessions?　　1　2　3　4　5

6. To what extent do you need your supervisors to ask you to think about strategies that might have been done differently or that may be done in the future?　　1　2　3　4　5

7. To what extent do you need your supervisors to function as teachers who are instructing you?　　1　2　3　4　5

8. To what extent do you need to give value judgments about your clinical behavior?　　1　2　3　4　5

9. To what extent do you need your supervisors to demonstrate how to improve your performance?　　1　2　3　4　5

10. To what extent do you need discussions with your supervisors to be focused on clients' behaviors rather than on your behavior?　　1　2　3　4　5

11. To what extent do you need your supervisors to be willing to listen to your professional problems?　　1　2　3　4　5

12. To what extent do you need to use conference time to provide information about the clinical session to your supervisors?　　1　2　3　4　5

13. To what extent do you need your supervisors to tell you the weaknesses in your clinical behavior?　　1　2　3　4　5

14. To what extent do you need to ask many questions during your conferences?　　1　2　3　4　5

15. To what extent do you need your supervisors to give a rationale for their statements or suggestions?　　1　2　3　4　5

From Larson, L. (1982). Perceived supervisory needs and expectations of experienced vs. inexperienced student clinicians. (Doctoral dissertation, Indiana University, 1981). *Dissertation Abstracts International, 42,* 4758B. (University Microfilms No. 82–11, 183)

16. To what extent do you need your supervisors to be the superiors and you the subordinate in the relationship?   1   2   3   4   5

17. To what extent do you need your supervisors to give you the opportunity to express your opinions?   1   2   3   4   5

18. To what extent do you need your supervisors to use conference time to discuss ways to improve materials?   1   2   3   4   5

19. To what extent do you need your supervisors to be willing to listen to your personal problems?   1   2   3   4   5

20. To what extent do you need to state the objectives of your conferences?   1   2   3   4   5

21. To what extent do you need your supervisors to help you set goals for your client?   1   2   3   4   5

22. To what extent do you need your supervisors to be supportive of you?   1   2   3   4   5

23. To what extent do you need your supervisors to motivate you to perform at your highest potential?   1   2   3   4   5

24. How often do you need your supervisors to meet with you for an individual conference?

    Please check each applicable time and then rate only those times checked according to your level of *need*.

    1 — most needed
    5 — least needed

    _____ weekly throughout practicum   1   2   3   4   5
    _____ weekly at beginning and end of practicum   1   2   3   4   5
    _____ at your request   1   2   3   4   5
    _____ at supervisor's request   1   2   3   4   5

25. What information sources have influenced your responses to the previous questions?

    Please check all applicable sources and then rate only those sources checked according to level of *influence*.

    1 — most influential
    5 — least influential

    _____ peer group (students at same training level)   1   2   3   4   5
    _____ graduate student clinicians (at more advanced level than you)   1   2   3   4   5
    _____ clinical supervisors   1   2   3   4   5
    _____ academic courses   1   2   3   4   5
    _____ training program policies (i.e. practicum manual)   1   2   3   4   5
    _____ other (please specify)

    _____   1   2   3   4   5

26. Do you have any supervisory needs which have not been covered in the previous questions? If so, please specify in the space below.

From Larson, L. (1982). Perceived supervisory needs and expectations of experienced vs. inexperienced student clinicians. (Doctoral dissertation, Indiana University, 1981). *Dissertation Abstracts International, 42*, 4758B. (University Microfilms No. 82–11, 183)

Appendix B:
A Rating Scale for Measurement of Attitudes Toward Clinical Supervision
Thomas W. Powell

This scale is designed to measure attitudes toward clinical supervision. Please read each item carefully and circle the response which best describes your attitude for that item.

> **SA** = *Strongly Agree*
> **A** = *Agree*
> **U** = *Undecided*
> **D** = *Disagree*
> **SD** = *Strongly Disagree*

1. Supervisees should analyze their own behavior.   SA   A   U   D   SD

2. The supervisor and the supervisee should strive for a collegial relationship rather than a superior-subordinate relationship.   SA   A   U   D   SD

3. The supervisor should be more responsible for the client than the supervisee.   SA   A   U   D   SD

4. Supervisees should play an active role in the supervisory process.   SA   A   U   D   SD

5. The supervisee should be subordinate to the supervisor.   SA   A   U   D   SD

6. The supervisee should be more responsible for the client than the supervisor.   SA   A   U   D   SD

7. Written feedback should consist of the supervisor's opinions.   SA   A   U   D   SD

8. The supervisor and the supervisee should plan jointly for the supervisory conference.   SA   A   U   D   SD

9. Self-analysis by the supervisee is more important than the supervisor's analysis of the supervisee.   SA   A   U   D   SD

10. The supervisor should dominate the supervisory conference.   SA   A   U   D   SD

11. The supervisory conference should focus on the supervisee rather than on the client.   SA   A   U   D   SD

12. The supervisory conference should focus on the client's behavior.   SA   A   U   D   SD

13. The supervisor should select goals for the supervisee.   SA   A   U   D   SD

14. Problems in therapy should be solved by the supervisor.   SA   A   U   D   SD

15. Supervisee's ideas are less important than the supervisor's ideas.   SA   A   U   D   SD

From Powell, T. (1987). A rating scale for measurement of attitudes toward clinical supervision. *SUPERvision, 11,* 31–34.

Directions for Administration and Scoring of the Clinical Supervision Attitude Scale

1.   Respondents should be asked to read each item and mark whether they strongly agree, agree, are undecided, disagree, or strongly disagree with the statement.

2. For positively worded items (i.e., items 1, 2, 4, 6, 8, 9, 11), assign values as follows:
    5 points: Strongly Agree
    4 points: Agree
    3 points: Undecided
    2 points: Disagree
    1 point: Strongly Disagree

3. For negatively worded items (i.e., items 3, 5, 7, 10, 12, 13, 14, 15), assign values as follows:
    1 point: Strongly Agree
    2 points: Agree
    3 points: Undecided
    4 points: Disagree
    5 points: Strongly Disagree

4.   Once point values have been assigned to each item, sum the points across all 15 items. The total should be between 15 (lowest possible score corresponding to one point per item) and 75 (highest possible score corresponding to five points per item.)

Appendix C:
Individual Supervisory Conference Rating Scale (ISCRS)
Kathryn J. Smith

Name_____ Date_____

Name of Supervisor or Student Clinician_____

Circle one: individual client   group

Please give your assessment of what happened in the conference just completed by rating the following items. Circle the number that best represents the level of occurrence of the activity suggested by each item. You can rate each item anywhere from one to seven.

	Definitely no	Neutral				Definitely yes
1. The clinician is reluctant to ask questions.	1 2 3 4 5 6 7
2. The supervisor provides justification for statements or suggestions.	1 2 3 4 5 6 7
3. The conference time is used to discuss ways to improve materials.	1 2 3 4 5 6 7
4. The supervisor offers suggestions on therapy techniques during the conference.	1 2 3 4 5 6 7
5. The supervisor uses the clinician's ideas in discussion during the conference.	1 2 3 4 5 6 7
6. The supervisor ignores problems presented by the clinician.	1 2 3 4 5 6 7
7. The conference time is used to provide feedback to the clinician about the clinical session.	1 2 3 4 5 6 7
8. Supervisors and clinicians participate in a teacher-student relationship.	1 2 3 4 5 6 7
9. The supervisor uses a supportive style.	1 2 3 4 5 6 7
10. The supervisor helps the clinician set realistic goals for the clients.	1 2 3 4 5 6 7
11. The clinician verbalizes needs.	1 2 3 4 5 6 7
12. The conference time is used to discuss weaknesses in the clinician's clinical behavior.	1 2 3 4 5 6 7
13. The supervisor presents value judgments about the clinician's clinical behavior.	1 2 3 4 5 6 7
14. A written summary of the supervisor's observations is given to the clinician during the conference.	1 2 3 4 5 6 7
15. Supervisors and clinicians participate in a superior-subordinate relationship.	1 2 3 4 5 6 7
16. The supervisor states the objectives of the conference.	1 2 3 4 5 6 7

From Smith, K. (1978). Identification of perceived effectiveness components in the individual supervisory conference in speech pathology and an evaluation of the relationship between ratings and content in the conference. (Doctoral dissertation, Indiana University, 1977). *Dissertation Abstracts International, 39*, 680B. (University Microfilms No. 78–13, 175)

Appendix D:
The Wisconsin Procedure for Appraisal Of Clinical Competence (W-PACC)

In 1971, the clinical staff of the Department of Communicative Disorders, University of Wisconsin—Madison assigned themselves an in-house research project: to make explicit the processes by which students in clinical practicum are appraised and graded. In serial studies over three years, this research has yielded information in three areas: (1) a working conception of clinical supervision and the appraisal process, (2) a procedure for summative appraisal of clinical competence, and (3) an aggregate of descriptive information on correlates of supervisory processes and clinical competence.

The purpose of this Applications Manual is to train potential users in the summative appraisal procedure titled: *The Wisconsin Procedure for Appraisal of Clinical Competence* (W-PACC). Information on both the conception of supervision underlying this procedure and reliability and validity data are presented in detail elsewhere. However, the following section is a brief summary of critical assumptions underlying application of W-PACC.

ASSUMPTIONS ABOUT CLINICAL SUPERVISION AND APPRAISAL

Figure 1 is a conception of basic elements in the supervisory process and appraisal. Subsequent sections of this manual will clarify terms and concepts expressed in Figure 1 and those which are incompletely developed here. Essentially, W-PACC is based on the following three working assumptions:

1. In its fullest sense, clinical practicum competence is currently assessable only through the individual "filters" of a supervisor. This is comparable to the academic freedom given to faculty in the classroom situation. "Objective" competency criteria for the full range of clinical skills and professional behaviors have not been (and may never be) universally adopted by working professionals.
2. Assessment of clinical skills involves two types of judgments. Is the clinician effective in a given skill? To what extent is effectiveness independent of the need for supervisory input?
3. Several factors may delimit the effective/independence scores achieved during any term of supervision; however, an adjustment for both entry characteristics and "process" characteristics (i.e., rate of clinician's learning and nature and quantity of a supervisor's input efforts can be made when assigning a grade.

From Shriberg, L., Filley, F., Hayes, D., Kwiatkowski, J., Schatz, J., Simmons, K., & Smith, M. (1974). *The Wisconsin procedure for appraisal of clinical competence (W-PACC)*. Madison, WI: Department of Communicative Disorders, University of Wisconsin-Madison.

335

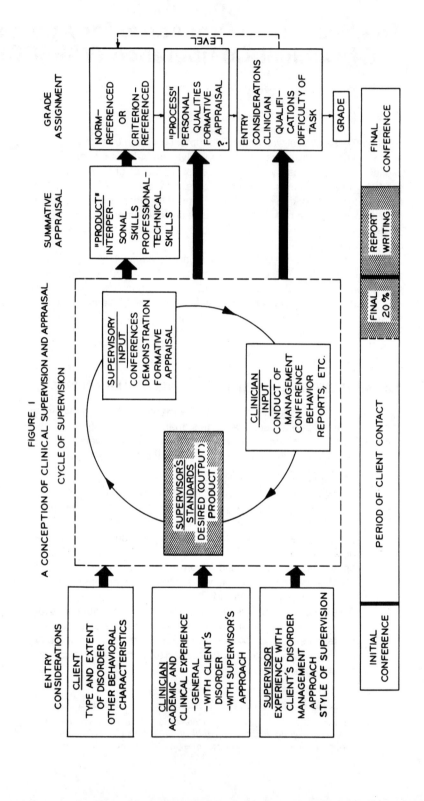

FIGURE I

A CONCEPTION OF CLINICAL SUPERVISION AND APPRAISAL

In W-PACC, each supervisor is given both the right and the responsibility to appraise the output "product" (e.g., clinician effectiveness during the last 20 percent of a semester, quarter, etc.) of his/her "supervisory-cycle" efforts. Summative product appraisal then is based on the extent to which effectiveness is demonstrated to be independent of supervisory input, and grades can be assigned from normative or criterion-referenced product score tables which adjust for the entrance characteristics of each trainee.

OVERVIEW OF THE WISCONSIN PROCEDURE FOR APPRAISAL OF CLINICAL COMPETENCE (W-PACC)

Subsequent pages of this manual are organized as a series of *Guidelines* which roughly correspond to the chronology of application of W-PACC. Following the assumptions just reviewed, W-PACC is a quantitative framework for appraisal of clinical trainees. Importantly, it allows the flexibility needed to accommodate individual differences across supervisors, practicums, and clinicians. Hence, the *Guidelines* to follow include choice points for the supervisor. The chronology of W-PACC administration is as follows:

Step	Procedures	W-PACC Manual Reference
1	During the initial conference(s) the supervisor assigns the clinician to a Level.	Fig. 1 (entry considerations) Guideline 1
2	During the initial conference(s) with the clinician, the supervisor reviews all pertinent information in this manual, including item descriptors for the practicum. The clinician should be fully aware of the basis for appraisal and grading.	Fig. 1 All Guidelines All Appendices
3	Supervision proceeds in the customary mode for the practicum, including use of formative appraisal instruments, observational analyses, etc. Filling out a Clinician Appraisal Form (CAF) at mid-term is optional.	Fig. 1 (cycle of supervision)
4	At the completion of the term the supervisor fills out a CAF, based on the clinician's performance during the last 20 percent of the term, i.e., appraisal of the "product" of supervision.	Fig. 1 (appraisal) Guidelines II, III, IV, V
5	Supervisor calculates interpersonal Skills, Professional-Technical Skills and "Average" Scale scores on CAF.	Fig. 1 Guideline VI
6	Supervisor assigns a grade.	Guideline VII

GUIDELINE I. ASSIGNMENT OF CLINICIAN TO LEVEL

Rationale

As indicated in Figure 1, a clinician's entrance characteristics for a practicum experience should be taken into account at the end-of-term grade assignment. To accomplish this, entry considerations have been formalized to four clinician Levels (Level I, II, III, IV). Each level (see Figure 2.—Criteria for Level Assignment) accounts for (1) a clinician's academic and clinical background relative to the practicum needs and expectations (e.g., client, task, supervisor) and (2) the total number of supervised clinical clock hours the clinician has accumulated. On this latter criterion, the assumption is that basic principles of and experience in clinical management are summative and generalizable.

When to Assign Level

At the *beginning* of the practicum assignment, the clinician and the supervisor should review the clinician's previous experiences (as below) and circle the appropriate level on the Clinician Appraisal Form (CAF).

How to Assign Level (Refer to Figure 2)

1. Under the column titled "Experience," find the Level at which the clinician meets the total number of supervised *therapy* clock hours criteria (do not include observation hours).
2. Inspect the other criteria at that Level:
   a. If the clinician meets all of the criteria for the Level as required under the column titled "Requirements," assign the clinician to that Level.
   b. If the clinician does not meet the required criteria, move back one level only and assign the clinician to this Level (even though some of the requirements will be exceeded). Note that if the clinician does not meet the criteria listed under "Academic or Equivalent Information" listed for Level III and Level IV, move back *only one level*.

GUIDELINE II. STRUCTURE OF THE CLINICIAN APPRAISAL FORM

The Clinician Appraisal Form (Appendix A) consists of: (1) a face sheet for summarizing pertinent information; (2) an Interpersonal Skills Scale (10 items); (3) a Professional-Technical Skills Scale (28 items); (4) a Personal Qualities Scale (10 items). Completion of face sheet information (Appendix A) is self-explanatory; calculation of Scale scores is discussed in Guideline VI.

LEVEL	REQUIREMENTS	EXPERIENCE	NUMBER OF CLIENTS	IMMEDIATE PRACTICUM	ACADEMIC OR EQUIVALENT INFO.
I	STUDENT CLINICIAN MUST MEET TWO OR MORE CRITERIA	LESS THAN 20 THERAPY CLOCK HOURS OF PRACTICUM WITH 1/4 TIME SUPERVISED OR MORE THAN 20 WITH LESS THAN 1/4 TIME SUPERVISED	NONE PREVIOUSLY OR FIRST SEMESTER OF PRACTICUM	PAST EXPERIENCES, NUMBER OF CLIENTS, OR CLINICAL PREPARATION IS INSUFFICIENT IN SUPERVISOR'S JUDGMENT	IS OR IS NOT PREPARED, IN SUPERVISOR'S JUDGMENT
II	STUDENT CLINICIAN MUST MEET OR EXCEED ALL CRITERIA	AT LEAST 30–40 THERAPY CLOCK HOURS OF PRACTICUM WITH 1/4 TIME SUPERVISED	AT LEAST 2 CLIENTS AND/OR THE EQUIVALENT OF A SEMESTER'S THERAPY EXPERIENCE	FIRST CLIENT WITH THIS PROBLEM	HAS OR IS CURRENTLY RECEIVING, IN SUPERVISOR'S JUDGMENT
III	STUDENT CLINICIAN MUST MEET OR EXCEED ALL CRITERIA	AT LEAST 90–100 THERAPY CLOCK HOURS OF PRACTICUM WITH 1/4 TIME SUPERVISED	AT LEAST 5–6 CLIENTS AND/OR A STUDENT TEACHING EXPERIENCE	FIRST CLIENT WITH THIS PROBLEM OR FIRST EXPERIENCE WITH THIS SPECIFIC MANAGEMENT APPROACH	*HAS OR IS CURRENTLY RECEIVING, IN SUPERVISOR'S JUDGMENT
IV	STUDENT CLINICIAN MUST MEET OR EXCEED ALL CRITERIA	AT LEAST 150–200 THERAPY CLOCK HRS. OF PRACTICUM WITH 1/4 TIME SUPERVISED	AT LEAST 8-10 CLIENTS	APPROXIMATELY THE SAME MANAGEMENT APPROACH USED WITH AT LEAST ONE OTHER CLIENT	*HAS OR IS CURRENTLY RECEIVING, IN SUPERVISOR'S JUDGMENT

* IF THE STUDENT CLINICIAN DOES NOT MEET THIS CRITERION, MOVE BACK ONLY ONE LEVEL

FIGURE 2. CRITERIA FOR ASSIGNMENT OF CLINICIAN LEVEL

Interpersonal Skills Scale

The 10 items in this scale appraise the clinician's ability to relate to and interact with the client, the client's family, and other professionals in a manner which is conducive to effective management.

Professional-Technical Skills Scale

The 28 items in this scale are nominally divided into four subdomains:

Developing and Planning: (8 items) — the clinician's approach to the task
Teaching: (9 items) — the clinician's ability to modify behavior
Assessment: (7 items) — the clinician's ability to assess behavior and make recommendations
Reporting: (4 items) — the clinician's ability to formulate oral and written reports

Personal Qualities

The 10 items of this scale provide additional information about the clinicians' general responsibility in clinical tasks. Clinicians' scores on this scale have been found to be statistically unrelated to effectiveness decisions. However, this information is available for grading decisions (see Guideline VII).

GUIDELINE III. INTERPRETATION OF CAF ITEMS

Background

The following statements about interpretation of items on each Scale (Interpersonal Skills, Professional-Technical Skills) on the Clinician Appraisal Form (CAF) are important to an understanding of the appraisal procedure:

1. At first inspection, some items on the CAF may appear to be appraising similar behaviors. In part, this is due to the necessary brevity of description for each item. Each of the items *is meant to* tap a *different* sub-skill within a Scale domain or sub-skill domain.

2. In keeping with the conception of supervision described, some items are interpreted differently by different supervisors — or the same supervisor may need to interpret an item differently for different practicum sites. Hence, explicit "Item Descriptors" are needed.

3. Appendix B is a list of Item Descriptors contributed by supervisors who have had considerable experience with the CAF. These descriptors should both *clarify item wording* and indicate *item flexibility*; they are suggestive rather than exhaustive.

Recommendation

Each supervisor who uses the CAF should derive *his/her own* descriptors for CAF items, using the descriptors presented in Appendix B *only as possible guidelines*. This suggestion is critical because:

1. Preparing descriptors for items will force an explicit understanding of how each item relates to the Scale domain (and for Professional-Technical Skills items, to sub-skill domains).

2. Items which initially seem similar can be differentiated.

3. Different practicums may warrant different descriptors for the same item.

4. Both test-retest stability and consistency in scoring items across students will be enhanced.

5. Supervisors have found such pre-determined descriptors to be extremely helpful in conferencing with students,—both as initial guidelines to appraisal domains and for end-of-term feedback (see Overview of W-PACC—Step 1).

GUIDELINE IV. MATCHING CLINICIAN BEHAVIORS TO NUMERICAL VALUES

Supervisors should adopt some explicit scheme for matching clinician behaviors to numerical values—i.e., the "decision" process. Scoring a CAF requires that a number from 1–10 be circled for each item (or "Does Not Apply" can be used for any of a number of reasons). Data (available elsewhere) indicate that supervisors *can* use this 10-point system reliably. Each of the following two schemes has been used successfully. *Scheme 2 may be particularly useful when a supervisee has more than one client.*

SCHEME 1. *A DESCRIPTIVE/QUANTITATIVE SCHEME*

Figure 3 contains the information and the sequence of decisions used in application of this scheme. For *each* item on the CAF, essentially two sequential decisions are made:

First decision: Referring to the column headings on the CAF (as reproduced in Figure 3) the supervisor first decides which of the four column headings best matches the clinician's behavior for *70% of the time or occasions*. Recall that this decision is made on the "product" of supervision, i.e., clinician behavior during the last 20% of the supervisory term. If clinician behaviors appear to warrant placement *between* either of two column headings, select the number next to the boundary which best quantifies the level of assistance needed—and no second level decision is necessary.

Second decision: The decision as to which of the numbers within a column heading best matches clinician behavior is next made by applying the descriptors listed under each column heading (Figure 3).

SCHEME 2. *A PROPORTIONAL/QUANTITATIVE SCHEME*

Figure 4 is an alternative scheme for matching clinician behaviors to a numerical value. This scheme accounts for the "proportion" of time or occurrences which a clinician needs assistance from the supervisor. It assumes that clinicians will need varying amounts of assistance only in *adjacent* column headings. To use this procedure:

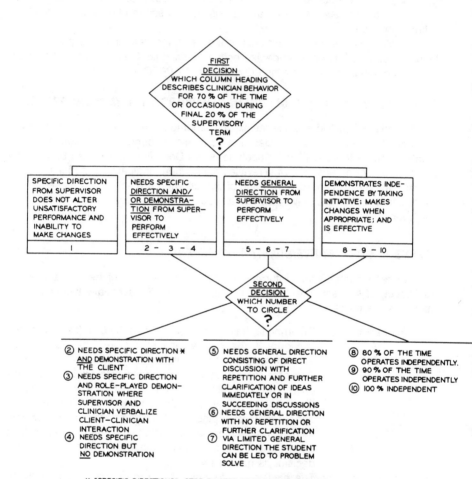

FIRST
DECISION
WHICH COLUMN HEADING
DESCRIBES CLINICIAN BEHAVIOR
FOR 70 % OF THE TIME
OR OCCASIONS DURING
FINAL 20 % OF THE
SUPERVISORY
TERM
?

SPECIFIC DIRECTION FROM SUPERVISOR DOES NOT ALTER UNSATISFACTORY PERFORMANCE AND INABILITY TO MAKE CHANGES	NEEDS SPECIFIC DIRECTION AND/ OR DEMONSTRA-TION FROM SUPER-VISOR TO PERFORM EFFECTIVELY	NEEDS GENERAL DIRECTION FROM SUPERVISOR TO PERFORM EFFECTIVELY	DEMONSTRATES INDE-PENDENCE BY TAKING INITIATIVE; MAKES CHANGES WHEN APPROPRIATE; AND IS EFFECTIVE
1	2 - 3 - 4	5 - 6 - 7	8 - 9 - 10

SECOND
DECISION
WHICH NUMBER
TO CIRCLE
?

② NEEDS SPECIFIC DIRECTION ✱ AND DEMONSTRATION WITH THE CLIENT
③ NEEDS SPECIFIC DIRECTION AND ROLE-PLAYED DEMON-STRATION WHERE SUPERVISOR AND CLINICIAN VERBALIZE CLIENT-CLINICIAN INTERACTION
④ NEEDS SPECIFIC DIRECTION BUT NO DEMONSTRATION

⑤ NEEDS GENERAL DIRECTION CONSISTING OF DIRECT DISCUSSION WITH REPETITION AND FURTHER CLARIFICATION OF IDEAS IMMEDIATELY OR IN SUCCEEDING DISCUSSIONS
⑥ NEEDS GENERAL DIRECTION WITH NO REPETITION OR FURTHER CLARIFICATION
⑦ VIA LIMITED GENERAL DIRECTION THE STUDENT CAN BE LED TO PROBLEM SOLVE

⑧ 80 % OF THE TIME OPERATES INDEPENDENTLY.
⑨ 90 % OF THE TIME OPERATES INDEPENDENTLY
⑩ 100 % INDEPENDENT

✱ "SPECIFIC DIRECTIONS"–STEP-BY-STEP REVIEW OF EVERY ASPECT OF THE PROBLEM

FIGURE 3. A DESCRIPTIVE/QUANTITATIVE SCHEME FOR MATCHING CLINICIAN BEHAVIORS TO NUMERICAL VALUES

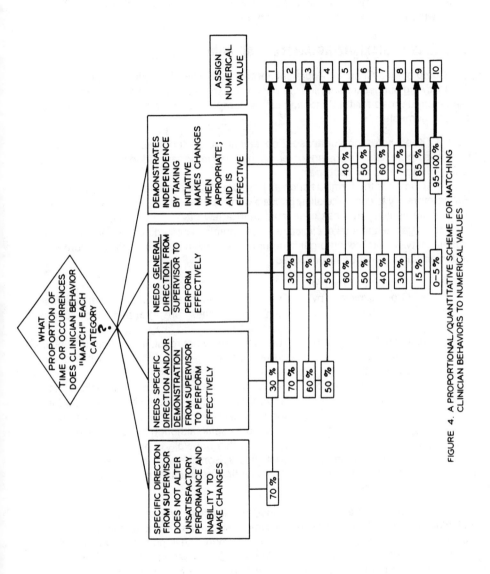

FIGURE 4. A PROPORTIONAL/QUANTITATIVE SCHEME FOR MATCHING CLINICIAN BEHAVIORS TO NUMERICAL VALUES

1. For *each* CAF item, decide the proportion of time or occurrences for which a clinician requires the type of assistance described by the four column headings.
2. Then, using the conversion values in Figure 4, circle the number on the CAF which corresponds to that proportion.

GUIDELINE V. MAXIMIZING RELIABLE SCORING

Completing a Clinician Appraisal Form should average 20 minutes per student. The following suggestions, which are based on experience and extensive discussion, are recommended for the "mechanics" of completing the forms at the conclusion of each semester:

1. Keep notes on supervisory observations, conferences, lesson plans, and formative appraisals. This is endorsed as the *most* important aid to making valid and reliable judgments for each item.
2. Complete the forms *as soon as possible* after the term of therapy has ended. Furthermore, try to complete all appraisals within a relatively short space of time, i.e., try to avoid spacing the task over more than a few days.
3. Organize the total of clinicians to be appraised according to *some* sub-group commonality. The following organizing principles, listed here in decreasing order of endorsed value, have been employed:

Grouping Principle	*Comments*
a. Group clinicians by practicum site	This is by far the most useful principle; students from similar sites are grouped and scored sequentially.
b. Group clinicians by similar client disorders	This may or may not result in a grouping similar to the above, e.g. group all clinicians who worked with stuttering, etc.
c. Group clinicians of similar Levels	Grouping by Level, e.g., all Level 1 clinicians, then all Level II etc. may at first appear logical. However, supervisors have found the two principles above to be more useful, although for some supervisory situations this principle is preferred.
d. Group clinicians by similarity in overall clinical skills	Some supervisors prefer to appraise their "best" clinicians first, regardless of Level, etc.

A *combination* of these grouping principles may be most useful, with one principle being used for the first organization into sub-groups, and a second principle for further sequencing of clinicians for scoring within each group. The important recommendation is for supervisors to adopt *some* organizing principle for scoring a group of clinicians, rather than filling out CAF's in a non-specified or chance sequence.

GUIDELINE VI. COMPUTATIONAL PROCEDURES FOR DERIVING SKILL SCALE PERCENTAGES

After having circled values for each item chosen for appraisal, the supervisor can calculate Scale scores on Interpersonal Skills, Professional-Technical Skills, and an "Average" of these two Scales. These values, expressed as percentages (to adjust for unscored items) are entered in the appropriate boxes on the face sheet of the CAF (see Appendix A). For each Scale, completing the following procedure will yield the Scale percentage:

1. Add the values circles for each item used. This total becomes the NUMERATOR.

    Example: If a student received five "7"s and three "8"s on the Interpersonal Skills Scale (two items were not scored) the total equals: 35 + 24 = 59

2. Multiply only the number of items actually used by 10. This product becomes the DENOMINATOR.

    Example: For the student above, only eight items were used, hence: 8 × 10 = 80

3. Divide the NUMERATOR by the DENOMINATOR; move decimal point two places to the right; round to a whole number (move any decimal .5 or above to the next highest *whole number*)

    Example: As above 59/80 = .7375
    = 73.75
    = 74%

4. Record each of the percentages obtained, Interpersonal Skills and Professional Technical Skills, in the appropriate boxes on the face sheet. An "Average" of these two scores (i.e., the sum of the two scores divided by two) is also entered in the appropriate box on the face sheet.

GUIDELINE VII. SUGGESTIONS FOR GRADE ASSIGNMENTS

Discussion

A conception of the elements of grade assignment is presented in Figure 1 (see Summative Appraisal and Grade Assignment). The working assumption is that a grade can be derived from a three-way weighting of "product" information, "process" information, and "entry characteristics" considerations. Both the function of "clinical" grades and the contingencies for receiving a specific grade in a particular setting should influence weighting and grading decisions. For example, grades can be used (1) to certify skill, (2) to predict success, (3) to suggest entry points for subsequent practicums, (4) as feedback to clinicians, (5) to compare the outcomes of different groups, and (6) to allow continuation in a clinical program (the customary academic contingency). Functional differences among grades of A, AB, B, BC, C, D, for example, might vary according to the purpose(s) above for which a set of grades is used. As with previous Guidelines, the suggestion is that *some* explicit framework for grade assignment must be developed by a supervisory team. Three suggestions for grade assignment are presented here.

SUGGESTIONS FOR GRADE ASSIGNMENT

Procedure 1: Non-Specified

Some supervisors or supervisory groups may prefer to use the CAF skill scores (Interpersonal, Professional-Technical, "Average") and Personal Qualities Summary solely as advisory input to grading decisions. Some supervisors prefer to avoid unwarranted use of "numbers" to characterize clinician competence. Following this procedure, which might be closest to a subjective approach to grading, the supervisor weighs (1) the CAF skill scores, (2) the "process" information, and (3) the student's level and difficulty of the client—and in some *non-specified* fashion, determines an appropriate grade. Such procedures are defensible to the extent that grading decisions obtain the same validity, on any of the six purposes for grading listed above, as that obtained by supervisors using more explicit quantitative procedures.

Procedure 2: Individual-Supervisory Norms

Procedures 2 and 3 are each in turn, subdivided into two options. These options refer to two possible ways of converting Interpersonal Skills or Professional-Technical Skills scores (or the "Average") to tentative letter grades.

OPTION A—NORMATIVE-REFERENCED

Step 1. Each supervisor plots the distributions of scale scores[1] obtained by her supervisees at each Level (or each Level by Practicum Site), for the current term and cumulatively over several terms.

Step 2. A tentative letter-grade is assigned based on a clinician's performance in comparison with peers. Either natural "breaks" in the distribution or frequency percentages can be used, similar to grading practices in some large academic courses.

Step 3. The final grade assignment may be derived by weighting the tentative letter grade derived above against information on "process" characteristics, personal qualities, and difficulty of task (other than as already adjusted for by Level assignment—see Figure 1, Grade Assignment).

Comment: Such norm-referenced grading generally promotes competition rather than cooperation among clinicians and is counter to the objectives of skills competency training

OPTION B—CRITERION-REFERENCED[2]

Step 1. In criterion-referencing grading, the distribution of scores is *not* used for grade assignments. Rather, each supervisor has a particular CAF score in mind which corresponds to a specific letter grade. (For example, in one practicum a supervisor may decide that a Level II clinician will need to obtain a CAF Professional-Technical Skills score of 88 or above to be considered for an "A". In normative-referenced grading, a clinician's grade depends on how well the other clinicians in the practicum performed; in criterion-referenced grading such comparisons are *not* relevant.) These decisions may not be possible to make until a supervisor has had several terms of experience with W-PACC and CAF data.

---

[1]Appendix C presents sample grade assignments aggregated over several supervisors. As evident in the assumptions about supervision and appraisal reviewed (pp. 1-3), Option B has been of greatest interest to the authors of this manual.

[2]Of the three scores, Interpersonal, Professional-Technical, and "Average", Professional-Technical appears to correlate highest with subjective grades.

Step 2. Grades may again be weighed against "process" information, personal qualities summary, and difficulty of task—final grading may be adjusted up or down accordingly.

Procedure 3: Group Supervisory Norms

The steps to apply each of the two options in Procedure 3 are essentially the same as those reviewed for Procedure 2 above. However, in Procedure 3, *grouped* supervisory CAF scores are used for all clinicians, rather than each supervisor's individual distribution of scores.

OPTION A—NORMATIVE-REFERENCED

Step 1. The CAF skill scores (Interpersonal, Professional-Technical, and "Average") from *all* clinicians in a training program are arranged in distributions for each Level or Level by Practicum Site.
Step 2. Based on this frequency distribution, the supervisory *group* determines which scores will be considered for "A's", which scores will be considered for "B's", etc.
Step 3. Each supervisor may adjust these tentative grades of the clinician she supervised up or down, according to "process" information, personal qualities summary, and difficulty of task considerations.

OPTION B—CRITERION-REFERENCED

Step 1. The supervisory *group* determines the CAF score that is required for each tentative letter grade at each Level or Level by Practicum site.
Step 2. Each clinician is assigned a tentative letter grade, according to the CAF skill scores obtained.
Step 3. Each supervisor adjusts grades by the other three considerations as above.

CLINICIAN APPRAISAL FORM (CAF)

Clinician's Name _____ Date _____ Circle:

Class Standing—JR. 1st sem., JR. 2nd sem., SR. 1st sem., SR. 2nd sem., GRAD. 1st sem., GRAD. 2nd sem.,

GRAD 3rd sem., Other _____

| Clinician Level |
| 1 2 3 4 |

Practicum Site _____

Type(s) of problem(s) _____

Problems in addition to communication _____ Age(s) of client(s) _____

Total number of therapy sessions _____ Supervisor _____

Comments:

*Interpersonal Skills Scale | | | |

*Professional-Technical Skills Scale

Average $\dfrac{(IS + PTS)}{2}$ = | | | |

Personal Qualities Summary

No. of "Satisfactory" items | | |

No. of "Inconsistent" items | | |

No. of "Unsatisfactory" items | |

No. of "Lack information" items | |

No. of "Does not apply" items | |

Total (should = 10)

*Percentage Score = $\dfrac{\text{Sum of scored items}}{\text{Number of items scored} \times 10}$

Interpersonal Skills	Does not apply	Specific direction from supervisor does not alter unsatisfactory performance and inability to make changes	Needs specific direction and/or demonstration from supervisor to perform effectively	Needs *general* direction from supervisor to perform effectively	Demonstrates independence by taking initiative; makes changes when appropriate; and is effective
1. Accepts, empathizes, shows genuine concern for the client as a person and understands the client's problems, needs, and stresses.		1	2 — 3 — 4	5 — 6 — 7	8 — 9 — 10
2. Perceives verbal and non-verbal cues which indicate the client is not understanding the task; is unable to perform all or part of the task; or when emotional stress interferes with performance of the task.		1	2 — 3 — 4	5 — 6 — 7	8 — 9 — 10
3. Creates an atmosphere based on honesty and trust; enables client to express his/her feelings and concerns.		1	2 — 3 — 4	5 — 6 — 7	8 — 9 — 10
4. Conveys to the client in a nonthreatening manner what the standards of behavior and performance are.		1	2 — 3 — 4	5 — 6 — 7	8 — 9 — 10
5. Develops understanding of teaching goals and procedures with clients.		1	2 — 3 — 4	5 — 6 — 7	8 — 9 — 10

349

Interpersonal Skills	Does not apply	Specific direction from supervisor does not alter unsatisfactory performance and inability to make changes	Needs specific direction and/or demonstration from supervisor to perform effectively	Needs *general direction* from supervisor to perform effectively	Demonstrates independence by taking initiative; makes changes when appropriate; and is effective
6. Listens, asks questions, participates *with* supervisor in therapy and/or client related discussions; is not defensive.		1	2 — 3 — 4	5 — 6 — 7	8 — 9 — 10
7. Requests assistance from supervisor and/or other professionals when appropriate.		1	2 — 3 — 4	5 — 6 — 7	8 — 9 — 10
8. Creates an atmosphere based on honesty and trust; enabling family members to express their feelings and concerns.		1	2 — 3 — 4	5 — 6 — 7	8 — 9 — 10
9. Develops understanding of teaching goals and procedures with family members.		1	2 — 3 — 4	5 — 6 — 7	8 — 9 — 10
10. Communicates with other disciplines on a professional level.		1	2 — 3 — 4	5 — 6 — 7	8 — 9 — 10

Professional-Technical Skills	Does not apply	Specific direction from supervisor does not alter unsatisfactory performance and inability to make changes	Needs specific direction and/or demonstration from supervisor to perform effectively	Needs *general* direction from supervisor to perform effectively	Demonstrates independence by taking initiative; makes changes when appropriate; and is effective
Developing and Planning					
1. Applies academic information to the clinical process.		1	2 — 3 — 4	5 — 6 — 7	8 — 9 — 10
2. Researches problems and obtains pertinent information from supplemental reading and/or observing other clients with similar problems.		1	2 — 3 — 4	5 — 6 — 7	8 — 9 — 10
3. Develops a semester management program (conceptualized or written) appropriate to the client's needs.		1	2 — 3 — 4	5 — 6 — 7	8 — 9 — 10
4. On the basis of assessment and measurement can appropriately determine measurable teaching objectives.		1	2 — 3 — 4	5 — 6 — 7	8 — 9 — 10
5. Plans appropriate teaching procedures.		1	2 — 3 — 4	5 — 6 — 7	8 — 9 — 10

Professional-Technical Skills	Does not apply	Specific direction from supervisor does not alter unsatisfactory performance and inability to make changes	Needs *specific direction and/or demonstration* from supervisor to perform effectively	Needs *general direction* from supervisor to perform effectively	Demonstrates independence by taking initiative; makes changes when appropriate; and is effective
6. Selects appropriate stimulus materials (age and ability level of client).		1	2 — 3 — 4	5 — 6 — 7	8 — 9 — 10
7. Sequences teaching tasks to implement designated program objectives.		1	2 — 3 — 4	5 — 6 — 7	8 — 9 — 10
8. Plans strategies for maintaining on-task behavior (including structuring the teaching environment and setting behavioral limits).		1	2 — 3 — 4	5 — 6 — 7	8 — 9 — 10
Teaching					
9. Gives clear, concise instructions in presenting materials and/or techniques in management and assessments.		1	2 — 3 — 4	5 — 6 — 7	8 — 9 — 10
10. Modifies level of language according to the needs of the client.		1	2 — 3 — 4	5 — 6 — 7	8 — 9 — 10

Professional-Technical Skills	Does not apply	Specific direction from supervisor does not alter unsatisfactory performance and inability to make changes	Needs specific direction and/or demonstration from supervisor to perform effectively	Needs general direction from supervisor to perform effectively	Demonstrates independence by taking initiative; makes changes when appropriate; and is effective
11. Utilizes planned teaching procedures.		1	2 — 3 — 4	5 — 6 — 7	8 — 9 — 10
12. Adaptability—makes modifications in the teaching strategy such as shifting materials and/or techniques when the client is not understanding or performing the task.		1	2 — 3 — 4	5 — 6 — 7	8 — 9 — 10
13. Uses feedback and/or reinforcement which is consistent, discriminating, and meaningful to the client.		1	2 — 3 — 4	5 — 6 — 7	8 — 9 — 10
14. Selects pertinent information to convey to the client.		1	2 — 3 — 4	5 — 6 — 7	8 — 9 — 10
15. Maintains on-task behavior.		1	2 — 3 — 4	5 — 6 — 7	8 — 9 — 10
16. Prepares clinical setting to meet individual client and observer needs.		1	2 — 3 — 4	5 — 6 — 7	8 — 9 — 10

353

Professional-Technical Skills	Does not apply	Specific direction from supervisor does not alter unsatisfactory performance and inability to make changes	Needs specific direction and/or demonstration from supervisor to perform effectively	Needs general direction from supervisor to perform effectively	Demonstrates independence by taking initiative; makes changes when appropriate; and is effective
17. If mistakes are made in the therapy situation, is able to generate ideas of what might have improved the situation.		1	2 — 3 — 4	5 — 6 — 7	8 — 9 — 10
Assessment					
18. Continues to assess client throughout the course of therapy using observational recording, standardized and nonstandardized measurement procedures and techniques.		1	2 — 3 — 4	5 — 6 — 7	8 — 9 — 10
19. Administers diagnostic tests according to standardization criterion.		1	2 — 3 — 4	5 — 6 — 7	8 — 9 — 10
20. Prepares prior to administering diagnostic tests by: (a) having appropriate materials available (b) familiarity with testing procedures.		1	2 — 3 — 4	5 — 6 — 7	8 — 9 — 10

Professional-Technical Skills	Does not apply	Specific direction from supervisor does not alter unsatisfactory performance and inability to make changes	Needs specific direction and/or demonstration from supervisor to perform effectively	Needs *general direction* from supervisor to perform effectively	Demonstrates independence by taking initiative; makes changes when appropriate; and is effective
21. Scores diagnostic tests accurately.		1	2 — 3 — 4	5 — 6 — 7	8 — 9 — 10
22. Interprets results of diagnostic testing accurately.		1	2 — 3 — 4	5 — 6 — 7	8 — 9 — 10
23. Interprets accurately results of diagnostic testing in light of other available information to form an impression.		1	2 — 3 — 4	5 — 6 — 7	8 — 9 — 10
24. Makes appropriate recommendations and/or referrals based on information obtained from the assessment or teaching process.		1	2 — 3 — 4	5 — 6 — 7	8 — 9 — 10
Reporting					
25. Reports information in written form that is pertinent and accurate.		1	2 — 3 — 4	5 — 6 — 7	8 — 9 — 10
26. Writes in an organized, concise, clear, and grammatically correct style.		1	2 — 3 — 4	5 — 6 — 7	8 — 9 — 10

Professional-Technical Skills	Does not apply	Specific direction from supervisor does not alter unsatisfactory performance and inability to make changes	Needs specific direction and/or demonstration from supervisor to perform effectively	Needs *general direction* from supervisor to perform effectively	Demonstrates independence by taking initiative; makes changes when appropriate; and is effective
27. Selects pertinent information to convey to family members.		1	2 — 3 — 4	5 — 6 — 7	8 — 9 — 10
28. Selects pertinent information to convey to other professionals (including all nonwritten communications such as phone calls and conferences).		1	2 — 3 — 4	5 — 6 — 7	8 — 9 — 10

Personal Qualities	Does not apply	Lack information	Unsatisfactory	Inconsistent	Satisfactory
1. Is punctual for client appointments.					
2. Cancels client appointments when necessary.					
3. Keeps appointments with supervisor or cancels appointments when necessary.					
4. Turns in lesson plans on time.					
5. Meets deadlines for reports.					
6. Turns in attendance sheets on time.					
7. Respects confidentiality of all professional activities.					
8. Uses socially acceptable voice, speech, and language.					
9. Personal appearance is appropriate for clinical setting and maintaining credibility.					
10. Appears to recognize own professional limitations and stays within boundaries of training.					

SAMPLE ITEM DESCRIPTORS

(See Guideline III for perspective on these descriptors.)

Interpersonal Items

1. Accepts, empathizes, shows genuine concern for the client as a person and understands the client's problems, needs, and stresses.

   The clinician demonstrates openness, acceptance, supportiveness, and honesty through verbal and non-verbal language. (The clinician does not make parent-like statements or reassurances such as "Don't feel that way; Don't worry; Everything will be all right; You should. . .; You shouldn't. . .," etc.)

   During the session, the clinician demonstrates acceptance, empathy and concern for the client. During conferences with the supervisor the clinician discusses the client, reflects these feelings and understanding of the client; thoughtful preparation for session is one indication of concern.

2. Perceives verbal and non-verbal cues which indicate the client is not understanding the task; is unable to perform all or part of the task; or when emotional stress interferes with performance of the task.

   The clinician demonstrates this by (1) making attempts to alter the task or terminating the task, (2) using language which indicates that he/she is aware the client is unable to perform the task. (This statement is made either to the client or to the supervisor, or to both.)

   The clinician's behavior indicates an *awareness* of the client's difficulty although he/she may not have the professional-technical skills to make the most appropriate and effective changes during the session.

3. Creates an atmosphere based on honesty and trust; enables client to express his feelings and concerns.

   Verbal and non-verbal responses of the client are included. The clinician does not "turn off" client questions, knows limits of knowledge and can say "I don't know" and listens to client.

   Look to the behavior of the client to measure the clinician's interpersonal skill. Does the *client feel* the clinician is accepting, interested, concerned for the client as a person, and understanding of the client's needs, problems, and stresses?

   The client's behavior is interpreted as a reflection of the atmosphere created by the clinician.

4. Conveys to the client in a non-threatening manner what the standards of behavior and performance are.

   In a positive manner the clinician indicates acceptable behavioral limits, verbally and non-verbally by manner and facial expression.

   The language of the clinician reflects a willingness to confront undesirable behavior and talk about it objectively and constructively.

   The clinician is able to state expectations in a positive manner, and to handle unacceptable behaviors in such a way that the client feels that a positive relationship with the clinician is not in jeopardy.

Applies only to interactions which occur *after* the client has performed inappropriately.

5. Develops understanding of teaching goals and procedures with client.

The clinician informs the client of immediate and long range goals, explains the sequencing of tasks and procedures, and questions the client for his ideas regarding teaching objectives and therapy procedures.

The client is made aware of his purpose in therapy to the extent to which it is appropriate at any point in time. He is led to understand the goals and procedures and recognize them as something he can accomplish.

6. Listens, asks questions, participates *with* supervisor in therapy and/or client related discussions; is not defensive.

The clinician contributes to discussion at a level commensurate with academic background and clinical experience and "teams" for problem solving with the supervisor.

The clinician is candid with the supervisor. The clinician discusses successes and failures and attempts to look for alternatives to deal with problems about teaching objectives and related clinical issues.

7. Requests assistance from supervisor and/or other professionals when appropriate.

The clinician recognizes when he/she needs assistance. The clinician indicates when he/she is unsure about teaching tasks or behavioral expectations and checks with the supervisor regarding any changes made on the lesson plans.

The clinician is willing to ask for assistance as soon as possible to insure that teaching is continuously effective.

8. Creates an atmosphere based on honesty and trust enabling family members to express their feelings and concerns.

Look to the behavior of the parents to measure the clinician's interpersonal skills. Do the parents feel that the clinician is accepting of and concerned for their child and for them? Can the parents openly discuss their feelings and concerns without feeling defensive?

9. Develops understanding of teaching goals and procedures with family members.

The clinician's manner is straightforward and self-assured. The clinician respects the desire of family members "to know."

The clinician clarifies goals and procedures without being judgmental. The clinician encourages and rewards parent involvement.

10. Communicates with specialists in other disciplines on a professional level.

The clinician exhibits professional self-confidence. The clinician attempts to understand the background of other professionals involved and adapts his/her language accordingly.

The clinician respects the integrity of specialists in other disciplines when there is an exchange of information.

Professional-Technical Items

1. Applies academic information to the clinical process.

   This item includes the application of classroom information as well as supervisory information given during the current assignment.

   As a result of attending class, group meetings, and discussions with supervisors, the clinician demonstrates an understanding of (1) the psychology of fear, (2) use of the DAF, (3) use of problem solving, and (4) stuttering behavior (these are only *some* examples.)

2. Researches problems and obtains pertinent information from supplemental reading and/or observing other clients with similar problems.

   The clinician actively seeks additional information. The clinician reads and evaluates materials recommended by other sources including the clinical supervisor.

3. Develops a semester therapy program (conceptualized or written) appropriate to the client's needs.

   The development of a therapy program is an ongoing procedure which extends throughout the clinician's assignment with the client.

   Within the first half of the semester the clinician defines long and short range goals.

4. On the basis of assessment and measurement can determine measurable teaching objectives.

   The clinician uses information obtained through formal and informal assessment procedures to determine appropriate teaching objectives.

   As a result of analyzing the client's speaking behavior and expressed feelings and attitudes, the clinician can identify the problems and determine appropriate objectives to alleviate these problems.

   The clinician can delineate which aspects of behavior on which to keep data.

5. Plans appropriate teaching procedures.

   Teaching procedures reflect knowledge of what the client might be able to do and at what level he is functioning.

6. Selects appropriate stimulus materials (age and ability level of client).

   The clinician makes good use of commercial materials; altering them is necessary to meet the client's needs, and/or creatively devises his/her own materials.

   The clinician respects limits imposed by motor development and interest.

7. Sequences teaching tasks to implement designated program objectives.

   The clinician knows base-line behaviors for task requirements and places the client's ability along the continuum.

   The clinician teaches various tasks using a hierarchy of difficulty format. He/she does not start with a difficult level of performance before client demonstrates ability to perform at a lower level.

8. Plans strategies for maintaining on-task behavior (including structuring the teaching environment and setting behavioral limits).

   The clinician explores alternate teaching environments and strategies for maintaining on-task behavior in order to provide structure for the client's progress.

   The clinician knows when it is important to keep the client on task and when it is important to deal with something else. The clinician helps define criteria for acceptable or successful speech behavior at a particular stage.

   The clinician can deal effectively with client behaviors such as inattentiveness, hyperactivity or distractibility.

9. Gives clear, concise instructions in presenting materials and/or techniques in therapy and assessment.

   The clinician demonstrates adequate preparation which eliminates the need to reword instructions or redesign materials during the session.

   The clinician uses language that is clear, specific and concise and is not redundant when giving directions or explanations.

10. Modifies level of language according to the needs of the client.

    The clinician uses active rather than passive language. The clinician uses "doer" language ("You are pressing your lips together"), and descriptive language rather than labels such as pullouts, cancellations, etc.

    By use of his/her words, the clinician indicates his/her understanding of the concept of the "total child," i.e., does not talk down to the child yet uses words which can be understood.

    The clinician provides a verbal model which is within the client's comprehension and/or modifies his/her speaking behavior so that the client's fluency is not adversely affected.

11. Utilizes planned teaching procedures.

    The clinician knows in advance the planned teaching procedures. He/she does not have to refer extensively to written lesson plan.

    The clinician demonstrates knowledge and purpose of the teaching procedure. The clinician uses this knowledge to: a. identify and describe those behaviors which facilitate the client's use of the procedure; b. monitor the client's behavior as it relates to achieving the objective.

12. Adaptability—makes modifications in the teaching strategy such as shifting materials and/or techniques when the client is not understanding or performing the task.

    The clinician overplans by having alternate procedures and materials available in case they may be needed. He/she knows base-line behaviors and can spontaneously return to these or to more advanced behaviors as appropriate within the session.

    This item deals with how the clinician reacts in *one particular session*, e.g., ability to see that, for that particular day, the material is too complex and is therefore able to modify the material; ability to modify a particular technique that is not effective (change from pullouts to cancellations, change from modifying real blocks to faked blocks, etc.).

13. Uses feedback and/or reinforcement which is consistent, discriminating, and meaningful to the client.

    The clinician's own verbal and non-verbal behaviors are used as reinforcement for desired verbal and non-verbal client behaviors.

    The clinician positively reinforces *on-target* behavior. The clinician positively reinforces attitudes and feelings that the client verbalizes that are conducive to progress.

14. Selects pertinent information to convey to the client.

    The clinician includes information related to the client's problems with communication and knows when to extend the information. The clinician keeps the client informed of progress during each session.

    The clinician demonstrates the ability to give information that is relevant to the client's problems, questions, etc.

    The clinician explains teaching strategies and expectations for progress to the client, i.e., this item may be particularly applicable to school age and adult clients.

15. Maintains on-task behavior.

    The clinician is consistent in maintaining set behavioral standards.

    The clinician facilitates client concentration or attentiveness to task.

16. Prepares clinical setting to meet individual client and observer needs.

    The clinician uses appropriate furniture for the client and places chairs so observers can see the client's face; arranges supplies including personal notes and books so they are available, but not cluttered; and respects the client's wishes regarding observers.

    Setting is interpreted to include not only physical elements (furniture; materials) but people as well. When teaching in a group situation, the clinician prepares seating arrangements which recognize the needs of individual children in relationship to the needs and behavior of other children.

17. If mistakes are made in the therapy situation, is able to generate ideas of what might have improved the situation.

    In conferences with the supervisor the clinician indicates an understanding of his/her mistakes and can creatively plan alternative procedures to meet problems which were unsuccessfully dealt with during the session.

    The clinician can independently verbalize future modifications in the therapy format.

18. Continues to assess client throughout the course of therapy using observational recording, standardized and non-standardized measurement procedures and techniques.

    The clinician recognizes goal achievement and moves the client through a systematic progression of designated objectives.

    The clinician recognizes when the client should add another goal, or when a particular goal needs to be emphasized. (For example, desensitization procedures; identification of stresses, etc.)

    The clinician keeps systematic data on measurable aspects of behavior.

19. Administers diagnostic tests according to standardization criterion.

   (no descriptors)

20. Prepares prior to administering diagnostic tests by: (a) having appropriate materials available; (b) becoming familiar with testing procedures.

   The clinician knows how to administer various diagnostic tests. He/she does not become overly absorbed in test materials and procedures and so miss interpersonal contact with the client.

21. Scores diagnostic tests accurately.

   (no descriptors)

22. Interprets results of diagnostic testing accurately.

   (no descriptors)

23. Interprets results of diagnostic testing accurately in light of other available information to form an impression.

   (no descriptors)

24. Makes appropriate recommendations and/or referrals based on information obtained from the assessment or teaching process.

   (no descriptors)

25. Reports information in written form that is pertinent and accurate.

   The clinician includes information which enables the reader to understand goals and procedures. The clinician effectively summarizes the information rather than detailing it.

   The clinician's first draft of the final report reflects a knowledge of client's behavior, teaching objectives, and clinical procedures.

26. Writes in an organized, concise, clear, and grammatically correct style.

   The clinician is able to write, using language which will be meaningful and useful to people outside the Speech and Hearing Clinic.

27. Selects pertinent information to convey to family members.

   The clinician selects relevant facts from therapy sessions or other observable aspects of behavior to share with family members.

28. Selects pertinent information to convey to other professionals (including all non-written communications such as phone calls and conferences).

   The clinician selects relevant facts from therapy sessions or other observable aspects of behavior to share with allied professionals. The clinician knows when to initiate contact with these professionals.

SAMPLE GRADE ASSIGNMENTS

The table below summarizes the correspondence between the "product" scores and grade assignments obtained over one group of supervisors (n = > 400 appraisals). Briefly, the values for each scale represent the *mean* value obtained by clinicians who would "subjectively" have been given the corresponding letter grade. Obviously, no claim is intended or should be inferred that these values are the recommended "norms" for grade assignments. Recall that the authors of this manual have been most interested in developing criterion-referenced norms at the *individual* supervisory level (again, the values below have been aggregated over *several* supervisors solely for the purposes of summary inspection). Moreover, in addition to reflecting "product" or scale scores, an individual grade can be adjusted *upwards* or *downwards* by a supervisor in consideration of (1) "process" information (up or down), (2) Personal Qualities Summary information (usually down), or (3) "Difficulty of task" information (usually up).

Level	Grade	Interpersonal Skills	Professional-Technical Skills	"Average"
1	A	92	85	88
	AB	81	72	76
	B	78	65	72
	BC	—	—	—
	C	48	41	45
2	A	94	88	90
	AB	88	81	84
	B	76	67	72
	BC	—	—	—
	C	—	—	—
3	A	96	93	95
	AB	92	86	89
	B	80	76	78
	BC	—	—	—
	C	81	61	71
4	A	98	96	97
	AB	96	89	93
	B	92	87	89
	BC	98	66	82
	C	—	—	—

Appendix E:
The Pre-Conference
Observation System
Frances K. Block

EXAMPLES OF SHORTHAND TECHNIQUES FOR WRITING TEXT OF LESSON

Symbols Used
+   Clinician thought response was good
−   Clinician thought response was not good
∕   Student evaluated own response
0   Someone else in the group other than the clinician evaluated the response
X   The model was repeated
IM Immediate Model
DM Delayed Model
NM No Model
⊕   Supervisor thought response was good   } These symbols are only needed if the supervisor
⊖   Supervisor thought response was not good } disagrees with the judgment of the clinician

Additional Techniques
Clinician talk versus client talk can be distinguished by differential placement on the page. For example:
Clinician talk can always be started at the margin.
Client talk can always be indented.

Shorthand Examples
1. shoe + good

2. under the table − no

3. book − X − X +

Equivalent Longhand Explanations
1. Child said *shoe*
    Clinician thought it was a correct response
    (+)

2. Child said *under the table*
    Clinician thought it was an incorrect response
    (−)
    Clinician told child it was an incorrect response (no)

3. Child said *book*
    Response was incorrect (−)
    Clinician repeated model (X)
    Second response was incorrect (−)
    Clinician repeated model again (X)
    Third response was correct (+)

Block, F. (1979). The preconference observation system: Supervisor's point of view. Paper presented at convention of American Speech-Language-Hearing Association.

4. red − − $\overset{\ominus}{+}$

5. I throw the ball ✓ − +

6. foots 0 − X ✓ − + good

7. a. The boy was walking
    b. walking
    c. No, tell me the whole
       thing
    d. The boy was
       walking +
       good
    e. The boy was eating
    f. boy was
       eating—not
       quite

8. She is happy ✓ +

    Him is looking ✓ + 0−

    X ✓ + 0+

4. Child said *red*
    Response was incorrect (−)
    Child said *red* again, with no intervening
        model, but response was incorrect (−)
    Child said *red* again with no intervening
        model and clinician said response was
        correct (+)
    Supervisor thought response was incorrect
        ($\ominus$)

5. Child said *I throw the ball*
    Child self-monitored response & indicated
        that it was incorrect (✓ −)
    Child corrected response without an
        intervening model (+)

6. Child said *foots*
    Another child in group indicated that the
        response was incorrect (0−)
    Clinician or another child in group repeated
        model (X)
    Child self-monitored response and indicated
        that it was incorrect (✓ −)
    Child repeated response without an
        intervening model.
    Response was correct (+)
    Clinician said good

7. Clinician's comments are along the margin
    Child's responses are indented

    Line d: + good at end meant clinician said
        good
    Line f: − not quite at end meant clinician said
        "not quite"

8. Child said *She is happy*. Child indicated that
        own response was correct (✓ +)
    Child said *Him is looking*. Child indicated that
        own response was correct. (✓ +)
        Someone else in group said the
        response was incorrect (0−)
    Correct model was repeated (X). Child said
        response was correct (✓ +). Another
        child in group said response was correct
        (0+)

9. reach $\overset{\ominus}{+}$ good

read $-$ X $\overset{\oplus}{-}$

9. Child said *reach*
   Clinician thought response was correct (+)
   Supervisor thought response was incorrect
   ($\ominus$)
   Child said *read*
   Clinician thought response was incorrect ($-$)
   and repeated model (X)
   Clinician thought response was incorrect ($-$)
   Supervisor thought response was correct
   ($\oplus$)

Sample Lesson #1

Clinician's Goals: Correct production of /s/ in words
Abbreviations: C = Clinician, D = Drew, P = Paul (fourth graders).

1. *C* — We're going to play a basketball game today. (Explained how to play) Spin. If you get a 1, take 1 card. If you get a 3, take 3 cards. Drew, you go first. *Say the word after me.*
2. D — yardstick + toast + glasses +
3. *C* — OK, that's 3
4. P — desk +, basket +
5. D — nest +, bicycle +, vest +
6. P — whistle +
7. D — toaster +
8. P — pencil +, baseball +, mustache +
9. *C* — Don't jerk your head forward
10. D — tricycle +, astronaut +
11. P — newspaper +, mask +
12. *C* — Good, your head's not going forward
13. D — icicle +
14. P — police car +, glasses +
15. D — bicycle +, basketball +
16. P — horseshoe +
17. D — spaceship +, seesaw +, whisper +
18. P — glasses +, Christmas tree +, icicle +
19. D — lasso +
20. P — sewing basket +
21. D — baseball bat +
22. P — bicycle +
23. D — policeman +, castle +
24. D & P — explained how to change game next time they play it
25. *C* — There were some good /s/'s when you told me how to redo the game. Want to start another game? Score is 2–0. Paul starts this time. *Say the word after me again.*
26. P — baseball +, tricycle +, toaster +

27. D — rooster +, ghost +
28. P — nest +, question mark +
29. D — whispering +
30. P — yardstick +, haystack +, mustache +
31. D — tricycle +, astronaut +, holster +
32. P — holster +, yardstick +
33. D — toast +
34. P — glasses +
35. D — desk +, basket +
36. P — nest +
37. D — bicycle +, vest +, whistle +
38. P — icicle +, police car +, glasses +
39. D — horseshoe spaceship
40. P — seesaw whispering
41. *C* — You just scored, now it's 2–2. Time's up. Next time we'll put more rules in.

Sample Lesson #2 (Traditional Approach)

A supervisor observes the same lesson as in example #1. The following comments could be made:

■ Explain goals of lesson, not just how to play the game.

■ You haven't given any reinforcement.

■ Clients don't do any self-monitoring.

■ Getting a lot of responses from them.

■ All responses are correct—need to go on to harder level. They don't need to repeat the words after you—try no model or short sentences.

■ These changes can be made *during* your lesson—don't need to wait until the next lesson to change goals.

■ Vocabulary is too repetitive—they know how to say the words, why keep repeating?

■ At the end of the lesson, there was no wrap-up concerning how well they did with their /s/'s. Count the number of correct and incorrect responses or have them count so that they know what they accomplished.

Sample Lesson #3

Clinician's Goals: Mike and Steve — *Correct production of /θ/ and /ð/ in all vocalic positions in sentences.*

Abbreviations: **C** = Clinician, **M** = Mike, **S** = Steve.

(Lesson has already begun)
1. C — That baby doesn't have any teeth
2. S — That baby doesn't have any teef — OK
3. C — Watch me. teeth
4. S — teeth + That sounded much better. I heard a good sound and your tongue wasn't pointed, it was flat.
5. C — Every Thursday I watched TV.
6. M — Every Thursday I watched TV. ⤶ +
7. C — It sounded good to me too. The earth is a large planet.
8. S — The earth is a large planet. ⤶ + It was good.
9. C — It sounded good to me too. It was so good, let me hear it again.
10. S — (Repeats) ⤶ + 0+
11. C — I thought so too. Pick a part to put on. Don't leave your toys in the bathtub.
12. M — Don't leave your toys in the bathtub. ⤶ + good
13. C — My brother was three today.
14. S — My brother was free today. — OK
15. C — Stick your tongue out, and make it flat. Look at the mirror. three
16. S — three + good
17. C — three
18. S — three + good
19. C — three
20. S — three + good
21. C — I thought I got lost
22. M — I thought I got lost + good
23. C — Put two points down. Father is very thin.
24. S — Father is very fin. — OK
25. C — Father is very thin.
26. S — fin — OK
27. C — Use the mirror. Make sure your tongue is very flat. Father is very thin.
28. S — Father is very thin. + good. Father is very thin. ⤶ +
29. C — Great. That was two good th's. The children thought the trip was fun.
30. M — The children thought the trip was fun.

What Sample Lesson #3 Would Look Like All in Shorthand

IM for all sentences

S   That baby doesn't have any teeth — OK X + That sded much better. I hrd gd sd and yr tongue wasn't pted, but flat.

M   Every Thurs. I watched TV. ⤶ + Gd. to me too.

S   The earth is a lrge planet. ⤶ + It was gd.

C   Gd to me too. again

S   ⌐ + 0+

M   Don't leave yr toys in the bathtub. ⌐ + good

S   My brother was free today. — ok   Stick yr tongue out, make it flat. Look in mirror.
    X + good   X + good   X + good

M   I thought I got lost   + good   Put two pts down.

S   Father is very fin — OK X — OK   Use the mirror. Mk sure yr tongue is flat.
    X + good. X ⌐ +   Grt. Two gd. th's.

M   The children thought de trip was fun. — OK   Let's try *the*

Sample Lesson #4

*Clinician's Goal — To elicit **I've got** in structured sentences*
                    Model criteria schedule of reinforcement—not listed

Abbreviations: ***C*** = Clinician, **A** = Andy.

1. *C*—We have a surprise, a treasure
    box. Reach in, and when you pick
    it, say, I've got a _____.
2. A — I got a seal.
3. *C* — Tell me something about it.
4. A — Animal
5. *C* — Big or little?
6. A — Big, 2 feet
7. *C* — How many eyes?
8. A — 2 eye
9. *C* — 2 eyes. Pick again.
10. A — Car
11. *C* — Tell me a whole sentence.
    That is a car.
12. A — That is a car.
13. *C* — Try saying the /ð/ in *that*. Stick
    your tongue out. (took out mirror.)
14. A — That - - - - -
15. *C* — Try *the*
16. A — The +
17. *C* — Now *that*
18. A — That +

19. *C* — Nice job. Pick something else. I've got. . .
20. A — I got
21. *C* — I've got. . .
22. A — I got a cup. Drink in a cup.
23. *C* — Don't you drink out of a cup?
24. A — (nods head)
25. *C* — What do you drink?
26. A — Water
27. *C* — Pick again.
28. A — Plate (/fweit/)
29. *C* — Plate
30. A — /fweit/
31. *C* — Okay. Pick another.
32. A — Mailbox
33. *C* — What goes in it? What do you do with it?
34. A — Put in there
35. *C* — Pick again.
36. A — Saw, cut woods
37. *C* — Wood
38. A — Yeah, cut saw
39. *C* — Have you ever used a saw?
40. A — Yeah
41. *C* — What did you cut?
42. A — Green machine

Appendix F:
Kansas Inventory of Self-Supervision (KISS)
Brenda L. Mawdsley

SELF-ASSESSMENT: OVERUSE OF "OK"

Clinician _____
Date _____

When supervising beginning students in speech-language pathology, it becomes apparent that many tend to say "OK" an excessive number of times during the management session. Four main types of "OK" responses seem to be the ones overused. They are "OK" used as (1) a filler, (2) a positive reinforcer, (3) corrective feedback and (4) tag question. The definitions are as follows:

"OK" as a filler—This happens when the clinician says "OK" for no reason throughout the session. For example "OK, now let's turn to the back page."

"OK" as a positive reinforcer—This is used after the client has given a correct response. Used in this manner, it can often appear as if clinicians are really not committing themselves as to the client's production.

"OK" as corrective feedback—This often occurs when beginning clinicians are afraid to commit as to the correctness or incorrectness of a response. After an error the clinician would say "OK" instead of giving rich descriptive feedback.

"OK" as a tag question—An example of this is "Pull your tongue up and back, OK?" or "Let's get out our speech books, OK?" The addition of "OK" makes a statement into a nonassertive request.

During a 20-minute session, count the number of times each of the following types of "OK" are spoken by the clinician.

TYPE	DATA
"OK" used as a filler	
"OK" as positive reinforcer	
"OK" as corrective feedback	
"OK" used as a tag question	

Total number of "OK"s _____

Mawdsley, B. (1987). Kansas inventory of self-supervision. In Farmer, S. (Ed.) (1987). *Clinical supervision: A coming of age*. Proceedings of a conference held at Jekyll Island, GA: Las Cruces, N.M., New Mexico State University.

After listening to the tape, set a realistic goal for reducing the incidence of "OK." Audio or video sessions weekly until the goal is met.

SELF-ASSESSMENT: POSITIVE REINFORCEMENT

Clinician _____
Date _____

Positive reinforcement is a tool which is utilized daily by speech-language pathologists. This form assists the beginning clinician in categorizing the various types of positive reinforcement used, and in examining sequences of positive reinforcement. For example, the clinician might say "Good talking," then smile at the client, then give him a token. Three types of positive reinforcement have been utilized and now can be categorized and counted. The clinician can analyze the type and amount of reinforcement being used, examine the amount of progress the client is making and adjust the reinforcement sequences accordingly.

Utilizing the coding system below, tally the type of positive reinforcement given the client after a correct response in the blank matrix, placing only one code per box. (Note: For a young client who needs maximum reinforcement, one may chart type of positive reinforcement used after any response.)

RESPONSE CODE
C = correct response
I = incorrect response

FEEDBACK CODE
PV = positive verbal
NVP = non-verbal positive
      (smiling, nodding,
      leaning)
PT = positive touch
T = token reinforcement
E = edible reinforcement

Total number of responses (C+I) = _____

Percentage of correct responses $\dfrac{C}{C + I}$ = _____

Examine the matrix and circle the sequences of positive reinforcement used. For example, a correct response followed by a smile, positive touch and a token would have a sequence code of C/NVP/PT/T. (Slashes indicate "followed by" in sequence counts). List the sequences and the number of times that sequence is used during the session.

SEQUENCE COUNTS

Sequence	# of Events
C/PV	
C/NVP	
C/T	
C/E	
C/PV/NVP	
C/PV/NVP/PT/T	
etc	

SELF-ASSESSMENT: CORRECTIVE FEEDBACK

Clinician _____
Date _____

Corrective feedback is defined as the type of corrective measures the clinician will utilize after the client has made an incorrect response. Beginning clinicians have historically demonstrated difficulty in this area by (1) using ambiguous feedback resulting in confusion for the client as to whether the response was correct or incorrect and (2) using feedback lacking descriptive qualities such as modeling, phonetic placement and motokinesthetic techniques. This critique form looks at types and sequences of corrective feedback used, then asks the clinician to review the percentage of correct responses to determine if the corrective feedback techniques utilized resulted in maximum gain by the client.

Utilizing the coding system below, tally the type of corrective feedback given the client after an incorrect or approximated response. Place the code for each event in one box of the matrix working left to right.

RESPONSE CODE
I = incorrect response
A = approximated
 response
C = correct response

FEEDBACK CODE
NR = no response from
 clinician
VN = verbal negative, e.g.
 "No, try again."
M = model
VC = visual cue
PP = phonetic placement
 e.g. "Put your tongue
 up and back."

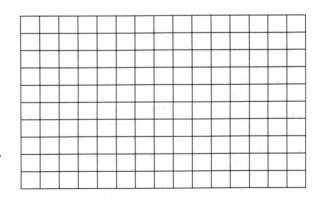

MC = motokinesthetic
cue, i.e. giving
tactile cues.

Total number of responses (I + A + C) = _____

Percentage of correct responses $\dfrac{C}{I + A + C}$ = _____

Examine the matrix and circle the sequences of corrective feedback. In the space below list the sequences and the number of times each sequence occurred in the session. The slash indicates "followed by" in sequence counts.

SEQUENCE COUNTS

Sequence	# of Events
I/NR	
I/VN	
I/VN/PP/M	
I/MC/PP/M	

SELF-ASSESSMENT: GROUP MANAGEMENT ROTATION RATES

Clinician _____

Date _____

Group management is not the norm in most practicum sites for speech-language pathology. Therefore, when the beginning student is faced with teaching two or more children at the same time, he often does not understand how to rotate from child to child quickly in order to keep all children as involved as possible and behavior problems at a minimum. With this self-assessment form student clinicians can assess, in minutes and seconds, the amount of time spent with each child in a group management session. This not only gives information regarding how quickly the SLP rotates from child to child, but this count will also yield a total amount of time spent with each individual child so the clinician can note if more time is being spent with one client than the others.

Below write out the session task for each child. This will help in the analysis since, for example, in articulation management more time may appropriately be spent with a client at the level of conversation versus a client at the word level of remediation.

Task for Child A _____

Task for Child B _____

Task for Child C _____

Task for Child D _____

Using the matrix below, figure in minutes and seconds the time spent with each child for "his turn" during the speech session. Compute the total amount of time spent with each child.

TURN

	1	2	3	4	5	6	7	8	9	10	11	12
Child A												
Child B												
Child C												
Child D												

Total time spent with Child A _____
Child B _____
Child C _____
Child D _____

$$\frac{\text{Total time with all children}}{\text{Total number of turns}} = \text{Mean length of each turn} = \underline{\qquad}$$

SELF-ASSESSMENT: RESPONSE RATE

Clinician _____
Date _____

The response rate form was developed so the clinician can self-assess how many responses per minute are being elicited from the client. When a supervisor says that the pace of the session is too slow, the supervisee can count responses to see if this is an area which needs to be improved. The clinician can accumulate baseline data and attempt to improve number of responses per minute until the supervisor and supervisee agree the number of responses per session is appropriate.

To figure response rate, add together correct and incorrect responses and divide by the number of minutes of direct management. For example, if in an individual management session the client had 37 correct and 24 incorrect responses, add these scores together for a total of 61. Then divide by the time involved in direct drill, e.g. 20 minutes. The response rate for the session would be:

$$\frac{61 \text{ total responses}}{20 \text{ min. direct drill}} = 3.05 \text{ responses per minute}$$

An example of figuring group response rates would be:

Child A has 12 correct and 43 incorrect for a total of 55
Child B has 29 correct and 12 incorrect for a total of 41
Child C has 42 correct and 9 incorrect for a total of 51

Add these totals together to find a total number of responses for the session. In this example the total equals 147. Next divide total responses in the session by the time involved in direct drill, 23 minutes.

$$\frac{147 \text{ responses}}{23 \text{ min. direct drill}} = 6.4 \text{ responses per minute}$$

Client	Task	# Correct	# Incorrect	Minutes of Drill	Resp. per Minute

Comments:

SELF-ASSESSMENT: CLINICIAN RESPONSE TO CLIENT SOCIAL COMMENTS

Clinician _____

Task _____

Date _____

As you listen to the audio- or videotape, after each social comment from the client note the category of the clinician's next remark by placing a checkmark in the appropriate space. Next note the effect your behavior had on the child in the column marked "Consequence." Indicate the topic of the "Client Social" by paraphrasing the comment in a few words, i.e., "recess fight."

Client Social (Comment)	Clinician			Consequences
	Social	Bad Evaluation	Return to Task	
Example 1. "Mary hit Tom"—recess fight				Client returned
2.				
3.				
4.				
5.				
6.				
7.				
8.				
9.				

Comments regarding the data: _____

_____

_____

_____

_____

_____

_____

_____

SELF-ASSESSMENT: CLINICIAN VS. CLIENT TALK-TIME

Clinician _____

Task _____

Date _____

For this self-analysis, you will need to have two stopwatches. As you listen to the audio- or videotape, measure the clinician's talk-time with one stopwatch and the client's talk-time with the other.

Talk-time of the clinician _____

Talk-time of the client _____

Total talk-time for session _____

Percentage of clinician talk-time _____

(Clinician talk-time / total talk-time = % clinician talk-time)

Comments regarding the data: _____

_____

_____

_____

_____

_____

_____

_____

Appendix G:
McCrea's Adapted Scales for Assessment of Interpersonal Functioning in Speech-Language Pathology Supervision Conferences

Elizabeth S. McCrea

Five categories of interpersonal functioning are scored according to the following rules:

PROCEDURES

1. Generally you will begin by making two passes through the segment of audio recording that you want to analyze. The first time you will record the speaker and the first few words of his/her utterance. This information is the unit of coding. The second time you will:
   a. Decide the category/categories for the utterance.
   b. Rate each category.
   You may make several passes through the data if necessary.
2. A set of formal scoring procedures is unavailable. Scorers may use their own methods for recording scores..

GROUND RULES

1. The utterance is the unit of observation. An utterance changes when the speaker changes or the topic of conversation changes.
2. Generally, the pattern of transcription will follow the CHANGE IN SPEAKER. However, there are some exceptions to this rule:
   a. Background "umhmms," "oks," etc. will not be transcribed.
   b. "Umhmm," "ok," "right" that stand out as separate because of a break in the primary speaker's speech *will not be transcribed* if they appear to be a social lubricant, a filler, acceptance that the message is being received. They *will be transcribed* when they appear to be meant as *positive reinforcement* or *agreement*; this will, in part, be determined by context and/or nonverbal cues.
   c. In extended utterances, segments will change when they do not relate to or focus upon the previous segment.
   d. When within-speaker off-topic interjections occur: transcribe the original statement, transcribe the off-topic interjection, *do not* transcribe the concluding statement but bracket it with the preceding two statements.

From McCrea, E. (1980). Supervisee ability to self-explore and four facilitative dimensions of supervisor behavior in individual conferences in speech-language pathology. (Doctoral dissertation, Indiana University, 1980). *Dissertation Abstracts International, 41*, 2134B. (University Microfilms No. 80–29, 239).

    e.   In instances of parallel talk, transcribe each speaker's utterances separately. Do not try to keep track of the multiple overlaps in the transcript.

    f.   When utterances are completely unintelligible, transcribe with an _____ as unintelligible.

    g.   When utterances are partially unintelligible, transcribe the audible portion and utilize a _____ for the part that is not understood. This will allow coding and rating of the audible portion.

3.   Rate each utterance. A Level 5 represents a neutral statement, 6 and 7 add to the statement and below 5 subtracts from the statement.

$$1 \quad 2 \quad 3 \quad 4 \quad / \quad 5 \quad / \quad 6 \quad 7$$

             subtracts   neutral adds

4.   The following are general clues to aid category selection:

    a.   *Empathic understanding* is scored only when the supervisor deals with the supervisee's feelings.

    b.   With the exception of tag questions, all supervisor questions are scored at some level of respect. Negative and positive reinforcement of the supervisee is scored as *respect*.

    c.   *Facilitative genuineness* is scored when the supervisor is relating his/her opinion.

    d.   All supervisor statements are scored under *concrete*.

5.   Score the supervisor utterances in as *many* categories as apply.

6.   Supervisee self-exploration is scored only when the supervisee is discussing his/her own behavior or feelings. If a supervisee has no self-exploration, score the utterance as NA (i.e., not appropriate).

7.   In rating behavior categories, utilize Time Rule, i.e., in extended utterances when several ratings of a behavior seem to occur, only apply the rating associated with longest segment of the utterance.

SUPERVISOR CATEGORIES

Concreteness: Concreteness means being specific. It is often complementary to empathy because one needs to be specific to show understanding.

SCALE FOR MEASURING CONCRETENESS DURING A SUPERVISION CONFERENCE

1	2	3	4	5	6	7
Supervisor statement which is extremely vague, causes confusion and greatly detracts from the flow of the discussion.	Vague statements by the supervisor which have no focus on the topic being discussed.	Supervisor statements which are vague but have focus related to the immediate past utterance.	Supervisor statements that have a previous focus and include some specific terms along with some vague terms. A new supervisor statement which is general with some focus.	Supervisor uses no vague terms. No use of indefinite pronouns in place of nouns. Statements are specific.	Supervisor statements will be specific (like level 5) but will include example or reasons.	Supervisor statements must be specific with an example and a rationale.

Facilitative Genuineness: Facilitative genuineness is expressing one's self naturally and openly. It is revealing one's own feelings and thoughts rather than acting strictly in terms of one's role as supervisor. To be genuine is to be honest, real, or authentic. In the early stages, a relationship only requires an absence of phoniness. The Supervisor remains silent or refrains from communicating his judgments. Facilitative genuineness is being open when it is helpful to the Supervisee. However, higher levels of genuineness may require the Supervisor to give negative feedback to the supervisee. When negative feedback is necessary, the Supervisor tries to take out the hurt.

SCALE FOR MEASURING FACILITATIVE GENUINENESS DURING A SUPERVISION CONFERENCE

1	2	3	4	5	6	7
Supervisor's opinions are stated in a sarcastic or insulting manner.	An apparent discrepancy between the supervisor's intent and what he/she says.	Supervisor may teach about a disorder, technique, supervisory process, etc. Supervisor reinforces client behavior and/or the therapy activity.	Supervisor as teacher but he/she includes some of his/her feelings.	Supervisor requests feedback from the supervisee or gives a suggestion directed toward the supervisee. Veiled negative evaluation.	Supervisor gives opinion that disagrees with supervisee's. Supervisor gives positive and negative evaluation. If negative evaluation is hurtful score level 5. Veiled positive evaluation.	Supervisor takes a risk and evaluates with justification.

Respect: Respect involves accepting the Supervisee as a separate person with human potentialities, apart from any evaluation of his behavior or thoughts; a Supervisor may evaluate behavior or thoughts and still rate high on respect if it is quite clear that his valuing of the Supervisee is unconditional. The Supervisor must believe in the Supervisee's ability to deal with a problem constructively when given proper guidance. For example, the Supervisor does not give the Supervisee advice off the top of his head. By avoiding this and encouraging the Supervisee to offer his own ideas, the Supervisor conveys to the Supervisee that he believes the Supervisee has the ability to find his own solutions. Respect is rarely found alone in communication. It is frequently paired with responses in other dimensions.

SCALE FOR MEASURING RESPECT DURING A SUPERVISION CONFERENCE

1	2	3	4	5	6	7
Supervisor relates a clear lack of respect for the supervisee in a sarcastic manner.	Supervisor may deliberately put the supervisee off by changing the topic of discussion or by communicating a statement with no focus to the previous one made by the supervisee.	Supervisor may ask the supervisee for clarification of an activity on a client. Also coded at this level are information and self-answered questions. Questions which seek rote or mechanical answers. Statements of the type "yes, but ..." are level 3.	Supervisor may ask for clarification of the supervisee's behaviors or feelings. Questions which guide the clinician to a specific answer.	Supervisor provides clarification of supervisee's previous utterance. Supervisor mirrors supervisee's thoughts, ideas, etc. Supervisor asks open ended questions which ask the supervisee for analysis or opinion regarding therapy. Supervisor makes a suggestion.	Supervisor clarifies the supervisee's utterance and goes further to interpret the supervisee's evaluation. Supervisor gives positive opinion about supervisee's behavior.	Supervisor positively evaluates the supervisee and goes further to take a risk for the supervisee related to the positive evaluation.

Empathic Understanding: Basically this behavior communicates understanding. It involves more than the ability of the Supervisor to sense the Supervisee's private world; it involves both the Supervisor's sensitivity to current feelings and his verbal facility to communicate this understanding in a language attuned to the Supervisee's current feelings. The Supervisor does not need to feel the same emotions but he must demonstrate an appreciation for and sensitive awareness to those feelings.

SCALE FOR MEASURING EMPATHIC UNDERSTANDING DURING A SUPERVISION CONFERENCE

1	2	3	4	5	6	7
Supervisor denies the feelings reflected by the supervisee. Denial may be accompanied by a hurtful or sarcastic manner.	Supervisor ignores feelings reflected by the supervisee.	Supervisor communicates only partial awareness of the supervisee's feelings.	Supervisor recognizes the supervisee's feelings without accepting or refuting them.	Supervisor recognizes and accepts the supervisee's feelings. Exact repetition or reflection of supervisee's feelings.	Supervisor recognizes and elaborates upon the supervisee's feelings. This may include providing a label for the supervisee's feelings when the clinician him/herself may not have labeled his/her feelings.	Supervisor recognizes, labels, elaborates upon, and accepts the supervisee's feelings.

SUPERVISEE CATEGORY

Self-Exploratory: The ability to objectively talk about one's own behavior and its consequences.

SCALE FOR MEASURING SELF-EXPLORATION DURING A SUPERVISION CONFERENCE

1	2	3	4	5	6	7
Supervisee is dishonest about his/her feelings or behaviors.	Supervisee holds back or refuses to self-explore when the opportunity is presented.	Supervisee gives a limited direct response to the supervisor's question about his/her feelings.	Supervisee may report that his/her behavior had a certain effect on the client or the therapy activity. (e.g. cause and effect relationships)	Supervisee analyzes the consequences of his/her behavior with no reporting.	Supervisee analyzes his/her behavior and relates his/her feelings about the behavior.	Supervisee analyzes his/her *feelings* or elaborates on his/her feelings about his/her behavior.

Appendix H:
Smith Adapted MOSAICS Scale
Kathryn J. Smith

CATEGORIES

Speaker

S: Supervisor—The individual who has major responsibility for the conference.
C: Clinician —The individual who participates with the supervisor in the conference.

Pedagogical Moves

STR: *Structuring*—Structuring moves set the context for subsequent behavior by (1) launching or halting/excluding interactions between participants, focusing attention on a problem; or (2) indicating the nature of the interaction in terms of time, agent, activity, topic and cognitive process, regulations, reasons, and instructional aids. Structuring moves form an implicit directive by launching discussion in specified directions and focusing on topics and procedures. Structuring may occur either by announcing or stating propositions for subsequent discussion. In general, structuring serves to move the discussion forward.

SOL: *Soliciting*—Soliciting moves are intended to elicit (1) an active verbal response on the part of persons addressed; (2) a cognitive response (e.g., encouraging persons to attend to something); (3) a physical response. Soliciting moves may be questions, commands, or requests. Rhetorical questions are not counted as solicitations.

RES: *Responding*—Responding moves bear a reciprocal relation to soliciting moves and occur only in relation to them. Their function is to fulfill the expectation of the solicitation. Responses may be in the form of answers, statements of not knowing, etc. In general every solicitation must be intended to elicit a response, and every response must be directly elicited by a solicitation.

REA: *Reacting*—Reacting moves are occasioned by prior structuring, soliciting, responding, or reacting moves but are not directly elicited by them. Pedagogically, these moves serve to modify (by clarifying, synthesizing, or expanding) and/or to rate (positively or negatively) what has been said in the moves that occasioned them. Reacting moves may evaluate, discuss, rephrase, expand, state implications, interpret, or draw conclusions from a previous move.

RSM: *Summary reaction*—A summary reaction is occasioned by more than one previous move and serves the function of a genuine summary or review.

Substantive Areas (Content Analysis)

A. Instructional
    1. Generality
        S: Specific—Pedagogical moves that focus on the objectives, methods, or instructional interactions for the particular client(s) on which the

From Smith, K. (1978). Identification of perceived effectiveness components in the individual supervisory conference in speech pathology and an evaluation of the relationship between ratings and content in the conference. (Doctoral dissertation, Indiana University, 1977). *Dissertation Abstracts International, 39,* 680B. (University Microfilms No. 78–13, 175) supervision is based. These may be related to the client(s) in the past, present, or future.

G: General—Pedagogical moves that focus on generalized objectives, methods or instructional interactions. These may include generalizations, past experience, or applications of theory from speech pathology and audiology or related fields (e.g., child development, linguistics, psychology).

2. Focus

O: Objectives and Content—Expected therapy outcomes and the content or subject matter related to these outcomes.

M: Methods and Materials—Materials of therapy and strategic operations designed to achieve objectives.

X: Execution and Instructional Interactions—Interactions between clinician, client(s), and content or therapy, either as the execution of a particular therapy plan or unexpected interactions and critical incidents.

3. Domain

C: Cognitive—Pertaining to cognition, knowledge, understanding, and learning. The cognitive domain is here restricted to cognitive interactions between client(s) and therapy.

A: Affective—Pertaining to interest, involvement, and motivation. Affective interaction between client(s) and therapy.

D: Social and Disciplinary—Pertaining to discipline, control and social interactions. Interactions between clinician and client(s) or client(s) and client(s).

B. Related Areas (Discussion that does not focus on the analysis of instruction)

SBJ: *Subject*—Discussion of content and subject matter where the intent is to have the clinician understand the topic of discussion.

SPR: *Supervision*—Discussion of topics related to supervision, the supervisory process, and training of clinicians.

GRL: *General Topics Related to Speech Pathology and Audiology*—Discussion of topics such as school, other professionals, parent interactions, and referrals, which are only indirectly related to therapy interactions.

GNR: *General Topics **Not** Related to Speech Pathology and Audiology*—Discussion of topics unrelated to speech pathology and audiology such as the weather or sports.

Substantive-Logical Meanings (Logical Analysis)

A. Processes Relating to the Proposed Use of Language

DEF: *Defining*—A statement of what a word means, how it is used, or a verbal equivalent. Definitions may be in the form of the characteristics designated by a term or specific instances of the class designated by a term.

INT: *Interpreting*—Rephrasing the meaning of a statement; a verbal equivalent which makes the meaning of a statement clear. Interpreting bears the same relationship to statements that defining does to terms.

B. Diagnostic Processes

FAC: *Fact Stating*—Giving an account, description, or report of an event or state of affairs which is verifiable in terms of experience or observational tests. Included are statements of what is, what was, or what will be, as well as generalizations and universal statements.

XPL: *Explaining*—Explanations or reasons which relate one object, event, action, or state of affairs to another object, event, action, or state of affairs,

　　　　or which show relationship between an event or state of affairs and a
　　　　principle or generalization. Included are conditional inferences, explicit
　　　　instances of compare- and contrast, and cause- and effect-relationships.
EVL:　　*Evaluation*—Statements about the fairness, worth, importance, value, or
　　　　quality of something.
JUS:　　*Justification*—Justification or vindication of an evaluation. Reasons for
　　　　holding an evaluation; support or criticism for explicit or implicit opinions
　　　　and evaluations.
C.　Prescriptive Processes
SUG:　　*Suggestions*—Suggestions, alternatives, and possible actions and goals
　　　　which might be used or could have been used in therapy.
SGX:　　*Explanations of Suggestions*—Reasons for offering a suggestion;
　　　　relationships between suggestions and other objects, events, actions,
　　　　states of affairs, principles, or generalizations.
OPN:　　*Opinions*—Directives or opinions of what should be done or ought to have
　　　　been done in a given situation. A definite evaluative overtone is presumed.
OPJ:　　*Justification for Opinions*—Justification or vindication of an opinion;
　　　　reasons for proposing opinion; support or criticism for opinions.

SUMMARY OF MOSAICS SCORING

Speaker

S:　　Supervisor
C:　　Clinician

Pedagogical Moves

STR:　　Structuring, launching or halting move that directs the flow of discussion.
SOL:　　Soliciting, asking for a physical or verbal response.
RES:　　Responding, answering or fulfilling the expectation of a solicitation.
REA:　　Reacting, amplifying, qualifying, or making an unsolicited reaction.
RSM:　　Summary reaction to more than one move or a genuine summary or review.

Substantive Areas (Content Analysis)

Instructional
　Generality
　　S:　Specific, pertinent to the specific client(s) being discussed
　　G:　General, pertinent to generalized objectives, methods, theory or related fields
　Focus
　　O:　Objectives and content to be taught.
　　M:　Methods and materials, strategic and planned aspects of implementing
　　　　objectives.
　　X:　Execution, critical incidents, tactical and unexpected interactions.

Domain
  C: Cognitive, pertaining to knowledge, learning, information, understanding.
  A: Affective, pertaining to affective interactions—interest, motivation, attending.
  D: Disciplinary and social interactions.
Related
  SBJ: Content and subject matter to be learned by the clinician.
  SPR: Supervision and clinician-training.
  GRL: General topics related to speech pathology and audiology.
  GNR: General topics NOT related to speech pathology and audiology.

Substantive-Logical Meanings (Logical Analysis)

Processes Relating to the Proposed Use of Language
  DEF: Defining, definitions and verbal equivalents.
  INT: Interpretations and rephrasings.
Diagnostic Processes
  FAC: Fact stating, accounts, descriptions, or reports.
  XPL: Explanations, reasons, or relationships.
  EVL: Evaluations.
  JUS: Justifications, reasons for evaluations.
Prescriptive Processes
  SUG: Suggestions, alternatives, and possible actions.
  SGX: Explanations, reasons, and relationships for suggestions.
  OPN: Opinions, directives of what should or ought to be done.
  OPJ: Justifications for opinions, reasons, support, and criticisms.

RULES FOR SCORING MOSAICS

General Rules

1. Listen to tape and score: speaker and pedagogical move.
2. Rewind tape, listen and score: instructional or related substantive areas.
3. Rewind tape, listen and score: substantive-logical meanings.

Specific Rules

General Coding Instructions

A. Code from the viewpoint of an observer, with pedagogical meaning inferred from the speakers' verbal behaviors.
B. Grammatical form may give a clue, but it is not decisive in coding. For example, *SOL* may be found in declarative, interrogative, or imperative form. Likewise, *RES* may be in the form of a question, indicating a tentative answer on the part of the speaker.
C. Coding is done in the general context of the discussion. When two people are speaking at once, or when a person makes an interruption which is not acted upon (the interrupted party continues speaking on the original topic), the interruption is not counted and coding continues in the basic context.

D. When one individual is making an extended pedagogical move which is periodically encouraged by grunts and statements such as "uh huh" and "go on," without actually changing discourse or pausing for longer than two seconds, these interruptions are not counted as separate pedagogical moves.

Pedagogical Moves

A. *STR* moves from an implicit directive by launching discussion in specific directions and focusing on topics or procedures. The function of *STR* is either launching or halting-excluding, generally by the method of announcing or stating propositions. When a choice must be made between *STR* and *REA*, code *STR* for statements which move the discourse forward or bring it back on the track after a digression. For example, a new *SUG* or *OPN* is almost invariably found in a structuring move.

B. In general, internal or parenthetical shifts of topic or emphasis are not separately coded unless they constitute a relatively permanent change in the discourse. The discourse is coded in the overall context.

C. Checking statements (e.g., "follow me?") are not coded as *SOL* within the context of another move unless some cue indicating a desired *RES* is present.

D. Implicit in any *SOL* is the concept of knowing or not knowing. Therefore, code *RES* for any of the range of possible responses, including invalid ones and those indicating knowing or not knowing alone (e.g., "I don't know").

E. A *SOL* which calls for a face is coded *FAC*, but if the *RES* gives both a fact and an explanation, the response is coded *RES/XPL*. In the same way, complex responses to solicitations of *EVL, SUG*, and *OPN* are coded as *JUS, SGX*, and *OPJ*.

F. A speaker cannot respond to his or her own solicitation. An immediate self-answer to a question indicates that it was a rhetorical question, which is not coded *SOL* in the first place. If a speaker answers his or her own question after an intervening incorrect answer, the correction is coded as a reaction to the incorrect answer. If the speaker answers his or her own question after a pause, the answer is coded as a reaction to the absence of an expected response.

G. When a reaction to a previous move is followed by a genuine summary reaction (*RSM*), both moves are scored for the same speaker.

H. *RSM* frequently occurs when a unit of discussion is concluded by a speaker, who then turns to a new topic. The coder must determine when *RMS* ends and *STR* begins.

I. A reaction to a solicitation occurs only when the reaction is about the solicitation and not a response to the *SOL*.

J. A reaction may follow the absence of other reactions to a move such as *STR*. For example, a speaker may make a proposal and then react to the absence of any positive reactions from the other participants.

Substantive Areas

A. Coding of Substantive Areas is in terms of the main context of discussion. However, in nondirective discussions shifts of substantive area are common. In order to code these shifts, which are an important aspect of supervision, the following rules are observed:

B.   Code Instruction Areas in preference to Related Areas if a conflict arises. For example, if it is difficult to determine whether discussion of subject content (e.g., language) is in the context of objectives for the clients (*SOC*) or in the context of the understanding of the content by the clinician (*SBJ*), code *SOC* in preference to *SBJ*.

C.   Code Instructional Domain (*C*ognitive, *A*ffective, or *D*isciplinary-social) first. This is the most general of the content dimensions, it tends to persist longest in the discourse, and it is the most difficult to code out of context. If a conflict arises in coding, code *C*ognitive in preference to *A*ffective and *A*ffective in preference to *D*isciplinary-social.

D.   Code Instructional Focus (*O*bjectives and content, *M*ethods and materials, e*X*ecution) second. Significant shifts in these areas occur more frequently than changes in Instructional Domain. If a conflict arises in coding, code *O*bjectives in preference to *M*ethods and *M*ethods in preference to e*X*ecution.

E.   Code Instructional Generality (*S*pecific or *G*eneral) last. Moves commonly shift from *S*pecific to *G*eneral and back again. For a single move, code the area which occupies the most time or emphasis in the move, and code each move separately. If a conflict arises, code *S*pecific in preference to *G*eneral.

F.   Indicate the Substantive Area of each move even if it is not explicitly referred to.

Substantive-Logical Meanings

A.   Only when *DEF* or *INT* are the main focus of the discourse are they coded as such. They are not coded when they are in the immediate context of other Substantive-Logical Meanings.

B.   In a sequence of complex moves (*XPL, SGX, OPJ*, or *JUS*), individual simple moves (*FAC, SUG, OPN*, or *EVL*) are coded in the context of the complex moves. For example, in a series of explanations, a move stating a fact will generally be coded as *XPL* since one can consider the fact is intimately related to the inter-relationships among the other explanations. However, when *FAC* represents a definite shift to a new topic or when it is in response to *SOL/FAC*, it is coded as *FAC*.

C.   Complex moves (*XPL, SGX, OPJ*, and *JUS*) always involve relationships between their simple analogues (*FAC, SUG, OPN*, and *EVL*) and other factors, such as generalizations, other simple moves, etc. In the analysis of therapy, particularly for objectives and methods, it is often difficult to determine when relationships are actually involved and when the move represents merely an extended description. As a general rule, these substantive-logical meanings are coded as complex whenever relationships are made to clients or specific therapy situations. In most other situations these moves are extended descriptions and are coded as simple moves.

D.   When more than one Substantive-Logical process occurs within a single pedagogical move and the overall context or emphasis is unclear, code according to the following order of priority; *OPJ, JUS, SGX, XPL, OPN, EVL, SUG, FAC, INT, DEF*. In effect, this means that complex is coded in preference to simple, prescriptive in preference to diagnostic.

Scoring Sheet for Adapted *MOSAICS*

NAME _____ DATE _____ TIME _____ to _____

SPEAKER	MOVE	SUBSTANTIVE	SUBSTANTIVE-LOGICAL	NOTES
S,C	STR SOL RES REA RSM	S,G O,M,X C,A,D SBJ, SPR, GRL, GNL	OPJ, JUS, SGX, XPL, OPN, EVL, SUG, FAC, INT, DEF	

Subject Index

*A*uthor Index